THE FUTURE OF PSYCHOANALYSIS

THE FUTURE OF PSYCHOANALYSIS

The Debate about the Training Analyst System

edited by

Peter Zagermann

Routledge
Taylor & Francis Group
LONDON AND NEW YORK

First published 2017 by Karnac Books Ltd.

2 Park Square, Milton Park, Abingdon, Oxfordshire OX14 4RN
52 Vanderbilt Avenue, New York, NY 10017

Routledge is an imprint of the Taylor & Francis Group, an informa business

First issued in hardback 2019

British Library Cataloguing in Publication Data

A C.I.P. for this book is available from the British Library

ISBN 978-1-78220-381-0 (pbk)
ISBN 978-0-367-32796-5 (hbk)

Edited, designed and produced by The Studio Publishing Services Ltd
www.publishingservicesuk.co.uk
email: studio@publishingservicesuk.co.uk

CONTENTS

To the memory of Robert S. Wallerstein

ABOUT THE EDITOR AND CONTRIBUTORS

Emanuel Berman, PhD, is a training and supervising analyst at the Israel Psychoanalytic Society and Professor Emeritus at the University of Haifa. He is the international editor of *Psychoanalytic Dialogues* and editor of *Essential Papers on Literature and Psychoanalysis* (1993). He is the author of *Impossible Training* (2004), and the recipient of the Sigourney Award, 2012.

Harold P. Blum, MD, is a training and supervising psychoanalyst at the Institute for Psychoanalytic Education, affiliated with New York University School of Medicine, Department of Psychiatry. He is a Distinguished Fellow at the American Psychiatric Association and was Executive Director of the Sigmund Freud Archives from 1987 to 2014. He is also President of the Psychoanalytic Research and Development Fund (2008 to present), was editor-in-chief of the *Journal of the American Psychoanalytic Association* from 1973 to 1983, and Vice President of the International Psychoanalytical Association from 1993 to 1997. He authored more than 150 psychoanalytic papers and several books, is the recipient of numerous awards and lectureships, including the inaugural Sigourney Award, Mahler, Hartmann, and Lorand prizes; Sigmund Freud lectures in New York, London, Vienna, and Frankfurt;

Anna Freud, Hartmann, Brill, Friend and Sperling lectures, and two plenary addresses to the American Psychoanalytic Association. He chaired five Symposia on Psychoanalysis and Art in Florence, Italy. From 1972 to 2012, he was Clinical Professor of Psychiatry at the New York University School of Medicine.

Kenneth Eisold, PhD, is a practicing psychoanalyst and organizational consultant. Dr. Eisold is Past President of the International Society for the Psychoanalytic Study of Organizations and also a former Director of the Organizational Program at the William Alanson White Institute, which he helped to found and where he currently teaches, supervizes, and serves as a Fellow. For several years, he directed the A. K. Rice Institute's National Conference on Leadership and Authority. His papers and publications have focused recently on the psychodynamics of psychoanalytic institutions and the vicissitudes of the profession. They have been published in such journals as the *International Journal of Psychoanalysis, The Journal of the American Psychoanalytic Association, Psychoanalytic Psychology*, and *Contemporary Psychoanalysis*. He has also published in the *Harvard Business Review* and provided commentary for *The Wall Street Journal*.

Cláudio Laks Eizirik, MD, PhD, graduated in Medicine in 1969, concluded his psychiatric training in 1972, and his PhD in medicine in 1997, all at the Federal University of Rio Grande do Sul (UFRGS), where he became a professor of the Department of Psychiatry and Forensic Medicine in 1976. He concluded his analytic training at the Porto Alegre Psychoanalytical Society in 1987. He was editor of the *Revista de Psiquiatria do Rio Grande do Sul* (1979–1981), as well as chair of the Graduate Program in Psychiatry of UFRGS. He was also Head of the Department of Psychiatry and Forensic Medicine of UFRGS and Dean of the Medical School of UFRGS. He was subsequently President of the Latin American Psychoanalytic Federation and then became the first Brazilian to preside over the International Psychoanalytical Association (2005–2009). He is a member of the editorial boards of the *International Journal of Psychoanalysis, Brazilian Journal of Psychiatry, Docta* (from Argentina), *Portuguese Journal of Psychoanalysis*, the *Journal of Psychiatry of Rio Grande do Sul*, and the *Brazilian Journal of Psychotherapy*. In 2011, he received the Sigourney Award. He is the author of books, chapters, and papers on analytic training, analytic technique, the process of aging, and the relation of psychoanalysis and culture.

Gigliola Fornari Spoto, MD, is a training and supervising analyst of the British Psychoanalytical Society. She originally trained as a psychiatrist in Italy. Dr. Fornari Spoto has been involved for many years with the institutional aspects of the training process, including a recent spell of six years as the Chair of the Education Committee. She edited Eric Brenman's *The Recovery of the Lost Good Object* (Routledge, London, 2006).

Cesar Garza-Guerrero, MD, is a graduate of the School of Medicine of the Autonomous University of Nuevo Leon, in Monterrey, Mexico, where he received The Robbins Award of Medicine in 1967. He completed his psychiatric training at the Menninger School of Psychiatry, then located in Topeka Kansas (1969–1972), where he was honored with the Sigmund Freud award, and his psychoanalytic training at the Topeka Institute of Psychoanalysis (1970–1976). He is certified by the American Board of Psychiatry and Neurology, and the Board on Professional Standards of the American Psychoanalytic Association. He is an ex-Chairman of the Department of Psychiatry at the University Hospital of Monterrey, Nuevo Leon, Mexico (1993–2003), and a Latin American Co-Chair of the International New Groups Committee (1997–2005). He is the author of three books: *The Superego Concept in Psychoanalytic Theory and Practice*; *Organizational and Educational Crisis in Psychoanalysis: Contemporary Challenges*; and *Psychoanalysis: Requiescat in Pace? A Critique From Within and an Undelayable Proposal*. In addition, he is the author of thirty-five papers published in indexed journals, and, in 2003, received the International Sigourney Award for his contributions to psychoanalysis—the same year he was elected to the American College of Psychiatrists. Presently, he is Co-director of Conceptual and Clinical Research at the Center for Psychoanalytic Education and Research, and Professor of Psychiatry and Psychoanalysis at the Department of Psychiatry of the University Hospital in Monterrey, Nuevo Leon, Mexico.

Otto F. Kernberg, MD, is a Fellow of the American Psychiatric Association, Director of the Personality Disorders Institute at The New York Presbyterian Hospital, Westchester Division, and Professor Emeritus of Psychiatry at the Weill Medical College of Cornell University. Dr. Kernberg is a Past President of the International Psychoanalytical Association. He is also the Training and Supervising Analyst of the Columbia University Center for Psychoanalytic Training and Research. In the past, Dr. Kernberg served as Director of the C. F. Menninger Memorial Hospital, Supervising and Training Analyst of the Topeka Institute for Psychoanalysis, and Director of the Psychotherapy Research Project of the Menninger Foundation. Later, he was Director of the General Clinical Service of the New York State Psychiatric Institute, and Professor of Clinical Psychiatry at the College of Physicians and Surgeons of Columbia University. From 1976 to 1995, he was Associate Chairman and Medical Director of The New York Hospital Cornell Medical Center, Westchester Division. He is the author of thirteen books and co-author of twelve others.

Douglas Kirsner, PhD, is Emeritus Professor at Deakin University, Australia, where he previously held a Personal Chair in Philosophy and Psychoanalytic Studies. His publications include *The Schizoid World of Jean-Paul Sartre and RD Laing* (Other Press 2003) and *Unfree Associations: Inside Psychoanalytic Institutes* (Rowman and Littlefield, 2009), numerous journal articles, book chapters, and edited collections. He is Associate Editor of the *International Journal of Applied Psychoanalytic Studies* and *Organisational and Social Dynamics*, and Editorial Advisor to *Psychoanalysis and History*. He has lectured widely internationally. He founded the Annual Deakin University Freud Conference, which he directed for twenty years. He is an Honorary Member of the American Psychoanalytic Association.

Elias Mallet da Rocha Barros, PhD, is a training analyst and supervisor of the Brazilian Psychoanalytic Society of São Paulo, Fellow of the British Psychoanalytical Society and Institute, Recipient of the Sigourney Award 1999, Past Latin American Editor of the *International Journal of Psychoanalysis*, Latin American Chair of the IPA International Encyclopedia and Dictionary, Past Chair of the Nice Training Conference, and past member of the IPA Education Committee for six years.

Robert Michels, MD, is Walsh McDermott University Professor of Medicine and Psychiatry at Weill Medical College of Cornell University. Formerly, he was Chairman of the Department of Psychiatry and Dean and Provost for Medical Affairs. He is a training and supervising psychoanalyst at the Columbia University Center for Psychoanalytic

Training and Research. He is past Editor-in-chief of the *International Journal of Psychoanalysis*.

Luiz Meyer, MD, graduated in medicine in São Paulo, Brazil in 1956. He studied psychiatry in São Paulo, Paris, and Geneva. His psychoanalytic training was done in Geneva, São Paulo, and London. He has written papers on several different aspects of psychoanalytical issues and also on training analysis. He has published three books: one on psychoanalytic family therapy (*Familia: dinamica e terapia, uma abordagem psicanalitica*), one of his collected papers (*Rumor na Escuta*) and a book of poems (*Réu Confesso – poemas reunidos: 1968–2010*). He teaches at the Institute of his Society and directs group seminars. In his private practice, he works with adult patients, families, and couples.

Robert L. Pyles, MD, is a psychiatrist and psychoanalyst at the Psychoanalytic Society of New England, East, where he was founding member and first President from 1990–1993; he is also a training and supervising analyst. He was twice President of the American Psychoanalytic Association. From 2001 to 2003, he was Vice President, North America, of the International Psychoanalytical Association. He chaired several committees, from 1999 to 2002 the IPA Subcommittee on the Status of Psychoanalysis, from 2003 to 2005 the IPA Education Work Group, also from 2003 to 2005 the IPA Credential Work Group, and from 2005 to 2008 he was Chair of the IPA Committee on Professional Practice.

Robert S. Wallerstein, MD, (1921–2014) was Emeritus Professor and former Chair at the Department of Psychiatry of the University of California San Francisco School of Medicine, and Emeritus Training and Supervising Analyst, San Francisco Center for Psychoanalysis. He was former President of the American Psychoanalytic Association (1971–1972) and a former President of the International Psychoanalytical Association (1985–1989). He graduated from Columbia College (June 1941), the Columbia University College of Physicians and Surgeons (September 1944), and the Topeka Institute for Psychoanalysis (June 1958). He was Director of Research at the Menninger Clinic (Topeka, Kansas) until June 1966, and then Chief of Psychiatry at the Mount Zion Hospital, San Francisco (1966–1975). He was twice a Fellow at the Center for Advanced Study in the Behavioral Sciences at

Stanford, California (1964–1965, 1981–1982), a Fellow at the Rockefeller Foundation Study Center at Bellagio, Lake Como, Italy (1992), and was given the Mary Singleton Sigourney Award for outstanding contributions to psychoanalysis in 1991.

Sara Zac de Filc, MD, has been a training analyst at the Buenos Aires Psychoanalytic Association, APdeBA, for many years. She received her Masters in Psychology from Bank Street College, New York in 1955, and returned to Argentina to become Assistant Professor at the schools of psychology and education of Buenos Aires University until her resignation during the 1966 dictatorship. Dr. Zac de Filc pursued her medical studies at Buenos Aires University's School of Medicine (with honours) and trained as an analyst at the Argentine Psychoanalytic Association and later at APdeBA, where she has had a long and fruitful professional life as seminar instructor, vice president, and president, among other positions. She has also been actively involved in the IPA, where she was member of the Executive Council and chair of several committees (Interregional Conferences, Education, Ethics), and in the creation of new societies in different Latin American countries as chair of an array of site visit and sponsoring committees. Dr. Zac de Filc was recipient of the Sigourney Award in 2002 and of the IPA award for "Extraordinarily Meritorious Service to the Association" in 2005. Her essays have been published in various Latin American journals and in the *International Journal of Psychoanalysis*, and she is co-editor of two collections of essays, one of them published in English as *Challenges of Psychoanalysis in the 21st Century* (Kluwer Academic/Plenum Publishers, New York).

Peter Zagermann, PhD, studied psychology, art history, and ancient history at the University of Munich, Germany. He did his psychoanalytic training with the German Psychoanalytic Association (DPV/IPA), is a full member of the DPV, as well as of the German Psychoanalytic Society (DPG), and a psychoanalyst for children, adolescents, and adults in private practice in Munich. In 2010, he made the documentary film *Introduction to Psychoanalysis* with Professor Otto Kernberg, in German, English, and Spanish, to provide basic audiovisual information about psychoanalysis for use worldwide. His publications include two books and a series of papers on psychoanalytic subjects in German, and the Monograph *Psychoanalysis. A General Theory of Psychic Structure Formation and Pathogenesis*, which is in the process of publication.

SERIES EDITOR'S FOREWORD

The Publications Committee of the International Psychoanalytical Association continues, with this volume, the series "Psychoanalytic Ideas and Applications".

The aim of this series is to focus on the scientific production of significant authors whose works are outstanding contributions to the development of the psychoanalytic field and to set out relevant ideas and themes, generated during the history of psychoanalysis, that deserve to be known and discussed by present psychoanalysts.

The relationship between psychoanalytic ideas and their applications has to be put forward from the perspective of theory, clinical practice, technique, and research so as to maintain their validity for contemporary psychoanalysis.

The Publication Committee's objective is to share these ideas with the psychoanalytic community and with professionals in other related disciplines, in order to expand their knowledge and generate a productive interchange between the text and the reader.

The Future of Psychoanalysis. The Debate About the Training Analyst System, edited by Peter Zagermann with the contributions of fourteen eminent psychoanalysts from all over the world (and with different theoretical frames), is an original and engaging book which, in the words of the Editor, "would like to give a balanced account of the pros and cons of the positions at stake" as far as the current discussion on training within the IPA is concerned. The question of the psychoanalytic theoretical education and clinical training has always been at the core of any international debate upon the future of our discipline, and this volume provides analysts and students with an up-to-date, disenchanted and courageous review of all of the current ideas and proposals on what a future psychoanalytic training might look like. I have no doubt that this brilliant volume, which fully accomplishes what the IPA Publications Committee Mandate is, will encounter the interest of psychoanalysts and psychotherapists worldwide.

Gennaro Saragnano
Series Editor
Chair, IPA Publications Committee

FOREWORD

Stefano Bolognini

President of the International Psychoanalytical Association

No other theme, in recent years, has raised so many discussions inside the IPA as training.

There is an evident tension inside our international organization regarding this crucial topic, and, as the President, I am both sensitive and highly interested in that. Thus, when I received the text of this book my curiosity was naturally stimulated.

The names of the authors are so well known and internationally respected that their contributions also work as a special indicator of the many current thoughts and possible future trends on training: furthermore, many of them have had significant roles and offices at the highest level in psychoanalytic institutions, so that their personal experience and prestige allows them to express their own vision frankly, with no fear of possible accusations of incompetence or ignorance about the complexity of these problems.

Yet, a reader expecting from these pages some academic, traditional, reassuring confirmation of the previously existing educational mentality and processes in psychoanalysis could feel unexpectedly displaced and surprised by the content of some of these chapters: this book hosts a real, innovative debate among independent thinkers who are connected by a strong, genuine interest in transmitting psychoanalysis to future generations and who reflect, with no bias or prejudice, on the experiences of their own and of previous generations.

Should the International Psychoanalytical Association—a century old, highly structured organization—be disturbed by the variety of different opinions, criticisms, and suggestions for changes presented in these papers? Not at all, in my view.

The IPA has a long history of difficulties in representing and working through its internal processes regarding training: had the IPA been an individual, I would frankly say it would have been, for long periods, rather a disturbed one, since its capacity for recognizing officially (more or less, at the level of its own self-representation) the actual existence of more than one training model had been failing for some decades; for complicated internal vicissitudes, it took a long time for us to acknowledge and include the French and the Uruguayan models alongside the Eitingon in the IPA Bylaws, even if it was common knowledge how analysts were actually trained in those countries.

An alternation between denial and negation was at work there; I was a member of the IPA Board when the long, exhausting debate (a real controversy lasting for years . . .) came to a conclusion, with the dramatic and conflictual recognition of the two other, already existing, models.

That is history, and I can say I was there: I remember how conflictual it had been, for many colleagues, to recognize the reality, with the evident feeling of betraying some early, sacred assumptions and ideals: a dramatic change and consequent mourning, for some of them.

Not by chance, one of the most dramatic sessions of the debate on training happened in Utrecht, inside an ancient, dark, and severe Dutch church of the sixteenth century, where the Board representatives discussed for two days in a tense atmosphere comparable to that of the Trento Council, where fundamental sacred principles had been the subject of legendary religious battles.

Nevertheless, finally, we were able to discuss, to vote, to decide, and to modify some pre-existing fundaments that had affected our institution and that had seemed for years impossible, almost unthinkable, to change. More or less, a process comparable to what can happen in a good enough analysis.

If the recognition and acceptance of some unending, unavoidable conflictuality is a sign of relative health in an individual, the discussion emerging from this book (a sort of polyphonic chorus with remarkable differences and, sometimes, contrasts) shows the liveliness of the collective mind in our community.

Which is good.

At the same time, given the high level of thinking and competence of the contributors, such debate maintains a positive tension towards the common ideal of preserving psychoanalysis from risks of falsification, perversion, loss of energy, and possible decline.

"Passion" is the substantial factor which inspires all these authors and which motivates them to explore this area: passion for psychoanalysis, for transmitting to future generations a unique patrimony of scientific knowledge, of professional competence, of sophisticated technique, and, finally, of deep contact with the human complexity.

However, not only that. Another part of the patrimony to be transmitted during training should be a "communitarian" richness; as I wrote in my official note as President in the IPA Newsletter (IPA E-Newsletter, May 2014), psychoanalytic training should also include the capacity to work together, to share constant working through with colleagues, and to actively participate in institutional life.

I call this the "quadripartite model" of analytic education, adding this fourth part to the other traditional elements: analysis, supervision, and seminars.

Probably each of us cultivates his or her private fantasies and dreams about a possible model of "good enough" psychoanalytic training. My personal fantasy is not particularly dedicated to a model of training, but to a model of institutional functioning of the IPA regarding training: I would like to put the IPA in such a condition as to be able to explore, to represent, to discuss as widely and deeply as possible its reality, its needs, its tensions, its problems, its perspectives, and its possible projects.

Just as, when working with individuals as their analyst, I try to provide them with the best conditions for thinking and for exploring their internal conflicts, when working with a large institution I would like to create, together with my colleagues, a suitable working atmosphere for reflection and discussion.

This book offers, in my view, a wonderful opportunity for that.

Introduction: How do we want to train?

Peter Zagermann

This introduction is, as a matter of fact, a call to action with the aim of reaching a fundamental discussion within our worldwide psychoanalytic community about one question: *How do we want to train?* We should direct our minds back in time to the point in 1920 that marks the beginning of the Eitingon model and ask what psychoanalytic training should look like against the background of the experiences we have gained so far and the principles resulting from our science itself. This is about a—potential—new beginning that also requires from us the courage to relinquish existing structures, as the case may be, and refocus on our primary commitment with respect to scientific truth.

As Stefano Bolognini said in his Foreword, the question of psychoanalytic training is the hottest and most fiercely discussed topic of the current international controversies in psychoanalysis, up to the point that the American Psychoanalytic Association faced the danger of a split, as Robert Pyles describes shockingly in his contribution to this Reader. It highlights sharply that we are dealing with the crisis of a large-scale conflict that requires solution. The readiness for a break also shows, however, how vital it is to put our basic values as psychoanalysts over and above all other interests. This Reader, therefore, aims to offer a platform for the different points of views, their complexities, and individual merits, in order to find our way back to our common scientific identity via their discussion. For this reason, it is also important to us that through the authors of this Reader all regions of the International Psychoanalytical Association will be heard: *How do we want to train?*

The explosive dynamics of the current situation which precipitate in a manifest polarization can be described, above all, with reference to the controversy about the training analyst system: one side regards the "Eitingon syndrome" (Zusmann, 1988) of the "authoritarian self-perpetuating training analyst elite, with its paranoiagenic and infantilizing aspects" (Wallerstein, this volume, p. 283) as that aspect of the cause for the current crisis which lies in institutionalized psychoanalysis itself; on the other side, it is a psychoanalytically valid perspective to consider, also, that the depressive anxiety that this crisis gives rise to can generate persecutory reactions that might lead to the singling out of an internal "enemy" in the institution itself, such as the training analysts who want to preserve their power and influence. In view of the existential threat which psychoanalysis faces on all relevant levels, the suggestion of a persecutory depressive reaction has a realistic background. The suggestion alone, however, is unable to remove the objectively describable negative mechanisms of our training structure, as they cannot be ascribed to the investigators' mental condition. Could it be that this very persecutory depressive reaction of ours to the actual misery of psychoanalysis puts us in a position where we recognize and take seriously the circumstances of that pathology of dependency resulting from the training analyst system, in as far as this pathology of dependency produces the very same persecutory depressive reaction in candidates? In any case, one must ask how it is possible, in a scientific association, that, systematically, the objective character of these phenomena is not recognized, or, respectively, is being resolved in a subjectivization.

Some authors warn of a "horizontal model" that cannot acknowledge hierarchy and authority because of its opposition towards oedipal exclusion. In this case, too, as analysts, one must acknowledge the possible justification of the criticism, on the one hand. On the other hand, a significant number of those authors who critically concern themselves with the training analyst system base their criticism on a detailed examination of the effects of the structure of this system, in terms of the psychoanalysis of organizations. Such prioritization of the importance of structure is, however, not what one would associate with an egalitarian point of view, while, at the same time, the point of view that stresses hierarchy and authority often appears to be blind to the negative effects of the structure of the training analyst system as practiced. It surely must be food for thought when three former presidents of the International Psychoanalytical Association, in this volume, are speaking with one voice, taking up position for a horizontal and, in so far, anti-oedipal model of training, along the above lines of argumentation. In other words, a simple polarization does nothing to clarify the complex problems which must be resolved and analyzed in the diversity of how they really appear via a common discussion and discursive debate of the question: *How do we want to train?*

The central theme with which we must concern ourselves with respect to the question of retaining or dismissing the training analyst system is clearly expressed by Fornari Spoto in her contribution to this Reader: "The complexity of the analytical situation in the Eitingon model of training is also one of the reasons why higher levels of competence in the training analyst are deemed to be necessary" (p. 90). Two questions arise here: one, if this is indeed an idealization of qualification, that is to say, whether, from an overall perspective, the claim for higher levels of competence is being met or not. And two, whether the Eitingon model and the real dependency it induces in the candidate on the training analyst and the training analyst system creates the particular difficulties, which are then being used in order to justify the introduction of a special, supposedly very gifted, caste of analysts. The systematic problem that we have lost sight of thereby, in my opinion, is that by creating a two-class society in our institutes and societies we have produced an oedipal fixation of inclusion and exclusion which paralyzes institutionalized psychoanalysis by tying our attention to the internal conditions of power and power shifts. What results from this as from any fixation is potentially a neurotic self-limitation of psychoanalysis. This would be an important internal cause for the crisis in psychoanalysis. Reason enough to also seek scientific dialog here, and to move away from the mentality of trench warfare. The question, also in this respect, is *How do we want to train?*

This brings me to Robert Wallerstein, to whose memory this book, which is essentially about the future of psychoanalysis, is dedicated.

In fact, his essay in this Reader is the last scientific work that left his desk, at age ninety-three. It clearly represents his legacy to psychoanalysis and, thus, simultaneously, is a piece of psychoanalytic history writing. I quote from his letter dated 14 June 2014, which accompanied the essay when he sent it to me.

> The paper does trace the trajectory of my own involvement in these issues (i.e. the reform of the psychoanalytic training system), and changing my mind at several points over the decades of my psychoanalytic involvement (starting in 1949). I do end up with my current comprehensive overview which I no longer expect to be shifting. It presents a case for what I think must eventually evolve, the inclusion of psychoanalytic training as a discipline within the university ... It also makes a radical change in abolishing the whole required training analyst system with the personal analysis of the candidate to become a totally voluntary and private affair not involved in any way with the educational structure. I am sure that it will raise lots of questions and controversy. Here it is for you.

Wallerstein, in his plea for a university-based full-time training, by the way invokes Anna Freud who, *nota bene*, already in 1971, in her essay titled, "The ideal psychoanalytic institute: a utopia", amusingly declared, "The present part-time system seems as out-of-date to me as if church services were still conducted in catacombs since this is where the early Christians were obliged to meet" (p. 230).

How do we want to train? The integration of psychoanalytic training into the university is, for the time being, an unrealistic thought for most constituent organizations of the IPA, given that the current crisis in psychoanalysis is very specifically a scientific crisis, due to the fact that formal research in psychoanalysis is largely absent. But then we have the case of Germany, where, in the forseeable future, it might become a reality that within the framework of statutory health insurance into which psychoanalysis is integrated the training in psychoanalytic psychotherapy might, by law, become part of the university-based clinical–psychological training. In this case, we are faced head-on with the problem that the training analyst system and the university are incompatible, as we are dealing here with two differently justified hierarchical systems that mutually contradict each other.

Then again, an integration into the university might, for example, be combined with Otto Kernberg's proposition (2014) to tie the authorization to conduct analyses which are undertaken in connection with training to a general certification to which, ideally, all analytically active members of a psychoanalytic institute, or a society, respectively, would submit themselves five years after their final exam. All these analysts would then be freely available to the candidates, without any further formal involvement in the training context. What this comes down to essentially is a termination of the training analyst system according to the Eitingon model; also along these lines, Kernberg titled his 2014 work "The twilight of the training analysis system". The contribution to the present volume by Kernberg and Michels takes this concept further. In Israel, the introduction of a similar concept in 1996 has, meanwhile, led to a broad termination of the training analyst system, which seems to work well, as Emanuel Berman describes in his contribution.

For the last time: *how do we want to train?* As initially mentioned, it appears to me the most important and most difficult task we face is to mentally question the Eitingon model at all, as a first step, and with it the training analyst system to which it gave rise. I am of the opinion that this is only secondarily connected with the simple question of retaining power, which is so frequently mentioned. As psychoanalysts, we have all been trained and raised, so to speak, within this system, and the massive oedipalization it produces, which I briefly described earlier and will expand on in my chapter in ths book, leads to a very explicit identification with this system, so that we are all inclined to look upon it as the only conceivable option and a quasi-natural reality. It is against that background that the question of retention of power can be played out in a way which, for psychoanalysts, is often amazingly crude and unreflected because one feels full oedipal justification. The first step, therefore, must be to take a look at the training analyst system in the history of its development in the 1920s and to focus, especially, on its coming into being out of the unresolved transference relationship of the first generation of analysts towards Freud. Only such fundamental and necessary relativization and reflective distancing, if we can adopt it, will help us accept the validity of those arguments that are put forward against the training analyst system on the functional level from the part of organizational psychoanalysis, in order to then look for an alternative, better form of training. This is the aim this Reader serves.

References

Freud, A. (1971). The ideal psychoanalytic institute: a utopia. *Bulletin of the Menninger Clinic, 315*: 225–239.

Kernberg, O. (2014). The twilight of the training analysis system. *Psychoanalytic Review, 101*: 151-174.

Zusman, W. (1988). Our science and our scientific lives. *Israel Psychoanalytic Journal, 1*: 351–377, 2003.

CHAPTER ONE

Change from within in a traditional psychoanalytic institute: twenty-five years of debate and transformation at the Israel Psychoanalytic Society*

Emanuel Berman

The Israel Psychoanalytic Society and its training body, the Israel Psychoanalytic Institute, were founded by Max Eitingon in 1933–1934, shortly after he had to leave Berlin. The institute is actually named the Eitingon Institute, although this title is rarely mentioned nowadays. The Society became an IPA component society from its first days (Rolnik, 2012). For many years it was a rather traditional organization. In the past quarter century, however, it went through rather radical changes, some of which were reached by consensus, whereas others were the final outcome of fierce debates, and could be controversial to this day.

In this chapter, I will summarize some of these changes, starting roughly around 1990–when I was a junior faculty member at the Institute–and reaching the time of writing in 2015. Let me say at the outset that I make no claim to be objective. I was quite active myself in promoting several of these changes, and I view the process as constructive, against the background of my criticism of what I see as major pitfalls of traditional psychoanalytic training, which I will outline briefly.

---

* Dedicated to the memory of Helmut Thomä.

I am myself a graduate of the Israel Psychoanalytic Institute (IPI), having been trained between 1977 and 1984. This was my second analytic training, after graduating in 1976 from the Postdoctoral Program in Psychotherapy and Psychoanalysis at New York University (Berman, 2010). Returning to Israel from studies and work in the USA in 1976, to join the faculty of the University of Haifa, I knew that in order to become part of the local psychoanalytic community I would have to undergo additional training, as the NYU program does not belong to the IPA. I was welcomed by the IPI, my studies at NYU allowed me to be exempted from introductory courses, but, by and large, I went through a full training program again. I never regretted it. I learned more and benefited from a second analysis and from three new, stimulating supervisions. The comparison between my two training experiences was very instructive.

To give just one example of the contrast: at NYU, while I was a young beginning clinician, I became one of the representatives of the candidates to the program senate, its governing body, and, therefore, a partner in all decisions about curriculum, procedures and even faculty appointments. At the IPI, while being by that time the head of the clinical psychology program at the University of Haifa, I was clearly expected to be (as a Hebrew idiom says) "a small head", and we, the candidates, were never consulted about anything. So, whereas I appreciated the Institute and its faculty, some of my positions after joining the faculty myself could be seen as an effort to find a synthesis between the high quality and serious investment of a traditional IPA institute and the innovative and egalitarian spirit of the (non-IPA) NYU program (Aron, 1996), with which I identified.

The major pitfalls of traditional psychoanalytic training

The most widespread model of psychoanalytic training is based on the structure of the Berlin Institute, established by Max Eitingon in 1920. An earlier attempt by Sándor Ferenczi to start a psychoanalytic institute took place in Budapest in 1919 but was short-lived owing to political upheavals in Hungary. In view of Ferenczi's strong anti-authoritarian views, it is fascinating to speculate what the style of worldwide training would be today if his institute had retained its seniority. In reality, however, the "Eitingon model" became the dominant one, and Eitingon made active efforts to spread it around the psychoanalytic world (Schröter, 2002). In spite of continuous criticism since the 1940s, changes in this model appear to be slow and hesitant.

Historically, the debate on the damaging aspects of training was opened in London by Balint, Ferenczi's disciple. In Ferenczi's spirit, Balint (1948) clearly outlines the need for a critical view avoiding denial and strives to explain "the curse of strifes which seem to adhere inevitably to our training organizations" (p. 167). Balint's central concern is that candidates are "far too respectful to their training analysts", developing "submissiveness to dogmatic and authoritarian treatment without much protest" (p. 167). The secessions of Adler and Jung, Balint suggests, made Freud believe "that the new generation should learn to renounce part of their self-assertion and independence, to be educated to discipline and self-discipline and to accept an authority with the right and duty of instructing and warning" (p. 170).

Bernfeld (1962) attributes much of the rigidity of the Eitingon model to the "Prussian spirit which rather flourished among the founders of the Berlin Institute", and to the anxiety aroused by Freud's cancer and the imminent threat of his loss, which his colleagues dealt with by "establishing a solid dam against heterodoxy" (p. 467). The result was the introduction of rigid selection and the subjection of newcomers to "a coercive, long drawn-out trial period of authoritarian training" (p. 467). Traditional training, Bernfeld suggests, "distorts some of the most valuable features of psychoanalysis" (p. 458); "institutionalization does not encourage thinking" (p. 468), he adds.

Rustin (1985) studies the tension in psychoanalysis between intimacy and self-exposure, on the one hand, and formal regulation and institutionalization, on the other. He concludes, "Orthodox forms of analysis and also supervision require a structured inequality of relationships. The more orthodox the analytic practice, the more hierarchical the organizations through which it takes place" (p. 151). Zusman (2003[1988]) coins "the Eitingon syndrome", which he describes as the basis of sectarianism, religiosity, and abuse of power in psychoanalytic institutes. Lussier (1991; see Wallerstein, 1993) highlights the inherent contrast between the goal of encouraging candidates to search for the truth and the rigid setup of rules and rituals. Lussier calls for safeguarding the privacy of a candidate's personal analysis and advocates avoiding any regulation of that analysis by the institute, except for the requirement that the analyst be reasonably experienced (e.g., practicing at least five years after having graduated).

Kernberg (1986) starts his involvement in the debate by expressing concern about indoctrination, about uncritical discussion of Freud, and about the reluctance of teachers to present their clinical work. While our expected models for psychoanalytic education would seem to be either the art academy or the university college, he suggests that, in reality, our institutes are closer to technical trade schools where defined skills are taught without encouraging creativity, or to monasteries and religious retreats founded on faith (p. 810). Kernberg also published a humoristic study of "Thirty methods to destroy the creativity of psychoanalytic candidates" (1996), and a comprehensive critique of psychoanalytic education (2000).

My own critique of traditional training (Berman, 2000, 2004) focuses on the dangers of the utopian dimension in training and particularly of the utopian New Person fantasy often identifiable in the more ambitious rationales of analytic education. I compare these phenomena in psychoanalytic education to the high aspirations, which might result in a tendency to humiliate individuals seen as insufficiently adapted to the New Person fantasy, in various religious and ideological traditions in human history (the variation I studied most closely is the early kibbutz movement in Israel (Berman, 1988), but there are many more). I relate these aspects to the frequent tendency toward idealization of analysis and analytic training, to potential persecutory aspects, and to the "analytic false self" components that might emerge within a new analyst's identity, when fulfilling expectations, complying and identifying with authority figures substitutes for a genuine process of individuation and self discovery.

Several characteristics of the "utopian state of mind" could contribute to its risks. Its emphasis on desiderata, and constant comparisons with a valuable end-state, might interfere with the full appreciation of the complexities and inner contradictions of existing reality. Splitting between the flawed present and the yearned for improved future might imply blindness to the inherently paradoxical and conflictual nature of human existence. The seriousness, strictness, and moralism of utopianism might push aside humor and irony, often necessary preconditions for a "live and let live" flexibility. Attributing emotional needs to condemned sources (evil, sinfulness, greed, materialism, narcissism, etc.) might prevent tolerance of the unavoidable imperfection of individuals and rationalize a judgmental and persecutory attitude toward them. Believing that goals sanctify means, one may forget how means mold outcomes. In structural terms, a utopian state of mind is dominated by a perfectionistic ego ideal and a rigid superego, at the expense of ego and id alike.

Our training system, Balint (1948) says, contrary to its conscious aim of developing a strong critical ego, necessarily leads to "a weakening of these ego functions and to the formation and strengthening of a special kind of super-ego" (p. 167). "Idealization processes and an ambience of persecution are practically universal in psychoanalytic institutes", Kernberg (1986, p. 815) suggests. Among the topics idealized in our literature (Berman, 2004), I would list the notion of analyzability as an absolute attribute of the patient, the idea of a standard "correct technique", the belief in "being fully analyzed" or its later version of "structural change", the related sharp differentiation between psychoanalysis and psychotherapy, the belief that applicants for psychoanalytic training can be objectively screened, and the pressure for a continuous thorough evaluation of trainees, when "candidates are subject to a process of judgment which is necessarily experienced as a judgment of themselves as persons" (Rustin, 1985, p. 152). This is a major source of "the paranoid atmosphere that often pervades psychoanalytic institutes . . . [with a] devastating effect on the 'quality of life' in psychoanalytic education" (Kernberg, 1986, p. 803).

The training analyst as a superior analyst

A central idealization concerns the training analyst. Although many authors agree nowadays with Ferenczi and Rank (1924) that "the correct didactic analysis is one that does not in the least differ from the curative treatment" (p. 60), the image of the training analyst as a superior analyst is still prominent in the literature, and much has been written about the outstanding qualities expected of training analysts. Such descriptions are very appealing, but I have some doubts whether they fit the way any of us are described in informal conversations among colleagues or trainees.

Moreover, while the goal is to make sure that candidates benefit from high-quality analysis and supervision, it appears that the appointment of training analysts is very often influenced by transferences, political alliances, charisma, visibility, personal popularity, rumors, and other factors not necessarily related to quality *per se*. "Discretion, secrecy and uncertainty about what is required to become a training analyst, how these decisions are made, where and by whom" are listed by Kernberg (1996, p. 1039) as widespread phenomena that sabotage the creativity of faculty members and, subsequently, of candidates.

The belief that training analysts can be chosen as the best according to objective standards appears to disregard intersubjective emotional reality and social processes. Experience shows that views about most analysts vary, and even senior colleagues may be admired by some and criticized by others. Variations in theoretical approach and in preferences for different analytic styles appear to influence such gaps, in addition to purely personal likes and dislikes, which are easily rationalized and intellectualized. Awad (2009) describes situations in which the supposedly objective criteria for choosing training analysts rationalize favoring certain theoretical orientations while blacklisting colleagues holding other views.

In this respect, "objectively choosing the best analysts as training analysts" might be equivalent to "objectively choosing the best applicants to be admitted as candidates"; both beliefs convey disregard for the subjective and intersubjective nature of all interpersonal perceptions and attitudes. Moreover, as every one of us is likely to have in mind a "private list" of analysts we genuinely respect (those to whom we would refer a family member or a close friend), and these lists cannot all be identical with the "official list" of training analysts, the forced idealization of an official list could inadvertently lead to an actual devaluation.

The category of training analyst is itself being criticized by several authors. Bernfeld (1962) writes,

> We possess no way by which we can rationally rank our membership into Good, Very Good, and The Best Analysts. . . . By singling out a few members . . . implying that they are the best analysts, we confuse fantasy and magic with reality factors . . . [and] disturb perceptibly the transference in the personal analysis. (p. 481)

Lussier (1991; see Wallerstein, 1993) also feels that having a separate class of training analysts is destructive:

> Can the science of psychoanalysis, by definition, admit, without inner inconsistencies, of two classes of analysts: The High Priests and the ordinary ones? For the unconscious phantasy formation of any candidate, the fact of being analysed by a member of the select group cannot but feed the unconscious belief in a special magic power, the phallic power, with which his "special" analyst has been invested. . . . What a fertile ground for idealization, unconscious magical participation to a special power through identification, a pathogenic transferential relation that can hardly be analysed. (Lussier, 1991, p. 16)

Meyer created quite a stir in the 2001 IPA conference of training analysts when he described becoming a training analyst as a pursuit of status and power, and discussed training analysis as stimulating narcissistic gratification, fostering an atmosphere with paranoiac qualities, and creating a tyranny veiled in academic clothing. In his subsequent paper (Meyer, 2003), he further elaborates his devastating deconstruction of the "official" training analysis as a fetish and as an ideological structure, and suggests that "every discriminated category of analyses should be abolished" (p. 1257).

Outlining the history of training analysts and institutes, Zusman (1988) speaks of "The Eitingon syndrome". Eitingon treated Freud's work as sacrosanct and organized the Berlin Institute accordingly. "The Committee" running the psychoanalytic movement acquired the characteristics of a sect or a secret society, and these were transmitted to all institutes, training committees, and local societies.

> The Eitingon syndrome is a transference phenomenon defined by the transposition of a petrified bipersonal relationship (Eitingon/Freud) to the institutional level, where it then multiplies by "regenerating" the original pair in each training analyst and his or her candidate. (Zusman, 2003[1988], p. 361)

This observation parallels Benjamin's (1997) comment, "The seduction by knowledge as power remained the unanalyzed transference in the geneology of analytic training, the unconscious basis of authority that leads us back to our ideal father" (pp. 792–793).

The intrusion of institute dynamics into a candidate's personal analysis, most prominent in those institutes which practice some form of reporting, in spite of the serious arguments raised against it (e.g., Kairys, 1964, McLaughlin, 1967), has provoked Kernberg's (1986) critique of the "hypocrisy and dishonest manipulation" involved in "the dramatic contradiction between hiding one's personality in order not to influence the candidate's analysis while actually influencing the candidate's progression behind his back" (p. 817). McLaughlin (1967) suggests making "every effort to remove the analysis of our candidates, as far as possible, from any institutional connection" (p. 230). Thomä (1993) emphasizes the need to achieve "a climate of freedom, where the analyst is not obliged to supply any information or give an assessment" (p. 26), so that "the analysis proceeds as a private affair" (p. 17).

However, the issue is not limited to reporting. Another intense intrusion might occur when a candidate is admitted while already in analysis with an analyst who is not a training analyst. Some institutes require termination of the ongoing analysis and initiation of a new one with a training analyst, irrespective of the feelings of either the trainee or the original analyst. To me, this procedure suggests that the idealization of training analysts has led us to lose our respect for the integrity, continuity, and natural course of the analytic process. Consequently, we present a negative role model to our trainees. A second analysis is often a blessing (even when the first one was conducted by a senior training analyst), but our analytic experience indicates it should be chosen and timed by the analysand rather than forced by administrators.

Long-term impact of inhibiting elements in training

Undoubtedly, we all strive to achieve the best therapeutic results in our analyses and to reach the highest possible standards in training future psychoanalysts and psychotherapists. My criticism is not meant to undermine this goal. On the contrary, I am suggesting that perfectionism, unrealistic idealizations, and a rigid and persecutory atmosphere may lower quality in spite of the honest wish to raise it.

Our fantasy wish might be to find the really suitable professionals, to assign to them analyzable patients with whom they can practice correct technique until structural change is achieved, to let only carefully chosen training analysts analyze them, and to evaluate our trainees continuously to guarantee good results, but this wish involves risky utopian elements and, therefore, might backfire.

This fantasy wish might stray too far from our clinical experience and from our life experience (Berman, 2000, 2004). In reality, we know that all of us, analysts in all stages of professional growth, have our personal and professional strengths and weaknesses; that we all do well with some patients and poorly with others, and we rarely can predict this in advance; that in all levels of the professional hierarchy there are colleagues we respect and colleagues we have doubts about, and we rarely all agree on such judgments; that good analytic work is creative, individualistic, and never standard; that all analytic successes are partial and never preclude the need for more treatment in the future.

The inhibiting influences of traditional training do not easily evaporate after graduation. Klauber (1983) writes, "For many years the younger psychoanalyst functions—or at any rate I functioned—in part with an analytical false self . . . It took me a good ten years of full-time psychoanalytic practice to feel myself a psychoanalyst" (p. 46). Orgel (2002) describes, "In committee meetings, one frequently 'hears' his or her own analyst's voice in the opinions expressed by present and former analysands" (p. 428). Rustin (1985) suggests that the public life of the analytic community is inevitably "influenced by the pressures of the more primitive loyalties and claims on loyalty which arise from the particular relationships in which analysts are trained" (p. 145). Ross (1999) adds,

> At almost every stage of their progression, candidates and younger analysts found themselves subject to pathologizing interpretations and to severe rites of passage in the manifest form of successive certifications of competence. (p. 66)

Dulchin and Segal (1982), in a thorough sociological study of the life of a psychoanalytic institute, demonstrate how the informal "leakage" of information, originating in personal analyses of candidates and members, as well as of their relatives and friends, influences all participants in the system, and often inhibits them out of fear of a damaging exposure. One senior faculty member became much more open in a research interview after finding out that the interviewer was not in analysis (p. 32). "The analytic process involved all the junior

Institute members in a form of reporting on one another to their senior members" (p. 36).

In other words, the impingements of the training period leave their lasting mark and are also later reactivated in the relationships within the psychoanalytic community.

> During training, obviously, candidates are closely scrutinized and evaluated; after becoming fully-fledged analysts, this scrutiny becomes more subtle, but no less important, as selections are made to key teaching, supervisory and administrative roles. (Eisold, 1994, p. 790)

Such scrutiny could snowball in some institutes and psychoanalytic societies, until they become haunted by the demons of ruthless perfectionistic judgment, turning at times into character assassination. In such settings, narcissism and other diagnostic terms may play the same function that "sin" and "vice" play in fundamentalist milieus and "bourgeois individualism" in utopian socialist groups.

The important point raised by Rustin (1985) is relevant at all stages of the professional ladder, from applicant to training analyst:

> Where 'interpretations' become utilized in everyday life to control individuals or groups, they are often experienced as invasions of privacy, and inhibit instead of supporting the development of individual autonomy. (p. 147)

Individual autonomy is crucial in psychoanalysis, a profession in which the analyst's personality is the major tool, a discipline that teaches us constantly about the illusory nature of all generalized conventional truths, not reached through genuine personal experience. Our clinical effectiveness and our theoretical potency alike are dependent on flexibility, on creativity, on a capacity to use ourselves fully to observe emotional reality freshly, in ourselves and in the other, and to become attentive to our own blind spots and the rigidities that stand in our way. Increasing such capacities is a primary goal of psychoanalytic training, and the factors that hinder them must be of great concern to us.

Bernfeld (1962) suggests that writing regulations and enforcing them "takes the life out of psychoanalysis" (p. 479). Our choice, however, is not between rigid structure and anarchy (Wallerstein, 1993). A stable, containing structure need not be formalistic and impersonal. Unique individual needs of trainees can potentially be legitimized as a crucial element to be taken into account and accommodated by the structure, rather than being stigmatized as a rebellious defiance subverting it and needing to be suppressed.

I am aware, of course, that my thinking also runs the risk of arousing a utopian, perfectionistic idealization of its own, of painless psychoanalytic training, of a completely relaxed, free institute. Such perfection can never be achieved. Paranoid anxieties are ubiquitous. Learning new skills unavoidably arouses feelings of impotence and helplessness. Criticism may always be experienced as hurtful, but without criticism no growth can be accomplished. Psychoanalytic training can never be all fun and pleasure.

Yet, differences of degree and proportion are, at times, very important. Having graduated from two different institutes, and having taught in more than one, I can attest to significant variations. The atmosphere of an institute may shape the balance between anxiety and excitement, between gradually increased confidence and a sense of being castrated, between a desperate, defensive reliance on a false analytic self (the fantasized Real Analyst as a variation of the utopian New Person), and a better potential for developing an intrinsic analytic identity, which is unique to each of us.

In this respect, an exclusive focus on individual dynamics (conveyed in referring all difficulties "back to the couch" (Kernberg, 1996, p. 1038)) can be defensively abused to deny institutional dynamics and group processes. A personal analysis is naturally geared toward an individual–biographical emphasis; at worst, it may be abused to deny group dynamics, while, at best, it can acknowledge them without being able to influence them directly. Open forums for group discussion of candidates and faculty, at times jointly, might be more helpful in resolving training issues than are individual couches.

Psychoanalysis can be seen as a theory about the possibilities of psychic change and also about the limits of psychic change. It has also been applied to the study of potential change in institutions and organizations, and of the stumbling blocks on the way to such change. It can be self-critically applied to our training structures, allowing a new understanding of inherent difficulties. This understanding can be useful in contemplating reasonable and realistic reforms in our own institutions and in working through the anxieties and resistances any such reforms are likely to generate.

In many national, religious, and social movements, a gap tends to evolve between ideals and the structures created to implement them. This may have happened to us as well. A better understanding of individual and group regressive processes at our institutes may be an impetus for changes in the structure and climate of psychoanalytic training, allowing a better fit between institutional forms of training and its substantial goals of individual growth.

The Israeli experience

I can now return to the specific case I wish to explore, that of the Israel Psychoanalytic Society and its training institute. In past publications, I reported in detail the sequence of what I named "the Israeli controversial discussions" of 1992–1996 (Berman, 1998, 2004), and summarized the subsequent developments of 1996–2003 (Berman, 2004). For the present chapter, I chose another structure, focusing on several key issues and making a comparison between 1990 and 2015, a quarter of a century later.

At the time of writing, in 2015, the Israel Psychoanalytic Society (IPS) has around 250 members, and over 100 candidates undergo training at the Israel Psychoanalytic Institute (IPI). (This proportion guarantees the future of the Society for some decades, in contrast to societies in which the member–candidate proportion is much more skewed, implying an unavoidable gradual decrease in membership.) The classical theoretical orientation of the past has been gradually broadened, and today one can sense in the Society strong influences of Klein, Bion, Winnicott, Kohut, French psychoanalysis, and relational–intersubjective trends. There is no "mainstream" any longer. This heterogeneous picture, while it is a blessing in my view, also presents certain difficulties for candidates (Berman, 2014). The Society's home is in Jerusalem, but, in recent years, most activity and much of the training has shifted to the Tel Aviv area (the Institute holds one semester in Jerusalem and one in Tel Aviv), against the background of demographic and cultural changes.[1]

The continued success of the Institute, in spite of growing competition,[2] can be attested by the fact that twenty-four qualified applicants[3] asked to be admitted in 2015, of whom the Admissions Committee chose to admit a dozen, with the help of two in-depth interviews each one undergoes.

Let me review some of the major changes in the IPS and IPI during the past quarter of a century. Many of the changes are interrelated, so the division is a bit arbitrary, and the full picture will emerge gradually.

Leadership and climate

For many decades, the IPS had a strong permanent leadership, composed of a small group of training analysts. Office holders maintained their roles for many years. The IPI was run by a Director (who had to be a psychiatrist) and by a Training Committee, mostly composed of training analysts, which was quite secretive about its procedures, and was in charge of many aspects: admissions, evaluation of candidates, curriculum, decisions about graduation (or dismissal), appointment of training analysts, etc. The number of training analysts was very small and new appointments were rare.

Processes of democratization and decentralization started in the 1980s and reached greater momentum in the 1990s. The position of Institute Director was abolished, and new, separate committees were established for admissions and for proposing training analysts, thus reducing the absolute power of the Training Committee. A new Ethics Committee was created as well, and a Program Committee was elected, relieving the Society Board from this function. Rotation in all positions—IPS officers, committee chairs, and members—became mandatory, and no one could fill a position for more than three years, so a much larger proportion of the membership became involved in decision making. Chairs of the Admissions and Training Committees have to be training analysts, but many members are younger colleagues, some of them recent graduates. Although not stated in the bylaws, members in key positions never return for a second term later on, so the expectation is for "fresh blood" in important roles.

At times, this creates instability, when a newly elected committee reverses the policy of its predecessors. For example, one Training Committee changed the curriculum to an elective structure, with seminars composed of candidates at different stages of training; a later Training Committee reversed the curriculum to mostly mandatory courses that an incoming class takes together. Such major decisions are always approved by the full IPS membership, and the instability they might cause is counterbalanced by a genuine experience of a democratic process.

During the past twenty-five years, a tradition has also evolved at IPS of holding yearly meetings in which issues related to Israeli psychoanalysis and psychoanalytic training are openly and informally discussed by all members attending, part of the time in small groups. Parallel to that, the IPI candidates hold a yearly weekend meeting of their own, independently organized and planned, which includes presenting and debating papers as well as small group discussions. The candidates have their committee, which often meets with the Training Committee.

In 2014, when a raise in the regulated cost of supervision was announced, the candidates protested what they saw as an exaggerated financial burden during training. While some faculty members responded angrily and viewed the candidates as demanding, disrespectful, and defiant, the Training Committee chose to open a dialogue with them, consulted the IPS membership through internet discussions, and subsequently made some changes in the training program. These changes—although not radical, and not altering the substance of the Institute's requirements—could shorten to some degree the length of training and reduce its cost. I mention later on some of these recent changes, but above all I wish to emphasize the thoughtful process and the open dialogue with the candidates, which were not possible twenty-five years ago.

Evaluation, graduation, votes

A central characteristic of the IPI, for many years, was a very thorough evaluation of candidates by the Training Committee. Frequent reports were submitted by supervisors, and long meetings were dedicated to a discussion of the personal characteristics and dynamics of each candidate. Some candidates were expelled. This reality often aroused anxiety and paranoia, but by the early 1980s, attempts to expel certain candidates aroused stormy reactions. When the Training Committee considered terminating the training of candidates due to negative reports of a supervisor, other supervisors protested, disputing the negative evaluation, and the opposing views made a decision impossible. This new development was influenced by a greater heterogeneity of the faculty, signified lesser confidence in impartial objective authority, and became part of a more skeptical climate regarding the impact of strict institutional evaluation and control.

In recent years, the Training Committee of the IPI became much less preoccupied with evaluation of candidates, and more invested in attempting to improve training. Without any formal decision, the written evaluation forms were abandoned at some point, to the relief of candidates and most supervisors. Evaluation and feedback have been actually delegated to the three supervisors of each candidate, who have practically become the main representatives of the Institute *vis-à-vis* the candidate. Little formal reporting by supervisors and teachers takes place, in spite of some attempts to resume it. The subcommittee for evaluation changed its name, and now defines itself as a subcommittee accompanying candidates through their training.

Some faculty members have been expressing concern that evaluation is now insufficient, and look for ways to reintroduce more systematic evaluation, warning that otherwise "every new applicant we admit is assured of becoming a training analyst in due time" (this implies also criticism of the new procedure for becoming a training analyst, to be discussed later on). Other faculty members (including myself) believe that supervisors should be encouraged to give more critical feedback to their supervisees, but committee evaluation discussions can be reserved for specifically problematic candidates, and are not needed as a routine.

Personally, I do not observe any lowering of standards since evaluation was minimized. Most candidates appear highly invested in their training (which is still quite demanding in terms of time, money, and emotional energy) and very eager to improve their knowledge and skills. It seems that their personal superego functions are usually quite effective, even without formal external reinforcement. In addition, the attentive and thoughtful atmosphere among the candidates (e.g., in group supervision) appears to supplement the input of faculty in encouraging serious scrutiny of one's functioning as a beginning analyst.

Considerable changes were gradually introduced in the form of graduation, though its centrepiece—a written report about one of the analyses conducted during training, including a brief theoretical discussion—has remained the same. In the past, this report was read and evaluated by the whole Training Committee, and the final conclusions were reported to the candidate by the committee chairperson (so the candidate was not present in the discussion and never knew who said what). In recent years, an *ad hoc* reading committee of three members is appointed for each graduating candidate (another aspect of decentralizing power); an attempt is made to create heterogeneous reading committees, in which at least one member is identified with the particular candidate's own central theoretical emphasis. The case is discussed openly in a joint meeting of the committee and the candidate, enabling the candidate to respond directly to any critical comments and questions. After approval, or after making required corrections, the candidate presents the case publicly as a graduation event.

Writing the case report is still a source of considerable anxiety, even though it is no longer followed by a vote. It is experienced as one's *resumé*, and candidates are often afraid they will be seen as insufficiently competent. I suspect this fear is an unavoidable aspect of training. Anxiety often inhibits writing, and some candidates end up presenting their case a few years after they were allowed to submit it (which is when they complete the five-year sequence of coursework, and all three of their supervised analyses reach sufficient duration).

In most cases, the actual meeting with the reading committee is benign, and friendlier than the candidate's prior fantasies. Some reading committees are more critical, at times asking for sections of the report to be revised, or for some theoretical aspects to be explored more fully. There were, however, a couple of instances when reading committees refused to approve a report that appeared to them as too disappointing. Although in all these cases the candidate eventually graduated (after more revisions, appointment of a second reading committee, etc.), the rumors about these situations certainly increased candidates' fears and inhibitions, arousing the experience of being dependent upon a capricious and unpredictable authority, possibly torn by its own internal conflicts.

At times, differences of opinion about quality (the case being seen as satisfactory by the supervisor, and as weak by the committee) coincide with theoretical disagreements as to what constitutes a serious psychoanalytic treatment. The present heterogeneity of the Institute might, in this respect, become a threat to the candidates (Berman, 2014). What one supervisor—for example—sees as a welcome expression of analytic holding and provision, another faculty member frowns upon as a confusing boundary violation, and the candidate may be caught in the cross-fire.

On the other hand, in some instances supervisors confided that they were also critical of the candidate's work, and felt happy that their concerns—maybe not taken seriously enough by the supervisee—were reinforced by another group of analysts not involved in ongoing supervision and in its complex transference–countertransference dynamics.

With a much larger membership and a larger candidate group, general attendance in graduation events is no longer expected, and often the audience consists of the candidate's supervisors, friends, and classmates, with only a few "outsiders". Moreover, some candidates ask for a case presentation "by invitation only" for reasons of confidentiality, especially when the analysis discussed is of a mental health professional.

The most significant change regarding graduation is that the vote on admitting graduates of the Institute into the IPS, following their case presentation, was abolished in the early 1990s. Admission as a member of the IPS is now automatic upon graduating its Institute. Only graduates of other IPA institutes, if they wish to join the IPS, are accepted through a vote of the membership.

Around 1990, many Israeli analysts went through three secret votes during their analytic career, and had to receive a two-thirds majority in each—a major source of persecutory anxiety. The first vote was upon graduating the Institute, and, once passing this vote, the analyst became an Associate Member of the IPS. At least two years later, and after presenting a paper to the Society (later on it was decided that the paper can be replaced by a record of active contribution to the Society, for members who did not wish to write a paper), a second secret vote was held, to be accepted as a Full Member. Finally, Full Members wishing to become training analysts had, for several years, to go through a (third) secret vote for this role. This voting was abolished in 1996, a central topic to which I will return.

So, between 1996 and 2014, only one vote remained—the vote on becoming a Full Member. Not surprisingly, this single vote absorbed all the paranoia inherent in being evaluated by one's colleagues, with criteria that cannot be spelled out fully by anybody. The significance of becoming a Full Member rather than an Associate Member was never clear, but as only Full Members could become training analysts, this was the most significant implication of the vote. In the discussion preceding each voting, only positive views were typically heard. Colleagues described their long acquaintance with the person discussed, and gave him or her warm compliments. In most cases, however, some unexplained "no" or "abstain" votes appeared in the ballot. Guessing who cast them became an anxious preoccupation of the person voted upon. Whereas in most cases their number posed no problem, there were several instances throughout the years when the "yes" votes turned out to be insufficient for the two-thirds majority required in the IPS bylaws. For example, if a particular colleague received 60% "yes" votes, 10% "no" votes, and 30% "abstain" votes, they were not approved as Full Members—a painful narcissistic injury.

In recent years, this voting procedure became harshly criticized in IPS business meetings. Many members commented that the differentiation between being an Associate Member and a Full Member is meaningless, and the criteria for supporting or not supporting a particular person are extremely vague. With the growth of the Society, many members might not know directly the person voted upon, and they might abstain because they do not have a firm opinion, not as an expression of reservation. Not everyone attends the papers presented, and some of the papers might be rather impersonal, not saying a lot about the presenter. The feeling was that the voting mostly measures personal ties and popularity, and, on the other hand, indicates whether a particular member "stepped on the toes" of some colleagues in professional or personal matters.

Moreover, it was repeatedly pointed out, the vote became mostly a symbolic rite of passage. Most of the colleagues who failed to receive a two-thirds majority presented themselves for a second vote a year or so later. In the second vote, all of them received enough support to become Full Members (in one case, the same person was elected president of IPS a few years later). A possible interpretation is that those members who cast a "no" or "abstain" vote because of a personal grudge or theoretical opposition on the first occasion felt guilty about contributing to a public shaming of a colleague, and changed their vote to "yes" on the second occasion, or else avoided participating in the second voting altogether.

Still, some of the more conservative members expressed concern about abolishing the last remaining vote. They feared this would signify that quality of analytic work becomes irrelevant, and everyone could eventually become a training analyst. A few years ago, a special task force proposed abolishing the voting but instead creating a system of evaluating members' work before they could become training analysts. Many IPS members (including myself) felt, however, that the proposed system was likely to become burdensome, inhibiting, and persecutory, and the change would actually be "from the frying pan into the fire". Opposition was so strong that the proposal was not even voted upon.

After many such debates, the IPS Board proposed in 2014 to abolish the "last remaining vote", and to make presenting a paper a requirement for the next step—becoming a training analyst—without any evaluation process. They also proposed creating special seminars for beginning training analysts, to discuss issues of supervision and the unique aspects of analyzing trainees; such (voluntary) seminars were, indeed, started in Jerusalem, Tel Aviv, and Haifa. The Board hesitated between two options: either maintaining the differentiation between Associate Members and Full Members but basing it on factual criteria alone (mostly years since graduation), or giving it up altogether, as happened in numerous IPA societies. In an open vote, the second option won a majority, and the IPS now has only one category of membership. In my view, these decisions signify the successful culmination of an important long process of making the IPS and the IPI into more egalitarian organizations with much fewer elitist, hierarchical, and persecutory elements.

Interventions in the personal analysis of trainees

The IPI has adopted a "non-reporting" policy from an early stage of its existence. Nevertheless, the issue of the Institute's intervention in the personal analysis of its candidates came up in two forms.

First, the question of interrupting ongoing analyses of trainees was the main trigger of the stormy "controversial discussions" of 1992–1996, which almost led to a split in the Society. I described their sequence in full detail elsewhere (Berman, 1998, 2004) and will only summarize them here.

For many years, most of the applicants for psychoanalytic training in Israel are experienced psychoanalytic psychotherapists, mostly clinical psychologists. Many of the candidates come to the Institute while already undergoing a personal analysis. This has been very helpful in terms of their maturity as trainees, but has also intensified one particular problem: while, in most cases, their analysts have been experienced colleagues with good reputation, many were not training analysts. The traditional demand at this juncture, that the prospective trainee interrupt his or her ongoing analysis and start a new one with an official training analyst, has aroused much pain and anger among candidates and members alike (especially those whose analysands were "taken away"). Many have complained that this practice conveys lack of respect for the integrity and natural course of the analytic process, and poses a negative model for trainees. This complaint has been reinforced by the awareness that such a policy is not universal: "If the candidate is in analysis with a non-training analyst, he will, in some institutes, be required to transfer to a training analyst. In others every effort will be made to allow the candidate to remain with his analyst" (Sandler, 1982, p. 394).

The criticism within the Society regarding the anti-analytic implications of interrupting analyses led to a two-thirds majority vote (as required for changes in the bylaws), in May 1992, in favor of a resolution I introduced, allowing the Training Committee to "grant waivers", that is, the option to recognize any ongoing analysis with a member of the Society, on an *ad hoc* basis, as fulfilling the training requirement. However, in the following business meeting, many objections to the change came up, especially the concern that the possible exemption would erode the status of training analysts. In addition, the Training Committee expressed unwillingness to evaluate these individual cases. The debate was heated, and two camps clearly crystallized: those seeing firm structure as the first priority ("traditionalists") and those who put greater emphasis on flexibility and individual consideration ("reformists"). Eventually, it was decided to suspend implementation of the resolution, pending further discussion. This discussion required numerous meetings, took three and a half years, and continued to be quite heated.

In April 1994, I reintroduced my original "waiver" resolution, but another colleague (Raanan Kulka) proposed a more comprehensive and radical change: removing the personal analysis of candidates from the list of functions exclusive to training analysts. In addition to eliminating the need to interrupt analyses, this would give the candidate full responsibility for choosing her or his analyst. Experience indicates, he suggested, that candidates are very careful in choosing their analysts, being the individuals most influenced by the choice. They are eager to have the most profound analytic experience, and look for experienced and serious analysts irrespective of formal requirements.

In the vote, the more comprehensive reform won a large majority, and was accepted. The resolution stated: "Each candidate must undergo a personal analysis while going through training in the Institute. The analysis will be conducted by a qualified analyst who is a member of the Society". Spontaneous applause, quite unusual in the Society, followed the announcement of the results. In a brief discussion that ensued, some members expressed great satisfaction, while others gave vent to grave concerns about the quality of future training.

The months following that resolution were particularly stormy. Members alarmed by the change sought to mobilize help from abroad, suggesting that the new policy is incompatible with the regulations of the International Psychoanalytical Association. Supporters of the change saw no such incompatibility, citing the variability in training structures of various institutes recognized by the IPA. Moreover, consultations with IPA leaders made it clear that at the time the IPS resolution was approved only a consultation with the IPA about changing training rules was required, even though at a later date IPA bylaws were changed to require a formal approval (although, to the best of my knowledge, this requirement was never actually applied). In reality, the autonomy of the IPS was fully respected, and the IPA never intervened in the Israeli debates.

In view of the concern that the radical disagreements would eventually lead to a painful split, it was decided in 1995 to elect a Task Force, chaired by IPS president-elect Abigail Golomb, which would seek a compromise. The task force, in which all opinions in the Society were represented, made the following recommendations, approved by a business meeting of the IPS in January 1996:

1. Candidates are expected to undergo analysis and supervision with training analysts.
2. The procedure to become a training analyst will be made easier. All existing requirements are to be maintained (five years of

membership; full membership; continuous practice of at least three analyses, four times a week; interest in psychoanalysis and activity in the Society; ethical conduct), but the plenary personal discussion and secret vote on each new training analyst are abolished. The Society's board will approve all members who meet all criteria, a month after their names are circulated in order to allow members to raise objections.

3. Candidates who start training while already in analysis with a member who is not a training analyst are expected to switch to a training analyst within two years, prior to seeing their first analysand. If they wish to continue further with their present analyst, so as not to interrupt the analytic process, they may apply to the Training Committee for special permission.

These decisions calmed the atmosphere down, and they have been, indeed, applied by and large in the past nineteen years. Requests to continue an ongoing analysis with a non-training analyst are approved mostly when that analyst is rather experienced, and usually rejected when the analyst in question is a recent graduate of the Institute. A few years ago, a proposal was raised to legitimize the latter situations as well, while requiring such younger analysts to be supervised by a training analyst on the ongoing analyses of candidates, but this proposal was not approved.

In the past few years, the question of intrusions into personal analyses came up again in another version. The training bylaws have required, for many years, a four sessions per week analysis lasting at least 500 sessions during the period in which the candidate conducts analyses under supervision. A few years ago, the Training Committee asked that training analysts submit, before the candidate graduates, a written declaration that this requirement was, indeed, fulfilled. They suggested this procedure because of rumors that some candidates are not acting honestly; they only have a shorter analysis during the period of training, or see their analysts less than four times a week, so the facts have to be confirmed by the analyst.

This request aroused another stormy argument. Many training analysts (including myself) felt that this would violate the "non-reporting" policy by drawing the personal analyst into the official training structure; we argued that the issue was an educational issue, and should be dealt with through discussions of ethics, not through new regulations. Indeed, Thomä (2004) suggests—in line with his view that the candidate's analysis should be "an absolutely private matter"—that "training analysts would no longer be allowed to report how many sessions candidates had undergone and after how many sessions they consider the analysis to end" (p. 219).

Other colleagues agreed with the argument of the Training Committee, that "non-reporting" only applies to the content of the analysis, and to the evaluation of the candidate, but not to confirming the formal requirements, which must be defended. It was eventually decided to apply this procedure, but only to candidates admitted in the future, not to present candidates.

Recently, however, two developments changed the situation. First, the Society's Ethics Committee debated the issue extensively, and ruled that asking for the analyst's signed report does indeed violate the "non-reporting" principle. Roughly at the same time, it was decided to abolish the 500-hour regulation, and to write instead "an analysis of substantial duration".

The background of the latter change was the attempt I mentioned before to make training somewhat less burdensome, in response to protests of the candidates. One of the issues that came up was individual differences in the candidates' history as analysands. Some entered analysis the year before applying to the Institute, knowing that an analysis of at least one year was required for admission. These candidates were usually content with being in a four sessions a week analysis during their training, and the 500-hour rule (which implies about two and a half years) made sense to them. On the other hand, some other candidates entered analysis for personal therapeutic reasons, long before starting analytic training. In some cases, the candidate had already gone through seven or eight years of analysis by the time of admission. In many of these instances, both candidate and analyst felt that, at that stage, three sessions a week (or maybe even less) are quite enough, and the requirement is too rigid. (As I shall discuss shortly, more than a decade ago the Training Committee decided that, while two of the supervised analyses conducted by the candidate must be of four sessions a week, the third one can also be of three sessions a week. In the private practice of IPS members, analyses of three sessions a week are quite common.)

The Training Committee reached the conclusion that erasing the 500 session requirement from the bylaws will allow it to discuss more freely with each candidate the format of personal analysis suitable for their present individual needs. The wording "substantial duration" indeed appears in the IPA requirements for training, where no specific period or a cumulative number of sessions are listed. In consequence of this change and of the Ethics Committee's conclusion, the requirement that analysts sign a declaration regarding the candidate's personal analysis is no longer in effect. The candidates report to the Training Committee the length and frequency of their personal analysis, and the committee can discuss with them whether it appears to be satisfactory.

Analyses conducted by trainees: timing, selection, gender, frequency, length, supervision

Numerous changes also occurred regarding the analyses conducted by candidates under supervision. What remains consistent over the years is the requirement for three such analyses with three different supervisors, although, on some occasions, the idea was raised to reduce the number to two, as some other IPA societies require. This would, indeed, have made the training easier. Still, the general feeling (among faculty, members, and even many candidates) is that three analyses guarantee greater variability in the characteristics of the analysands, and three supervisions guarantee greater variance in analytic approaches to which the candidate is exposed.

In the past, these supervised analyses could begin after the candidate completed two years of introductory courses. When I was a candidate, one of the numerous hierarchies at the IPS and IPI was a division of the candidates into two subgroups: "junior candidates" in their first two years, and "senior candidates" in advanced years. Later on, this division was abolished, and, subsequently, it became possible to start analyses after three semesters. As part of the 2014 reform it was decided to allow starting supervised analyses after one academic year at the Institute. This development makes perfect sense in view of the fact that almost all candidates are experienced clinicians, typically in their forties and, at times, older, who have already studied psychoanalytic theory extensively before starting the Institute: in their clinical psychology internship, in psychoanalytic psychotherapy schools,[4] in private reading groups, etc. The truth is that they do not need introductory courses at all.

In 1990, and a few years later, too, the IPI had a system for screening potential patients to evaluate their analyzability. A candidate wishing to start supervised analysis with a patient (whether their own psychotherapy patient—a possibility discouraged in the past as "the transference was already contaminated by the face to face interaction"—a view which no longer exists, or a new patient seeking analysis) was expected to first refer the patient for a diagnostic interview. In each major city, a senior analyst was appointed to conduct the interviews, and these analysts had a final say. The criteria were mostly ego psychology criteria: ego strength, reality testing, tolerance of frustration, capacity for insight, lack of severe pathology.

Unlike some other changes discussed here, this practice was never formally abolished. It simply evaporated during the 1990s. Candidates (who, as I mentioned, are usually seasoned psychotherapists in their forties or older) now tend to find their own analysands, either from their therapeutic practice, or among new referrals they receive. They gradually stopped referring prospective analysands for screening ("there is often no other means of correcting such inexpedient laws than by boldly violating them", Freud, 1926e, p. 235), and instead started discussing the potential analysand with the supervisor who was to supervise the analysis. Nobody appeared to miss the old system, which often contributed to complications and split transference patterns (the interviewer as the real parental figure and the younger candidate/analyst as a substitute, etc.), visibly infantilizing the candidates.

After describing this change, Bar-Lev Elieli (2001, p. 31) asks,

> Does this mean that we trust our trainees more than before? Does it mean that we are afraid of losing any opportunity for an analysis? Does it mean that nowadays we feel more skilled in handling difficult cases in psychoanalysis, or that we have more trust in psychoanalysis? Are we more flexible, less rigid? ... Or are we operating as part of a wider cultural transition where youngsters can have a louder voice?

This shift can also be understood in the context of the growing doubts about the notion of analyzability, as an objective attribute of the analysand alone. Balint's argument "that any kind of technique and the criteria for selection are interdependent" (Balint, 1969, p. 101) has become more influential. Serious attention to countertransference and to intersubjectivity makes it clear that a patient unanalyzable by one analyst may prove to be analyzable by another analyst, with a different model, different personality, or a different supervisor. In other words, in our present theoretical climate, the goal is no longer objective assessment by an impartial expert (who must meet the analysand directly in order to bypass the candidate's possible distortions), but, rather, in-depth examination of the pros and cons of a potential analysis by the analyst and the supervisor, the two individuals who will be involved in the analysis for years, and whose actual subjective experiences may play a crucial role in its success or failure.

Personally, when approached by a candidate with such a question, I do not strive to make an objective diagnosis and prediction (I believe, in any case, that individuals with severe pathology can benefit from analysis), but, rather, to make sure that the candidate is aware of potential risks and complications and of countertransferential stumbling blocks, and does not start the difficult journey with naïve expectations, unsublimated rescue fantasies, or denied emotions. In most cases, I expect the candidates to make their own decision, after we have reached more clarity about the initial dynamics in the dyad and their relevance to a potential analytic process (Berman, 2014).

The change in this area is also related to the growing interest in the conversion of psychotherapy into psychoanalysis. The greater acceptance of this possibility is related both to pragmatic reasons (fewer patients who decidedly seek analysis), and to theoretical reasons, which include the lesser emphasis on "uncontaminated" anonymity in contemporary psychoanalysis, and the greater trust in working through analytically the patient's experience of the analyst's exposure and subjectivity.

In terms of the candidates, the different way of accepting analysands has increased their autonomy, and their trust in developing their own unique analytic identity (which may include preferences as to whom to analyze), rather than adopting some standard, "correct" way of analyzing ("analytic false self"). In addition, this change abolishes one source of "long periods of waiting in uncertainty" (Kernberg, 1996, p. 1032). In general, these changes weaken the control of the Training Committee over candidates, while empowering the individual supervisor as the actual representative of the Institute, and empowering the supervisor–candidate dyad (Berman, 2004).

Until recently, every candidate was required to treat analysands of both genders. This became another issue causing delays in graduation;

as we know, women seek therapy and analysis more than men, probably due to cultural norms of "masculine self-sufficiency". Numerous candidates found three female analysands, but got stuck in looking for a male analysand. As part of the 2014 reform, this requirement was transformed into a recommendation.

In 1990, as before, only analyses of four sessions a week were recognized for training. This created painful situations when an analysand wished to switch to three sessions a week, either for external reality reasons or for internal dynamic reasons, and the candidate opposed this wish vehemently in order not to lose the analysis as part of one's training requirements. This was a clear example of the way in which a rigid aspect of training pushed candidates to an authoritarian position *vis-à-vis* their analysands, remote from a more open climate of elasticity in an analysis, in which frequency of sessions can be negotiated by both partners rather than one-sidedly imposed. During the 1990s, the IPS Training Committee decided that one of the three required analyses can be of three sessions a week, as are many analyses conducted by IPS members (and most analyses in France and other countries). This helped prevent many of those problematic clashes.

For many years, only analyses lasting at least two years were recognized towards graduation. This created great tension in many analyses, when trainees became very worried that the analysand would drop out before twenty-four months are completed, and they would have to start another analysis from the beginning and delay their graduation. In some analyses I supervised, the quality of work miraculously improved from the twenty-fifth month on, when the threat was over. In another analysis I supervised, the patient wanted to terminate in the middle of the second year, but, having discovered on the IPS website that only analyses of at least two years are recognized for training, he told his analyst that in order not to sabotage him, he would leave the day the two years are over—which indeed happened. As part of the 2014 reform, the Training Committee now allows greater flexibility. If one supervised analysis ends after more than a year but less than two years, it can be recognized if the other two analyses last over two years, and if, in the supervisor's view, the candidate's work in that particular analysis contributed to the candidate's professional growth.

One more aspect of the 2014 reform is that after being supervised for three years on a particular analysis, candidate and supervisor can decide whether to switch to meeting once every two weeks rather than every week. Moreover, if the candidate starts a fourth analysis during training (numerous candidates do so), supervision can be by one of the existing supervisors, and the frequency can be chosen freely by candidate and supervisor.

The appointment of training analysts

Probably the most radical changes at the IPI during the past three decades have been in the area of choosing training analysts. Until the mid-1980s, these were decisions reached secretly by the powerful Training Committee. The number of training analysts remained very small, and some experienced colleagues who were in high demand as analysts and supervisors were denied the appointment for mysterious reasons; they were, at times, approved as *ad hoc* analysts for particular candidates, but not counted as part of the "chosen".

Towards the end of the 1980s, a process of democratic transformation has started in the IPS and in its Institute. An effort was made to allow a much larger proportion of the membership to become actively involved in decision-making and in administrative roles. Many members came to feel that too many functions had become concentrated in the Training Committee. The responsibility for recommending new training analysts was moved to another new committee. The latter committee was requested to reach its recommendations after examining the potential training analysts' professional credentials (the minimum being full membership, five years of membership, and the maintenance of a continuous analytic practice of at least three analyses) as well as their competence, and, if satisfied, to submit their names for a vote by secret ballot of all members (requiring a two-thirds majority). This reform was effective, leading to the selection of several new training analysts, after many years during which there had been no more than a dozen training analysts throughout Israel (Berman, 1998, 2004).

The new system created, however, new problems. Members of the new committee for screening training analysts reported great difficulty in conducting an objective evaluation of the quality of potential nominees. It was becoming gradually clearer that such evaluation is conducted in the absence of actual knowledge regarding a member's analytic skills, and is often influenced by transference feelings, charisma, visibility, personal popularity, political alliances, and so on. This realization eventually led to a more radical change.

In discussions held during 1995, many IPS members expressed open disgust with the persecutory and hostile atmosphere generated by the determination to discuss people's "merit", and subsequently voiced the desire to simplify the process of appointing training analysts, and to reduce its judgmental quality. It was also suggested that making it easier to become a training analyst would reduce the number of cases in which incoming candidates have to switch analysts, an issue that—as mentioned before—almost led to a split in the IPS. The task force headed by Abigail Golomb was asked to handle both issues, and, as I mentioned before, one of its recommendations, adopted by the IPS in 1996, was to change the procedure for appointing training analysts. All existing factual requirements were maintained (five years of membership; full membership; continuous practice of at least three analyses, four times a week; interest in psychoanalysis and activity in the Society; ethical conduct), but the plenary personal discussion and secret vote on each new training analyst were abolished. Ever since 1996, the Society's board approves all members who meet all criteria as training analysts.

As a result, the number of training analysts has considerably increased (to a little more than half of the IPS membership), allowing a real free choice of a personal analyst and of supervisors, who can also be switched by the candidate "with no questions asked". (Free choice has been the official policy for decades, but it was practically meaningless when the number of training analysts in each city was very small.)

It might be said that, with this change, the definition of a training analyst was altered from being evaluative to being factual, from an analyst of better quality to an active, experienced, older analyst. Issues of merit regarding training analysts were, therefore, withdrawn from collective Society or committee judgment, and handed over in practice to the serious personal consultations candidates usually initiate with senior analysts they trust. "Did we leave the control in the hands of our candidates? Yes! They, the consumers of our teaching and supervision, will choose", suggests Bar-Lev Elieli (2001, p. 33). But I would add that candidates make their choices on the basis of their great motivation to have the best analysis possible, and do not wish to just "go through the motions" and waste time, money, and emotional investment on an analysis which is not experienced as helpful.

This change also goes hand-in-hand with an intersubjective emphasis, which casts doubt upon absolute "objective judgment" of quality. Even the most senior analysts, we know, may be admired by some and disliked by others, and variations in theory and in style play a role in this heterogeneity: what one values as consistency another suspects to be rigidity; what one welcomes as flexibility another derides as impulsivity, and so on. Unlike committee or group votes, personal choice by the candidate gives full weight to the candidate's subjective preferences and intuitions.

My own subjective impression is that the quality of training analysts appointed in the IPS remained equally variable in all three stages: secret decision by the Training Committee, open debate and election by the Society, and appointment according to factual criteria.

In general, a vast majority of the IPS membership is happy with the present policy. One change approved a few years ago was to accept training analysts who conducted, after graduation, two four times a week analyses and one three times a week analysis (as is allowed for candidates), and to also accept training analysts whose three post-graduation analyses were not simultaneous, but took place over a longer period of time. Recently, with the decision to abolish the category of Associate Member, the requirement to present a paper to the Society, previously needed for Full Membership, was added to the demands of prospective training analysts. New training analysts are now encouraged to participate in seminars discussing supervision and the unique characteristics of analyzing candidates and other trainees and colleagues.

Conclusion

Although many stages in the quarter-century process I describe were tense and painful, when some of us enthusiastically fought for change and other colleagues attempted to stop it and expressed grave concerns about its results, my overall conclusion is optimistic.

Unlike numerous psychoanalytic organizations, the IPS did not split, and we saved our trainees the painful experience of choosing between—for example—a beloved personal analyst and an appreciated supervisor, who suddenly belong to two antagonistic organizations. In spite of forceful opposition by more conservative colleagues, transformations in almost all areas of training and organizational structure made the IPS and IPI less rigid, less hierarchical, and less persecutory. The emphasis on continuous evaluation at all stages of one's analytic career is greatly reduced, and, contrary to alarmist fears, I do not feel the quality of clinical work and of theoretical thinking has been lowered.

My feeling is that our present way of conducting training gives a better chance for individual development, for finding one's unique personal voice as a psychoanalyst, for creating a genuine analytic identity not predominantly influenced by imitation, identification with the aggressor, and aspects of a false analytic self.

It should be noted that the IPA never interfered in the changes described. I hope that this is an indication that the IPA no longer defines itself as a controlling authority, but, rather, as a voluntary alliance of psychoanalysts and psychoanalytic groups maintaining pluralism and respecting local autonomy and a multiplicity of voices.

Notes

1. Affluent, secular, and educated populations continuously move from Jerusalem to the greater Tel Aviv area in recent years, including many analysts. Jerusalem is becoming poorer and more ultra-orthodox, and the opportunities to practice analysis and psychoanalytic therapy in Jerusalem gradually diminish.
2. For many decades, the IPS was the only psychoanalytic organization in Israel, and the IPI offered the only option of psychoanalytic training. In 2000, a new body was created by experienced psychoanalytic psychotherapists, the Tel Aviv Institute of Contemporary Psychoanalysis (TAICP), which is also quite successful. In spite of much controversy within the IPS in respect of this matter, many of its training analysts also see in analysis and supervision TAICP candidates, or offer seminars as guest faculty at TAICP (Berman, 2004, pp. 149–152). On a few occasions, joint scientific meetings of the IPS and TAICP were held. In 2015, a third institute was created, the Human Spirit Institute (HSI), with a unique Kohutian–Buddhist orientation. Many of its founders are IPS members; some belong to TAICP. Neither TAICP nor HSI joined the IPA. These developments had a

complex impact on the IPS, but I do not view them as a central influence on the changes I explore in this chapter.

3. Until recently, only psychiatrists, clinical psychologists, and psychiatric social workers could apply. In recent years, the applications by psychiatrists decreased, and the majority of candidates are clinical psychologists. In 2014, the IPS decided to admit also school psychologists, developmental psychologists, medical psychologists, rehabilitation psychologists, creative art therapists, and bibliotherapists, if they have considerable supervised experience in practicing psychoanalytic psychotherapy. All applicants must be in analysis for at least one year at the time of application.
4. A unique feature of the therapy field in Israel is the existence and popularity of numerous postgraduate psychotherapy schools, mostly offering three-year introductory programs to psychologists, psychiatrists, social workers, art therapists, etc., as well as advanced programs (focusing on Winnicott, Klein, Kohut, relational psychoanalysis, and other orientations) to graduates of such introductory programs. Students in these programs conduct psychotherapy of one or two weekly sessions, and most programs have a clear psychoanalytic orientation. The IPS itself sponsors several such programs, and other schools (where many IPS members and advanced IPI candidates also teach) belong to universities and to private organizations.

References

Aron, L. (1996). *A Meeting of Minds: Mutuality in Psychoanalysis*. Hillsdale, NJ: Analytic Press.

Awad, G. (2009). Critical thoughts on choosing training analysts. *International Journal of Applied Psychoanalytic Studies, 6*: 263–265.

Balint, M. (1948). On the psychoanalytic training system. *International Journal of Psychoanalysis, 29*: 163–173.

Balint, M. (1969). *The Basic Fault: Therapeutic Aspects of Regression*. London: Tavistock.

Bar-Lev Elieli, R. (2001). Discussion of J. Schubert's paper on training models. *Psychoanalysis in Europe, 55*: 27–35.

Benjamin, J. (1997). Psychoanalysis as a vocation. *Psychoanalytic Dialogues, 7*(6): 781–802.

Berman, E. (1988). Communal upbringing in the kibbutz: the allure and risks of psychoanalytic utopianism. *Psychoanalytic Study of the Child, 43*: 319–335.

Berman, E. (1998). Structure and individuality in psychoanalytic training: the Israeli controversial discussions. *American Journal of Psychoanalysis, 58*: 117–133.

Berman, E. (2000). The utopian fantasy of a New Person and the danger of a false analytic self. *Psychoanalytic Psychology, 17*: 38–60.

Berman, E. (2004). *Impossible Training: A Relational View of Psychoanalytic Education*. Hillsdale, NJ: Analytic Press [Routledge].

Berman, E. (2010). My way. *Psychoanalytic Inquiry, 30*: 116–132.

Berman, E. (2014). Psychoanalytic supervision in a heterogeneous theoretical context: benefits and complications. *Psychoanalytic Dialogues, 24*: 525–531.

Bernfeld, S. (1962). On psychoanalytic training. *Psychoanalytic Quarterly, 31*: 457–482.

Dulchin, J., & Segal, A. J. (1982). The ambiguity of confidentiality in a psychoanalytic institute; third-party confidences: the uses of information in a psychoanalytic institute. *Psychiatry, 45*: 13–37.

Eisold, K. (1994). The intolerance of diversity in psychoanalytic institutes. *International Journal of Psychoanalysis, 75*: 785–800.

Ferenczi, S., & Rank, O. (1924). *The Development of Psycho-Analysis*. New York: Dover.

Freud, S. (1926e). The question of lay analysis. *S. E., 20*: 183–258. London: Hogarth Press.

Kairys, D. (1964). The training analysis. *Psychoanalytic Quarterly, 33*: 485–512.

Kernberg, O. F. (1986). Institutional problems of psychoanalytic education. *Journal of the American Psychoanalytic Association, 34*: 799–834.

Kernberg, O. F. (1996). Thirty methods to destroy the creativity of psychoanalytic candidates. *International Journal of Psychoanalysis, 77*: 1031–1040.

Kernberg, O. F. (2000). A concerned critique of psychoanalytic education. *International Journal of Psychoanalysis, 81*: 97–120.

Klauber, J. (1983). The identity of the psychoanalyst. In: E. D. Joseph & D. Widlocher (Eds.), *The Identity of the Psychoanalyst* (pp. 41–50). New York: International Universities Press.

Lussier, A. (1991). Our training ideology. Paper presented at Fifth IPA Conference of training analysts, Buenos Aires.

McLaughlin, F. (1967). Addendum to a controversial proposal. Some observations on the training analysis. *Psychoanalytic Quarterly, 36*: 230–247.

Meyer, L. (2003). Subservient analysis. *International Journal of Psychoanalysis, 84*: 1241–1262.

Orgel, S. (2002). Some hazards to neutrality in the psychoanalysis of candidates. *Psychoanalytic Quarterly, 71*: 419–443.

Rolnik, E. (2012). *Freud in Zion: Psychoanalysis and the Making of Modern Jewish Identity*. London: Karnac.

Ross, J. M. (1999). Psychoanalysis, the anxiety of influence and the sadomasochism of everyday life. *Journal of Applied Psychoanalytic Studies, 1*: 57–78.

Rustin, M. (1985). The social organization of secrets: towards a sociology of psychoanalysis. *International Review of Psychanalysis, 12*: 143–159.

Sandler, A.-M. (1982). The selection and function of the training analyst in Europe. *International Review of Psychanalysis, 9*: 386–398.

Schröter, M. (2002). Max Eitingon and the struggle to establish an international standard for psychoanalytic training. *International Journal of Psychoanalysis, 83*: 875–893.

Thomä, H. (1993). Training analysis and psychoanalytic education: proposal for reform. *The Annual of Psychoanalysis, 21*: 3–75.

Thomä, H. (2004). Psychoanalysis without a specific professional identity: a utopian dream? *International Forum of Psychoanalysis, 13*: 213–236.

Wallerstein, R. S. (1993). Between chaos and petrification: a summary of the Fifth IPA Conference of Training Analysts. *International Journal of Psychoanalysis, 74*: 165–178.

Zusman, W. (2003)[1988]. Our science and our scientific lives. *Israel Psychoanalytic Journal, 1*: 351–377. Originally presented to the Linden Hall Conference of the IPA.

CHAPTER TWO

Training analysis and the Psychoanalytic Institute

Harold P. Blum

Introduction

Psychoanalysis has always supported the concept of change in theory and clinical practice and, to a lesser degree, in psychoanalytic education. Freud initially thought that to become an analyst, to gain insight into unconscious mental life, one had only to analyze one's dreams. He soon realized that becoming an analyst required more than a lone journey on the royal road of dream interpretation.

So long as psychoanalysis flourished, so long as it had social status and influence in intellectual and academic spheres, psychoanalysts were both pleased and complacent.

Challenges to what seemed to be time honored and working well could be taken lightly and critics could be largely ignored. Indifference to, or disparaging attitudes toward, psychoanalysis in the community, in medicine, the behavioral sciences, and the humanities, however, were associated with a worldwide decline in clinical practice. With fewer patients and a corresponding decline in applicants for psychoanalytic training, dissatisfaction and disappointment intensified. Psychoanalytic institutes declined in size, scope, and morale.

There were growing concerns about creativity among our candidates and recent graduates.

Brief psychotherapies, psychopharmacology, group therapy and family therapy supplanted interest in psychodynamic psychotherapy. In the USA, cognitive–behavioral therapy is taught to students of psychiatry, psychology, and social work as a treatment of choice for many mental disturbances. The search for a quick fix and a culture of narcissism demanding immediate gratification and self-satisfaction augmented longstanding bias and belligerence toward psychoanalysis.

This decline in interest and prestige had a beneficial side effect; it led to examination of traditional analytic thought about analytic training, analytic organizations, and the future of psychoanalysis. This has included such issues as who might become candidates, assignment *vs.* selection of training analysts by candidates, selection of training analysts, whether the category of training analyst should even continue to exist, reporting to education committees by training analysts, graduation requirements, etc. Kernberg's (2000, 2004, 2013) incisive dissections of psychoanalytic education has contributed to awareness of the threats to psychoanalysis from internal as well as more easily recognized external sources. Kernberg (1986) delineated four models of psychoanalytic institutes, two positive and two negatives: (1) a trade school; (2) a monastery or religious retreat; (3) an art academy—to foster creativity; (4) a university—to foster scholarship and new knowledge. The first two models emphasized, respectively, becoming skilled practitioners and/or accepting received wisdom and unquestioned dogma. Aware that both had their own drawbacks (for example, of elitism and entrenched authority), Kernberg proposed utilization of the two positive models of the art school and the university. Universities had lagged behind psychoanalytic organizations in promoting women, accepting minorities, and criticizing stereotypes. From a psychoanalytic structural perspective, the institute can represent a collective superego that is either benevolent or prohibitive. Kernberg has long advocated eliminating a training analyst oligarchy along with consistent transparency in psychoanalytic institutions. Senior analysts should present their own clinical material instead of only scrutinizing and supervising the reports of their juniors.

I shall discuss various problematic and paradoxical issues in psychoanalytic training, as well as changes in training, with a particular focus on the USA (Reeder, 2004).

History of the training model

Training analysis has a long history and tradition in psychoanalytic education. Exactly how the training analyst category was created is embedded in the remote past; historical records have apparently been lost. It is not clear whether it was by Eitingon acting as Chairman or by a group vote including Rado and Horney that training analysis was proposed about 1920 in the burgeoning Berlin institute. The designation of the category and the process of training analyst appointment were related to insecurity about analytic competence and the representation of psychoanalysis in the external world. In its early years, psychoanalysis was under widespread attack as a form of quackery, of phrenology, of perverse sexuality, and as advocating unbridled sexual and antisocial behavior. In its pioneer period, psychoanalysis had to be protected from dilution and distortion, from "wild analysis" by wild analysts.

In 1912, in the midst of personal and group turmoil surrounding Freud's dispute with Adler, Stekel, and Jung, Adler and Stekel defected, and, in 1914, Jung resigned as president of the IPA (Freud, 1914d). In response, Ferenczi expressed the hope that a small psychoanalytic group could be personally analyzed by Freud so that they could represent pure analytic theory. Jung had probably been the first to recommend that each analyst should be analyzed by another analyst, foreshadowing training analysis. Jones suggested a secret committee, akin to the Paladins of Charlemagne, to monitor Jung, to report to Freud, to protect the kingdom of their master (Grosskurth, 1991). Freud, responding to the recommendation of Ferenczi and Jones, consented to the formation of this secret committee of his gifted devoted disciples. This committee can be recognized as the aristocratic parents of the family romance of the early psychoanalysts. Analysts were proud of their filiation and descent from Freud, who gave intaglio rings to the loyal pioneer analysts, Abraham, Ferenczi, Jones, Rank, and Sachs. The rings, derived from ancient seals, symbolized a pledge of unswerving allegiance to their aggrandized father figure, founder of the new science of psychoanalysis. The committee pledged to discuss internally any disagreement with the fundamentals of psychoanalysis before public disclosure of dissent. Jones chaired the committee and Eitingon was added to the committee in 1919. It is not clear when the secret committee of ring bearers, which functioned for some ten years, became known to the members of the International Psychoanalytical Association. In my view, the committee can be considered the precursor of the education committee which would later determine selection of training analysts, supervisors, the institute faculty, and the curriculum.

The prototype "Eitingon" model, designed as a tripartite structure in Berlin in1920, consisted of training analysis, supervision, and a teaching curriculum. This model became standard and has endured in most international psychoanalytic institutes. The category of "training analyst" was consolidated in 1925 by an international training commission, initially chaired by Eitingon. The process of selection of training/supervising analysts was left at that time to the few small local institutes.

Candidate requirements

Not only have there been changes in training as a result of reconsiderations, at least in part due to the critiques of psychoanalysis noted above, but requirements for becoming a candidate also changed, in part in response to the law of supply and demand, but also to the deepened understanding of analyzability. The idealization of the analytic institute itself had fostered ambivalence toward medicine, academic psychology, and universities; institutes were, for the most part, isolated independent entities. In the USA, successful litigation against the requirement of being a physician for training and membership in the American Psychoanalytic Association revoked the monopoly of physicians. (This requirement had been waived for a few particularly qualified non-medical candidates.) Non-medical psychotherapists and those attracted to psychoanalysis from other fields became welcome and their acceptance compensated for the corresponding decline of applications by physicians. Concerned about their loss of medical identity as well as their continuing debt from loans to finance their expensive medical training, physicians even less frequently sought psychoanalytic training. The flexibility of work schedules was particularly attractive to women, both medical and non-medical. Ultimately, training analyst committees had to limit their own monopoly of analytic education and to admit highly qualified non-medical analysts into their own ranks.

Training analyst

Against the background of decline in prestige, practice, and income, the traditionally exalted position of the training analyst has been challenged with accelerating debate. In the USA, diatribe has infiltrated analytic discourse, to the detriment of careful contemplation of the issues. Demands for the abolition of the training analyst category countered by insistence on preservation of the category have too often been the subject of inflammatory rhetoric rather than consideration of both pros and cons, advantages and disadvantages, of different training models. In the American Psychoanalytic Association the specter of litigation and splitting emerged within the Association, with interrelated abrasive debate regarding national *vs.* local institutions controlling the appointment of training analysts. The original secret committee was the precursor of the training analyst committee of the international training commission. The ruling oligarchy of training analysts was idealized in the structure of the International Psychoanalytical Association (IPA) Congress until relatively recent meetings. Beginning in 1965, the IPA fostered the development of psychoanalytic education with a pre-Congress restricted to training analysts. The side effects of the training analyst category and, later, of the pre-Congress of the IPA, however, were not taken into account. The elite training analyst groups of the various institutes had a special biannual conclave prior to the biannual Congress. Training analysis and educational issues were not in the program of the Congress itself. The format of the pre-Congress implied that mainly training analysts were interested in psychoanalytic education. At the end of the pre-Congress, many training analysts left, saturated with meetings and eager to begin family holidays. Thus, those analysts did not mingle with the non-training analysts and candidates attending the Congress. Eventually, the pre-Congress and then the Congress proved too expansive and expensive. I had previously pointed out to the IPA, when I was a vice president, the problematic isolation of the pre-Congress and the protracted duration of the meetings. The pre-Congress has now been radically contracted, promoting greater attendance within the Congress.

The development of the category of training analyst was originally intended to ensure that the best and brightest, the most experienced and resourceful analysts trained the next generation of analysts.

Actually, most of the psychoanalysts in the fledgling IPA were inexperienced and could have been categorized as novices by present day standards. They had little formal analytic training and relied upon, and profited from, Freud's personal instruction and his early papers on psychoanalytic theory and technique. They were drawn to what was then a revolutionary understanding of the human mind and its disorders. Dazzled by the illumination of new psychoanalytic insights, they were also self-selected, troubled, and drawn to a movement or "cause" with radical explanatory and therapeutic promise. The attraction to a movement or cause had social and political implications quite apart from a scientific discipline. Training analysts, presumably selected, among other attributes, for their greater cultural sophistication, were thought to have wider intellectual influence, more effectively representing psychoanalysis in the sciences and humanities. Many of the early analytic patients came from academia and the arts. Their choice of an eminent training analyst seemed to support the notion of respected superior analysts as ambassadors to the wider social and academic world. The two-class system of training and non-training analysts, those in power and those with less influence and status inside and outside the institute, would have long-range repercussions. The division of the institute and society into "haves" and "have nots", higher and lower status groups, was bound to lead to disappointment and discontent. The family romance and lineage of candidates and their training analysts is inherently interwoven with oedipal and narcissistic conflicts. The two-class system could be readily related to the exalted adoptive parents and the lower rank biological parents of the family romance. The training analyst might be unconsciously regarded as omnipotent. Arlow (1972) referred to miscarriages of training with master–apprentice relationships, repeated institute splits, and the family romance of training analysis. The training analyst carries the omniscience of God, like Moses with the commandments, or like the rebel Prometheus, who steals divine omnipotence. Arlow also noted the advance of favored candidates who were properly compliant and deferential to institute authority.

Admission to the upper class might elicit triumphant narcissistic fantasy gratification and rejection might evoke envy, jealousy, and aggression. Unrecognized and unanalyzed, as was not infrequently the case, the failure to become a training analyst represented castration and narcissistic humiliation for the aspiring analyst. After graduation from the institute, the analyst, in identification with his/her training analyst and supervisor, frequently desires elevation to the exalted training analyst society within the society and institute. If this is not achieved, the oedipal child has not completed identification with the idealized parent and might be left feeling inferior and castrated. Neither can the graduate who is not a training analyst parent the next generation of analysts. The older generation has stymied the development of the next generation. The question of inclusion or exclusion activates unresolved primal scene conflicts and narcissistic gratification or injury (Kernberg, 2013; Zagermann, Chapter Fourteen, this volume). Analytic identity is validated or impeded.

If the training analyst group is self-perpetuating and self-selects training analyst appointments, it is likely to become a self-indulgent, encapsulated, entrenched, narcissistic, controlling clique within the psychoanalytic institute and society. Moreover, a monopoly over the appointment of training analysts exacerbates group infantile omnipotence and economic advantages. Referrals are more likely to be given to the superior analysts and, in turn, candidates may depend on the largesse of the training analysts and their supervisors for patient referrals. If the number of training analysts is restricted without new appointments, a monopoly is maintained. The stage is set for submission and/or rebellion by the alienated non-training analysts. When a group of analysts splits off from its former institute, it intends and actually acquires the prerogatives of training analyst and faculty appointments in the new institute.

Through identification with their former, initially idealized, analysts, the new training group may lay claim to the myth of the superior knowledge of the training analyst. The original training group too often in the past expressed both a superior and vindictive attitude toward the rebels. Identification with the former training analyst could be identification with the aggressor. The rebels are then regarded as not having the knowledge or analytic expertise to create an institute that will preserve their presumed excellence as well as denial of any oedipal defeat. The rebels have supposedly been unable to constructively analyze or self-analyze their unresolved negative transference which they have enacted in the splitting of the institute. Aggression in the training dyad is particularly difficult to analyze (Orgel, 2003). It is also more difficult to analyze infantile transference, as well as muted narcissistic rage, in the psychoanalytic situation of the institute.

The out-groups had dared to challenge the omnipotent and oedipal authority of the in-group. The institute splitting corresponds to the internal splitting of idealized and denigrated self and object representations or, in other terms, splitting of internalized object relations. The splitting off of authority to the group of supervisors from the training analyst group posed the same power and privileged oligarchy in a new form.

Being a training analyst became the major representation of status within the analytic organizations and institutes, virtually a monolithic path to career prestige (Auchincloss & Michels, 2003). As institutes evolved, the training analysts dominated the education committee and, in turn, admissions, progression, and graduation committees, of which they were usually the chairs. The criteria of selection were initially hardly transparent. Power, control, and prestige were concentrated in a training analyst oligarchy (Zagermann, Chapter Fourteen, this volume). The older generation of training analysts may close ranks in a self-contained, self-serving authoritarian structure with determinants from all developmental stages. If the candidate cannot separate and individuate (Mahler et al., 1975) after termination, analytic independence and creativity are impeded.

Training analysis

There have been many conferences, seminars, and papers about training analysis and analytic education, especially following the revival of psychoanalytic institutes following the Second World War (e.g., Bernfeld, 1962). Debate about the assets and liabilities of training analysis has intensified, and a chorus of analysts has been vociferous in asserting that the category of training analyst be eliminated (Masur, 1998). The problems of training analysis in particular have been recently explored by Kernberg (2000) and Zagermann (Chapter Fourteen, this volume). My own assessment of training analysis is influenced in the main by clinical considerations, group psychology, and the historical and cultural context of psychoanalytic education in the USA.

A potential candidate might be required to transfer from a personal analysis to a training analysis. The candidate and former analyst might be wounded if the analysis was progressing well. A prospective candidate would be lost if he/she refuses to obediently transfer and decides to stay with the original choice of personal analyst. Clearly, this choice would be obviated if the special category of training analyst were eliminated. Current progressive policy in most institutes requires that candidates should be in their own analysis while undertaking the control analysis of others, but permission not to transfer to a training analyst generally remains an institute option. The assignment of a training analyst in the past was usually done by the education committee. Only gradually did this practice give way to candidate choice. Secrecy and reporting were initially regarded as commendable, with the main rationale of protecting psychoanalysis from unsavory and unstable personalities. Following much reassessment and consideration, however, reporting by the training analyst to the institute education committee about a candidate's progress or psychopathology has now been abandoned by almost all IPA institutes. Violating analytic confidentiality and neutrality, a report by a training analyst distorts the analytic process in a variety of ways, including inhibition of free association. Fortunately, this policy is now considered inappropriate, antiquated, and contrary to analytic principles. Reporting has also contributed to gossip among members within analytic organizations. A report by a training analyst would now be regarded as a report about the training analyst as much as about the candidate. The shift to non-reporting was initially gradual and gathered momentum in the last decades of the twentieth century

As an antidote to the too brief analyses of many of the training analysts prior to the Second World War, analysis became ever longer. Most analysts in the fledgling IPA were inexperienced and novices by today's standards. The IPA requested a minimum of three years of training analysis after the Second World War. Long analyses became commonplace, with little inquiry into the side effects. For candidates the very lengthy analysis increased the possibility of a narcissistic dyad, indoctrination, and abject dependency, and even the formation of a social/political bond. While some candidates benefited from the extremely long analyses with new growth and development, others remained vassals, sycophants, and subservient children. Meanwhile, the candidate aged, giving rise to the satirical comment, "sixty-five years old at graduation". In the USA, the trend toward ever increasing length of treatment has reversed; long analyses are less frequent and training analyses are shorter than in the preceding generation. Four sessions per week for training analysis and supervised cases is the mode rather than the earlier five sessions per week standard. These changes might also reflect a desire to attract training applicants, a recognition of economic pressures, and the realization that very prolonged analysis could foster institutionalized infantilization and regression rather than developmental progression. While some graduate analysts might successfully self-analyze the conflicts that were side-stepped in the training situation (particularly in the past, when analytic income was more assured), the problems inherent in a training analysis more often led to a second analysis. The first analysis was for training, the second analysis was personal.

The countertransference of the training analyst has dimensions that are not present in the analysis of non-candidates. While intergenerational conflict is often evident in a non-training analysis, it is primarily based on fantasy alone. In training analysis, there might be a realistic fear that the analyst does indeed have power and influence on the candidate's career. In a revival of the Oedipus complex of the child, the jealous parent can castigate and symbolically castrate the child. If the elderly training analyst has a waning ego and social function as well as physical decline, envy of the younger generation could be particularly activated. The very elderly analyst's health or hearing might be impaired, sexual passion diminished, with the increased possibility of depression following the loss of spouse, siblings, or friends. The revered elderly training analyst's slow decline might be overlooked while his/her jealousy and envy of the younger generation might be intensified. The training analyst, who might usually support the vigor and capacities of younger colleagues, might be unaware of his/her unconscious opposition (Zagermann, Chapter Fourteen, this volume). This aspect of intergenerational conflict could reactivate rivalry with children and with grandchildren, usurping children's affection and attention. A needy elderly analyst might cultivate the affectionate friendship of their patients without interpretation of its influencing the analytic process. Some training analyses might overemphasize issues of the institute and training at the expense of personal and familial issues. If there is an overemphasis on transferences in the training situation, the training analysis might be isolated from the rest of the candidate's conflicts at home and in his/her object world. Training analysis is then subverted to defending against personal analysis.

The training analyst and candidate may be associated with each other for better or worse in the psychoanalytic community, even if they are in different institutes. Termination in the ordinary personal analysis means that the analyst might not see the former analysand again and their real relationship is consciously terminated. Not so in training analysis. The dyad usually continues in interminable post-analytic contact and communication. After graduation, the former candidate and training analyst will meet in their national and international psychoanalytic associations. They might eventually be on committees or panels, working together, even voting for or against each other. Efforts to completely maintain the training analysis separate from the intrusion of the institute have been significantly improved, but a complete separation and total avoidance of professional intersection is not possible. The transference and real relationship might become enmeshed in unanalyzed vicissitudes of life in the analytic community. The training analyst might derive narcissistic gratification from the candidate's success, or embarrassment and narcissistic injury if the former candidate fails to live up to expectations or engages in unanalytic or unethical behavior. Unanalyzed vestiges of jealousy, rivalry, envy, and unresolved hate could combine and coexist with genuine affection and admiration. Moreover, after the analysis has formally terminated, problems of confidentiality and analytic neutrality might persist without the safeguards of the analytic situation and process. Unresolved conflicts could be beneficially attenuated, or could be reactivated and exacerbated in the organization's setting (Kairys, 1964).

After decades of argument and debate, the question of training analysis *vs.* personal analysis has not disappeared, but intensified. Is not a training analysis, after all, an analysis with the dyad engaged in an analytic process with the candidate free associating on the couch? In my view, training analysis tends to be a compromised analytic process. Free association in the analytic situation, and freedom of association with colleagues who might be out of favor could be inhibited if the training analyst can impinge on the candidate's career (Kirsner, 2009). The training analyst is better known to the candidate than to the non-candidate patient. He/she has heard about the analyst, might have seen the analyst at conferences, listened to the analyst's papers and discussions, and heard discussion about the training analyst's lectures, articles, classes, supervision, and criticisms. Anonymity, confidentiality, and neutrality are often compromised before treatment begins. The analyst might be charismatic and popular, or be known for short or long analyses, for particular positions in the institute or local and international societies. Candidates might have communicated with each other about their training analyst, as a supervisor or instructor. The training analyst might have extra-analytic knowledge of the candidate from other candidates and faculty, verbal and non-verbal, covert and overt. Training analysis has been satirized as analysis in a goldfish bowl.

Supervision and training analysis

In the pioneer period, it was thought that the candidate's analyst, able to analyze the candidates' countertransference and analytic immaturity, was best suited to be the first supervisor. However, subsequently, this policy was changed. Counter-identification with the conflicts of the candidates' control cases in a "parallel process" was initially overstated as an analytic and supervisory problem. Identification with the training analyst and supervisors is equally important in terms of a parallel process. The candidate's transferences to the patient, to the supervisor, to his/her own training analyst, and to the institute might be displaced from one to the other. The supervisors' countertransferences to the candidate (and, at times, to the candidate's patient) can be crucial to the candidate's course in the institute.

The initial supervised analytic cases of the candidates were called "control cases" in the USA, without analysis of the meaning of "control". Candidates could, indeed, be controlled, with an unspoken implication of reliance on the expertise of the supervisors and of submission to the authority of the supervisor. Control analyses were left to each supervisory dyad to determine the degree of candidate independence of the supervisor. The candidate might be more or less autonomous from the supervisor's clinical evaluation of the diagnosis, analyzability, and analysis of the control cases, as well as the duration of supervision. In evaluating the candidate, the supervisor might consider how long the candidate had been in his/her own analysis; whether the particular case was the candidate's first, second, or third control case; whether the candidate had lost prior cases; whether any cases were at or near termination. Of great significance are the attitudes of the supervisor and the candidate if they disagree about the analytic work and the way in which disagreement or dissatisfaction is resolved. The candidate is now frequently provided with the supervisor's report to the education committee, usually dominated by training analysts, and is, expectably, very concerned about the report. With a paucity of analytic cases, candidates are more dependent on supervisor referrals. Graduation depends on the imprimatur of the supervisors, who might feel burdened by their responsibility to the candidate, institute, and future patients. These responsibilities could activate intense supervisory countertransferences, which could be positive as well as negative, and could promote a candidate's graduation.

Supervision can foster the development of the candidate's own style and independence of the candidate from the training analyst. Or, under negative conditions of an archaic training analyst oligarchy, supervision can interfere with the development of candidate autonomy. It is important that candidates have freedom to choose supervisors and to change supervisors. As a training analyst, the supervisor might have knowledge about his/her supervisees from candidates who are their classmates. Neither the supervisor nor the supervisees are anonymous figures. The candidate might have had the supervisor as class instructor, and the supervisors might have heard comments about candidates from other training analyst instructors. This information could be beneficial or detrimental to the supervision. The supervisor might unwittingly or deliberately attempt to analyze the candidate in the guise of analyzing the candidate's countertransference to the control case. Friendship or rivalry with the candidate's analyst and/or with the candidate can be a knotty complication of supervision. Most supervisors/training analysts know each other and have their feelings and attitudes about their colleagues. When supervisors meet to collectively evaluate a candidate, they might learn more about the candidate and his/her progress in training than from analytic work with one control case. However, there is the danger of being influenced by senior training analysts and by a collective attitude, with concomitant impairment of objectivity and judgment. Candidate associations in the training analysis to control cases are fraught with cross-currents of transference and countertransference. Clandestine consultations outside the institute might be sought when there is strident dissatisfaction with supervision or with the training analysis.

Candidates' concerns about their progress might reverberate among their peers and among potential applicants (Blum, 2007).

When there is competition or collusion between supervisors or between supervisor and training analyst, the candidate might be co-opted as a messenger between them, or could be "convoyed", granted safe passage to graduation and, later, to becoming a training analyst. Again, the situation has analogies to the manifold problems of family relationships. Supervision can be friendly, engaging, and an enriching educational and extra-analytic experience, as it is rationally meant to be. It offers a counterweight to the candidate's training analysis and identifications with the style and theoretical frame of the training analyst.

Discussion

There are many obstacles to traverse on the road to graduation; they can become stop signs rather than stepping-stones to graduation and mebership. Some institutes required that a "control case" be terminated or near termination as a requirement for graduation. Other institutes require demonstration of analytic skills to the supervisors, who then report to a training committee. In some institutes, a paper might be required to be presented to the society, who could vote approval (or not) to society membership or, first, to associate membership. The question of inclusion or exclusion activates unresolved primal scene conflicts and narcissistic gratification or injury (Kernberg, 1996, 2013; Zagermann, Chapter Fourteen, this volume). If the candidate has a much delayed graduation, analytic identity is impeded, subjugation is fostered, and independence postponed (Meyer, 2003). Too often, the enthusiasm of the recent graduate is submerged and lost in prolonged waiting for recognition and advance within the institute hierarchy. Highly regarded contributions to the arts and sciences prior to analytic training might be treated with indifference or disdain by supercilious group countertransference of the elite oligarchy. Institutional inhibition of innovation was incisively satirized in Kernberg's (1996) critique: "Thirty ways to destroy the creativity of psychoanalytic candidates". Admission to the institute activates the family romance of adoption by new, superior parents. Little Oedipus does not attain stature until graduation and full membership in the psychoanalytic society.

All analyses are subject to the strengths, limitations, and match of the analytic dyad, as well as the inherent limitations of psychoanalysis. Many of the criticisms of the training committee's self-nomination and self-perpetuation, their control over faculty appointments and excessive requirements for candidates' progression and graduation have been corrected. A current problem of the long training situation which is not generally subject to a satisfactory solution involves "compassionate" and/or compelled graduation. A candidate who has spent a decade or more in training analysis, as well as in supervision and institute affiliation, might still be regarded by the education committee as deficient. The candidate may be graduated in tolerant compassion. If the candidate is asked to resign or face dismissal from the institute, litigation might ensue. An institute could be coerced into a compassionate graduation under legal and consequent financial threat. The graduated analyst might do no harm as a mediocre therapist, but does not meet the high standard of a training analyst. The graduate, however, would qualify as a training analyst if any analyst could analyze a candidate without further evaluation or certification.

A derivative problem concerns training analysts who are asked to resign from that position or from their institute. The underlying issues may concern ethics or competence and the protection of the analyst's patients. The thorny problem of litigation might arise. An impaired training analyst may be protectively and safely helped to get assistance and appropriately resume practice or, otherwise, retire. An unethical analyst presents legal, personal, and social difficulties, which require skillful management for all involved within and outside the institute. Minimizing damage to patients, and the entire institute, are quintessential priorities. What if the training analyst or ambitious graduate resigns and applies for membership and even training analyst status in another institute? The former institute might be coerced into relative silence under threat of extensive expensive litigation and intimidation. While it may be appropriate in ordinary circumstances to have training analyst status portable to other institutes, in some circumstances this would be unwise and detrimental to the profession and patients. Training analyst appointment can be contraindicated, and legitimately suspended or revoked.

Not all graduates are interested in becoming training analysts or want the burdens and responsibilities. Some institutes require low fees for training analysis and supervision, which might deter some analysts from becoming training analysts. Conflict between analytic and educational aims was described as the syncretic dilemma of training analysis (Lewin & Ross, 1960). Fifty-five years later, the more trenchant dilemmas concern the allegiance of training analyst to the candidate *vs.* the institute as well as personal *vs.* institutional conflicts.

All institutes require structure and valid authority with controls over abuse of power. An institute may, in fact, offer more protection against maltreatment than is available in personal analysis. Analytic education has largely become far more transparent and open to candidates' suggestions and criticisms than in the past. Despite the unforeseen complications and detrimental side effects of the traditional Eitingon model, psychoanalysis also provides the method for self-analysis and the analysis of group conflict within the institute. Institutes may be required or independently seek external consultation and evaluation, allowing for constructive criticism and developmental change. Just as clinical psychoanalysis is now remote from the pioneer period, analytic institutions have also progressively evolved. In some institutes, any graduate with the required five years of experience and "immersion" in analytic work may become a training analyst. Currently perfectionistic and nihilistic attitudes are more likely to be both scrutinized and analyzed. Psychoanalytic education and practice will be influenced by growing numbers of women, as well as increasingly diverse backgrounds among the candidates. Analytic education and clinical analysis will probably change at a more rapid pace than previously with unprecedented global analytic communication. International contemplation of ideas and issues is now possible in ways beyond the dreams of our analyst forebears. Neuroscience, analytic, and interdisciplinary research will also contribute to the psychoanalysis of the future. Of course, rapid change rather than careful, time-tested change has its own dangers.

Yet, the special problems, paradoxes, and complexities of the analysis of candidates persist. Unlike other patients, the candidate has to acquire clinical expertise, theoretical and developmental knowledge, and a reliable capacity for self-analysis. A standardized evaluation for certification as training analyst has been proposed in the USA; it seems to me unlikely that there would be agreement among different analytic frameworks with the American Psychoanalytic Association and IPA institutes about the form and content of the examination. One analytic group could view the analytic work of an institute of a different orientation as practicing psychoanalytic psychotherapy rather than psychoanalysis. A consensual agreement on an objective, standardized examination for training analyst certification is a noble concept that, one hopes, might be a future reality.

Are we confident that any analyst with about five years of independent analytic experience can deal with the complications of the analysis of a candidate and their reverberations within the institute? While I deeply appreciate the convergent, convincing critiques of training analysis, I wonder if it would not be wise to wait for greater consensus about replacing the training analyst system with a superior alternative. No wonder Freud (1937c, p. 248) noted psychoanalysis and education among the impossible professions (plus government).

Acknowledgement

I express my deep appreciation to Elsa J. Blum, PhD, for her editorial expertise.

References

Arlow, J. (1972). Some dilemmas in psychoanalytic education. *Journal of the American Psychoanalytic Association, 20*: 556–566.

Auchincloss, E., & Michels, R. (2003). A reassessment of psychoanalytic education: controversies and changes. *International Journal of Psychoanalysis, 84*: 387–403.

Bernfeld, S. (1962). On psychoanalytic training. *Psychoanalytic Quarterly, 31*: 453–482.

Blum, H. (2007). Talking about supervision: ten questions, one hundred answers. In: L. E. Elliott (Ed.), *Talking about Supervision: 10 Questions, 10 Analysts = 100 Answers* (pp. 23–27). London: Karnac.

Freud, S. (1914d). On the history of the psychoanalytic movement. *S. E., 14*: 7–66. London: Hogarth.

Freud, S. (1937c). Analysis terminable and interminable. *S. E., 23*: 211–253. London: Hogarth.

Grosskurth, P. (1991). *The Secret Ring*. New York: Addison-Wesley.

Kairys, D. (1964). The training analysis: a critical review and controversial proposal. *Psychoanalytic Quarterly, 33*: 485–512.

Kernberg, O. (1986). Institutional problems of psychoanalytic education. *Journal of the American Psychoanalytic Association, 34*: 799–834.

Kernberg, O. (1996). Thirty methods to destroy the creativity of psychoanalytic candidates. *International Journal of Psychoanalysis, 77*: 1031–1040.

Kernberg, O. (2000). A concerned critique of psychoanalytic education. *International Journal of Psychoanalysis, 81*: 97–120.

Kernberg, O. (2004). *Contemporary Controversies in Psychoanalytic Theory, Techniques and their Applications*. New Haven, CT: Yale University Press.

Kernberg, O. (2013). The twilight of the training analyst system. Plenary Address, American Psychoanalytic Association.

Kirsner, D. (2009). *Unfree Associations*. New York: Jason Aronson.

Lewin, B., & Ross, H. (1960). *Psychoanalytic Education in the U.S.* New York: Norton.

Mahler, M., Pine, F., & Bergman, A. (1975). *The Psychological Birth of the Human Infant*. New York: Basic Books.

Masur, C. (1998). The training analyst system: asset or liability? *Journal of the American Psychoanalytic Association, 46*: 539–549.

Meyer, L. (2003). Subservient analysis. *International Journal of Psychoanalysis, 34*: 1241–1262.

Orgel, S. (2002). Some hazards to neutrality in the psychoanalysis of candidates. *Psychoanalytic Quarterly, 71*: 419–443.

Reeder, J. (2004). *Hate and Love in Psychoanalytic Institutions*. New York: Other Press.

CHAPTER THREE

Psychoanalytic training: then and now

Kenneth Eisold

The heroic age and the domestic era

Looking at the landscape of psychoanalysis today, there are few signs remaining of the battles that swept across it until recently: the bitter schisms that rent many institutes, the proscribing of dissident ideas, banishment of colleagues, arrogant dismissals of alternative treatments, sharp competitive judgments of fellow analysts, as well as harsh attitudes towards outsiders. All of that characterized psychoanalysis in its "heroic" age, as it was struggling to establish itself as well as, in a period of decline, it was struggling to hold on to its self-image as the "gold standard" of psychotherapy.

Freud, a self-identified "conquistador" in his youth (Masson, 1985, p. 398), became in adulthood a "good hater" (Sachs, 1944, p. 117), surrounding himself with a band of "paladins" (Grosskurth, 1991). He demanded of his followers that they do battle with him against his enemies, and then there were colleagues who constituted in his eyes a particular danger to psychoanalysis because they had been disciples and followers at the start: Adler, and Jung, of course, then Ferenczi. Subsequently, conflicts in New York led to what Ernest Jones referred to as the "psychoanalytical civil wars", running roughly from 1931 to

1938 (Hale, 1995, p. 103; see also Frosch, 1991). This was followed by the outbreak of conflict in London between the local Kleinians and the émigré Freudians, intense in-fighting expressed, ultimately, in the Controversial Discussions that narrowly averted the splitting up of the British Society (see King & Steiner, 1991).

Moreover, after the Second World War, schisms occurred in Germany, Austria, France, Sweden, and Norway (Eckhardt, 1978). In France, the controversies surrounding Lacan produced at least four institutes: the Freudian School, the Fourth Group, the Paris Institute, and the French Psychoanalytic Association (Turkle, 1992). The record is not precise, but Gitelson (1983) also noted schisms in Spain, Brazil, Mexico, Argentina, and Venezuela, as well as, in the USA, in Washington/Baltimore, Philadelphia, Boston, Cleveland, and Los Angeles. Arlow (1972) refers to half a dozen splits in the American Psychoanalytic Association, and adds to the census of splits in the International Psychoanalytical Association Columbia and Australia.

Now, we are in a relatively tranquil "domestic era". Institutes that split apart in the past are negotiating mergers. Strict standards are being relaxed, while alternative methods are increasingly tolerated or, even, affirmed. Virtually anyone seeking training can find it today.

To be sure, we are also in a period of contraction, as fewer patients seek psychoanalytic treatment, with many analysts subsisting on reduced practices and slender reimbursements from insurance companies. Institutes can no longer afford to be uncompromising, and, indeed, they are reaching out to a wider variety of mental health professionals than at any time in the past to fill their classes. This has led them to offer training in alternative therapies, though it has not led them to experiment much with alternative methods of training.

Each institute, as in the past, still has its own faculty and its own set of analysts or supervisors dedicated to training candidates who have come up through the ranks of that institute and been vetted for their training roles by their senior colleagues. Rarely do the faculty members of other institutes have a hand in that training, and faculty members seldom work with candidates outside their own institutes. Such isolated, independent organizational structures are often called "silos", as they are self-sufficient containers, isolated from each other.

Moreover, each institute, each "silo", is virtually identical to the others. Their autonomy—and their isolation—has not led them to deviate significantly from the basic training model established in

Berlin almost one hundred years ago. Each candidate is required to undergo a "training analysis", to take courses offered by their own faculty, and to see patients under the supervision of designated senior colleagues. Moreover, in addition to following this "hallowed tripartite" model (Wallerstein, 1993, p. 175) each institute usually has a "training committee", sometimes called an "education committee", charged with evaluating candidates, approving courses, selecting faculty, and frequently selecting training analysts as well. They are monitored as they "progress" through the stages of training, and they are usually required to present their work as they approach the end of their training after completing a set number of treatments (see Kächele & Thomä, 2000).

This might not strike most analysts as strange, and the paradox of uniformity might not strike them as troubling. For us, it is familiar and normal, the way things have always been. But why is this so? Why have they not developed along different lines in response to differences in the composition of their members or cultural differences in their environment? If institutes do not interact with each other or exchange faculty, what has kept them so alike? Why have different theories of development or psychic structure not led to different forms of training? Is it possible that this basic model is the only conceivable one, and that it was born full blown in its current, perfected form?

To be sure, there are some differences among institutes, different courses candidates are required to take, and different procedures for determining the selection of training analysts. In addition, some institutes are subject to the regulations and rules of umbrella associations, such as the International Psychoanalytical Association and the American Psychoanalytic Association, which set and monitor standards and strive to keep them uniform. Although, by and large, this pattern of self-imposed uniformity is impressive, it is also stifling, as Otto Kernberg noted in his classic paper published twenty years ago, "Thirty methods to destroy the creativity of psychoanalytic candidates" (1996). When that paper was published, it elicited a buzz of recognition for his trenchant points. His spirit of irreverence was perhaps even more striking and a source of hope for reform. Little has changed, however, as a result.

The outstanding exception to this uniformity, of course, has been France, where Jacques Lacan, beginning by undermining the authority of the psychoanalytic fathers who "presume to know", went on to establish a radically different form of training based on the authority of candidates themselves—or, better, their need to establish themselves as authentic authorities in their own right. Within the French Institute, struggling to conform to the requirements of the IPA, it became increasingly clear that Lacan's practices were at variance with the orthodoxy it required (see Roudinesco, 1990; Turkle, 1992).

However one views Lacan's innovations, sessions of variable length, his willingness to enlist analysands in fulfilling personal needs, impromptu sessions in the middle of the night, and so forth, it would be fair to say that this was a serious attempt to break with standardized rules and to relate psychoanalytic practice more closely to theory. But it was unacceptable to the commission charged with investigating the French Institutes' suitability to become a component of the IPA, with the result that, eventually, Lacan was dropped from the list of training analysts (he referred to this as his "excommunication"), and it became clear that the French institute would not be accepted so long as Lacan was associated with it.

The fall-out from the IPA's rejection of Lacan and his innovations led to the creation of a number of other institutes and splinter groups, a chaotic situation, certainly chilling to any spirit of innovation. The subsequent conflicts might also suggest that the self-imposed uniformity of institutes had served the defensive function of keeping under control the latent competitiveness of analysts, who might otherwise have striven to depart from the standard model. At the very least, that uniformity can be seen as containing the anxiety inherent in deviation and experimentation.

There are other possible explanations. The uniformity can also be seen as the product of an "apostolic age" (Arlow, 1982), in which disciples of Freud spread throughout the world with word of his discoveries: the dynamic unconscious, transference, infantile sexuality, the Oedipus complex, and so forth. This process, spurred on by the diaspora of analysts fleeing Nazi Germany, was informed by the desire of the refugee analysts to replicate the professional world they had lost, and so it was little surprise that they recreated the training model they knew.

Yet, even before the diaspora, it was clear that Freud and his disciples had strenuously sought to control the movement and prevent alternative views from taking hold (Grosskurth, 1991). The "secret committee", formed after Jung's "defection", was designed, in part, to ensure that Freud's loyal sons would faithfully sustain his theories while monitoring and restraining their own competitiveness. And, arguably, when training was first set up in the 1920s, the institution of the training analysis incorporated that task as well.

The end of this embattled "heroic age" has brought with it the fear that psychoanalysis itself would die, and, indeed, the world of psychoanalysis is suffering a decline, at a time when psychotherapy and interest in mental health are growing. Indeed, the current decline of psychoanalysis (see Eisold, 2007; Hale, 1995) is all the more disturbing and poignant given the upsurge of interest in psychotherapy and the proliferation of other treatment methods.

But today, fewer candidates apply for training as fewer patients seek psychoanalytic treatment. Some institutes are chaffing under the restrictions of traditional standards as the general decline of our field has exacerbated competition for members. The lowering tide is stranding many ships.

One response within many institutes has been the development of training programs in psychotherapy, informed by psychoanalytic thinking about transference and the layering of unconscious motivations. Another response has been to minimize the focus on training altogether, emphasizing the individual development of existing members through presenting papers and offering workshops—the new primary mission of the many other umbrella organizations that are proliferating in this pluralistic era: the Academy of Psychoanalysis, the Division of Psychoanalysis of the American Psychological Association (Division 39), the International Association for Relational Psychoanalysis and Psychotherapy (IARPP), the American Association for Psychoanalysis in Clinical Social Work (AAPCP), the International Association for Psychoanalytic Self Psychology (IAPSP), the International Federation of Psychoanalytic Societies (IFPS), the International Forum for Psychoanalytic Education (IFPE). This impressive array of professional associations primarily provides opportunities to present papers and panels, keeping analysts busy developing their ideas, talking to each other, and, I suspect, diverting their attention from the general decline of the field as a whole.

Increasingly, in the umbrella organizations that do focus on training, the International Psychoanalytical Association and the American Psychoanalytic Association, alternate "models" are being proposed and accepted. Moreover, one hears frequently that, at times, the "rules" are simply ignored by the component institutes and societies, chaffing under the restraints they impose while struggling to adapt to this new landscape.

Some of those umbrella organizations represent a further fragmentation of the field, being open only to sub-specializations in the field of mental health such as psychologists, social workers, and such newly established categories as mental health workers. Increasingly, as the industry of mental health treatment has expanded, the state has stepped in to establish new forms of certification independent of what many institutes have established for themselves. Indeed, an inflection point of absurdity was reached recently when, at the behest of a non-American Psychoanalytic Association institute, New York State established a "certificate in psychoanalysis", reflecting requirements that vary from what most institutes in the state offer. That law pushed several institutes to set up parallel programs to help candidates qualify for this new certificate, forcing them to compete, in effect, with their own certificate granting programs.

Embedded as we are in this paradoxical system of training, we tend not notice how strange this uniformity is. Indeed, as our institutes and associations adapt to changes induced by economic and social factors, our adherence to the standard model becomes even more fixed—and odd. We adapt, but we do not seem to change. Moreover, there continues to be little research on training. Twenty years ago, a meeting of directors of training in the American Psychoanalytic Association concluded, "empirical research [about training] was not thought appropriate" (Ahmed, 1994), and that attitude persists. This stance reflects the virtual absence of any research on many of the factors that shape training: the effectiveness of the designated training or supervising analysts, the selection of candidates, or the difference that frequency makes in an analysis—two, three, four, or five times weekly—though rules on frequency have often been the defining feature of bitter disputes among psychoanalytic factions. The field does not seem to want to investigate or explore what we have in common or what we tend to assume keeps us apart.

The great benefit of having such uniformity and certainty is that it leaves little room for questions about what training should be. It becomes, clearly, the inevitably "right way" to train. As psychoanalysts, of course, we are trained to suspect that such certainty in an individual masks anxiety and perhaps even conflict. Yet, on an institutional or group level, we are all too ready to accept such beliefs as normal and appropriate. This means that institutionally, though, we are less able to conceive improved forms of training. New ideas seldom have the opportunity to develop.

Obviously, this institutional sclerosis must have consequences for those in training or those beyond training who rely on their institutes to do an effective job with candidates in order to replenish the field. Indeed, there are some fairly objective signs of trouble, though they are not always linked to this paradox. Candidates do complain about their training, often particularly about the quality of the teaching to which they are exposed. Such complaints can sometimes be felt as too risky to voice loudly, but, then, graduates express their resentments in other ways: they often do not volunteer for committees or roles in training, or engage in institute affairs. They contribute less to fund-raising, and, even, sometimes fail to maintain their memberships in their institutes or graduate societies.

Data on this are hard to come by and are often murky, as alienation and disaffection are not easy to measure. Lack of participation in institute governance is sometimes explained away as practitioners are too busy to spare the time committee work demands, or too financially strapped to give away valuable time needed to make ends meet. And, to be sure, the traditional rewards of status and referrals that stemmed from taking such prominent roles in the governance of institutes are also in decline.

Indeed, the field is generally strapped for cash. Institutes struggle to cover expenses, seeking new ways to generate income. I mentioned above the proliferation of psychotherapy programs, and there are, in addition, specializations that are continually being designed and added to institute curricula: workshops and programs in parenting, eating disorders, attention deficits, trauma, sexual abuse, the arts, etc. Institutes have a decided advantage here, as trainings in various forms of psychotherapy are not generally available elsewhere. Medical schools long since stopped training residents in psychotherapy, partly because they have shifted focus to medications, partly also because there is little demand. Graduate schools, in addition, seldom offer training, apart from the narrow focus on specific techniques whose outcomes and effectiveness individual academic psychologists seek to measure. That approach offers advancement in academic careers for those who develop such treatments, theorizing them and researching them with their students. In all these cases, however, training for the sake of providing a public service or meeting a social need seldom figures in the thinking of those providing service.

Here, our institutes fill an important gap, fulfilling a need with which few others are concerned. Graduate programs in psychology as well as medical schools have priced themselves out of the market. They cannot afford to train students for psychotherapy practices, particularly in an era when insurers and providers are struggling to keep down the costs of medical care. The incentives are lacking.

What we have, then, is essentially a cottage industry of psychotherapy, centered around institutes that provide generally low-cost training, for practitioners subsisting on work that is no longer profitable for others to perform. It is up to each individual practitioner to make it work economically, to rent an office he or she can afford, to cover expenses, to create a niche that distinguishes them from others while promoting their services by word of mouth or social media, while the system keeps driving down the prices they can charge.

A sign of this is how, increasingly, institute listservs have turned into informal referral networks, as participants respond to requests for therapists who are on specific insurance panels, treating disorders in other neighborhoods or cities, or willing to work at unusual times or for low fees because the patient is interesting or deserving. They strive to join the network of "providers", even if they cannot provide the service themselves. To be sure, that could be seen as simply wanting to be helpful, and, no doubt, sometimes that is what it is. But it is also a way of promoting oneself as knowledgeable and potentially helpful even when unable to participate directly. It is the generosity of the poor, while continuing to affirm the identity of a "provider".

To be sure, our field is somewhat more stratified than this overview suggests. The reputation and standing of institutes vary, allowing some graduates to charge higher fees or benefit from more robust referral networks. And, generally, psychiatrists charge higher fees than psychologists, while social workers charge less, mental health workers even less than that. The more successful practitioners, by and large, are specialists who publish books on their area and offer talks and workshops.

If the analogy with eighteenth and nineteenth century weavers in England holds, the cottagers who held on to their livelihoods in the face of the Enclosure Acts, on the one hand, allowing landowners to confiscate the land on which their sheep grazed, and the mill owners, on the other, who built far more efficient equipment for weaving, we can be seen as awaiting a new technology that will finally put us out of business.

This is, of course, a considerable irony for psychoanalysts who not only once tried to distinguish the "pure gold" of psychoanalysis from the "alloy" of psychotherapy, as Freud once put it (Freud, 1919a). Few patients today seek out three or four times weekly treatments, featuring the couch and free association, though some analysts strive to maintain such traditional practices by offering reduced fees. For candidates who need to find several analysands for training, this is increasingly an obstacle. Time is in short supply in our work-driven culture, and patients find it difficult to make even their once or twice weekly psychotherapy appointments.

Apart from such problems that make it more and more difficult for institutes to offer their traditional training, there are more subtle problems that stem from our rigid training models and the ways in which we have been set up. One of the biggest is that our institutional "silos" trap practitioners within their institutes. There are two major costs of this. One is that they are deprived of the potential fertilization that comes from being exposed to different styles and practices. Those having developed within their own particular silos are conditioned to accept the *status quo*, including the idealizations sanctioned by the group mind. Existing practices are not challenged. Indeed, they are hardened.

An even greater problem, though, is that the interpersonal differences and difficulties, the transferences and conflicts that inevitably characterize organizations—and professional organizations in particular—have no outlet outside the institute. Internal politics can become more frustrating and bitter as individuals feel stuck in their organizations, unable to leave. Often, in the past, those differences led to schisms or the establishment of alternative institutes, but, as the field is contracting, now they lead to alienation and covert battles, political struggles, disaffection, and contempt. Unhappy teachers and supervisors often have little choice but to put up with those they do not like or respect, or with whom they disagree, or of whom they do not approve.

Battered and beleaguered, our institutional silos have become prisons, in effect. We cling to them, but they offer us no security, and often even little advantage in the marketplace. To be sure, we can leave them, stop paying dues and stop attending meetings—and we often do just that—but there is nowhere else to go. Other institutes, by and large, will not take us in.

Meanwhile, stuck inside our organizational silos, the slights and disappointments that inevitably arise among institute members, the recognition that comes to some, but not to others, the intellectual and political differences, the alliances and friendships, the gossip, the favoritism, the slights, perceived and otherwise—all of these have no external outlet. This emotional "noise" is comparable to what occurs in academic departments, notoriously the site of such personal hatreds, jealousies, and resentments. The academic world, however, offers more individual opportunity. Professorships might not be easy to find today, but a successful scholar will expect to get offers from other universities or be able to renegotiate a teaching load. Academics are less embedded in their academies than analysts in their institutes, freer to roam. Universities and other schools do not depend on the willingness of faculty to volunteer themselves as institutes do, and they charge higher fees and pay better salaries.

The future

Let me briefly summarize the dilemma. The numbers of those seeking psychoanalytic treatment as well as training in psychoanalysis are in decline, at a time when the demand for psychotherapy is rising and the need for mental health services is increasingly recognized. But our field seems unable to adapt to this change. We adhere to a "standard model" of training established 100 years ago, and have not shown much capacity for significant change.

Institutes do add on services in psychotherapy as well as provide exposure to specific treatments for particular disorders, but, at the core, they remain committed primarily to turning out "psychoanalysts" who see patients three, four, or five times weekly for prolonged periods of time. The demand for this service no longer exists as it did, certainly not sufficiently to support the array of institutes that have come into existence over the years.

Let me make it clear that I am not implying that traditional psychoanalytic treatments are no longer valuable or effective. On the contrary, I believe that wonderful work is being done. Many of my colleagues are thoughtful and effective, and I myself continue to be grateful for the training I received. But, as the management theorist Edward Demming once put it, "survival is not mandatory". Competition is putting more and more psychoanalysts out of work, as marketplace dynamics undermine the viability of our existing practices.

It might be argued that we should simply accept the fact that we will be working for fewer and fewer clients who will value our help and can pay for it. Under such circumstances, many institutes will go under, and the survivors will move on without being forced to compromise their integrity or modify their hard-won skills and identities.

The alternative argument is that we have something of great value that can be repackaged or repurposed. The unconscious, the repetition of old patterns of behavior, dissociation, and irrational beliefs will not cease affecting human behavior, but they might not require psychoanalysis as currently practiced to unearth and change. Is there a way we could adapt that knowledge respectfully and without compromise?

Our history suggests a lack of flexibility in our methods of training. We might not be troubled by the bitter conflicts and schisms of the past, as the sources of our current discontents are more buried, but we appear to be encased in an identity that prescribes what and how we must work as well as organizational structures that resist alteration.

Yet, necessity and opportunity can teach us, and our field has attracted brilliant and creative minds, many of whom could rise to the challenge. Let me propose some steps it might be possible to take.

Greater choice in the selection of training analysts and supervising analysts

At the core of the silo structure is the restrictions it imposes on choosing training analysts, and it seems obvious that greater choice is desirable as well as greater separation between training analysts and candidates.

This is actually more of a thorny problem than it may seem at first, but not for what is usually perceived to be the problem, the need to ensure quality. Existing systems for selecting training analysts and supervising analysts have not been rigorously evaluated. They are maintained, I believe, largely because they are familiar and sustain the illusion of control, not because they have proved more effective than "free markets".

The more troubling problem is that the training analyst system is a key element in developing and sustaining cohesiveness within institutes. Arguably, it would be better for candidates to be free to choose their analysts from a wider pool, and that would also help institutes circumvent the incestuous conflicts and tensions the current system inevitably arouses, along with the transferences and judgments that cloud perceptions on all sides.

One simple reform to help ensure the privacy of candidates and the confidentiality of their personal information would be to allow, and even encourage, training analysts from other institutes to conduct the analyses of candidates. A further reform would be to allow training analyses to be conducted by any graduate of any institute, on the presumption that the successful completion of training should be sufficient to ensure a competent analytic experience. This would also eliminate the tensions inherent in having two tiers of psychoanalysts in our societies: training analysts and graduates. There is little apart from anecdotal evidence to suggest that the selection of training analysts actually makes for superior candidate analyses, and significant evidence that the distinction between the two tiers promotes competition, envy, and alienation within institute faculties.

An analogous suggestion would be to invite graduates of other institutes routinely to teach courses. This would do much to overcome the isolation of our silos, bringing in new ideas and dissipating the stale atmosphere that inevitably characterizes seminars that are taught too frequently.

It can be argued, on the other hand, that the intense analytic relationships formed in training between analysts and analysands, supervisors and supervisees, bind many members of institutes together emotionally, forming a nexus that often makes faculty members want to work together and willing to volunteer the time required for teaching and committee work. Without that, institutes might be weakened even further. (This bonding obviously exists in parallel with the negative dynamics created in the "silos", the disturbing "noise" that leads to alienation and disengagement for many.)

Some candidates actually prefer to "play" the system, however, currying favor and avoiding confrontation with their more blatant problems while planning their future advancement. This is not an argument for retaining the system, but it does suggest an additional difficulty in changing it.

Expansion of training in psychotherapy, essentially fewer sessions over shorter periods of time than in traditional psychoanalysis

Clearly, there is a market for this in today's world, and, as I pointed out, institutes have moved in to capitalize on this need. However, they have been hamstrung in their willingness to take advantage of this opportunity, still viewing psychotherapy as the lesser form of treatment. Indeed, when they do set up such programs, they often view them as feeders for psychoanalytic training, hoping that students, once exposed to the benefits of dynamic psychotherapy, will want to go on to the "superior" training offered in psychoanalysis. The success of such programs is often measured by the numbers recruited for psychoanalytic training. Understandable as that may be, it compromises the psychotherapy programs in several important ways.

If the faculty views psychotherapy training as second best, students inevitably will pick that up, and sense a lack of commitment to excellence. Second, it will be more difficult to recruit the best teachers and supervisors to participate, as they will be reluctant to embrace a second-class status. Finally, the energy required for innovation and experimentation in psychotherapy will be inhibited or drained off.

The great advantage psychoanalysis has had from the start was our recognition of the role the unconscious plays in human motivation. Even today, in the psychotherapy programs that have been added on to institute offerings, those programs benefit from their proximity to a community of teachers, supervisors, and others steeped in an understanding of the unconscious. That would need to be a core element in the brands of dynamic psychotherapy we could develop and promote.

Our ability to do that would be profoundly enhanced by recent advances in neuroscience. Instead of viewing those discoveries as evidence that our theories have been correct all along, as we have tended to do, we might better mobilize them to develop new approaches that could be seen as more practical and scientific.

We would be aided in this immeasurably by the public knowledge that the existence of the unconscious is no longer just a theory, but has scientific backing.

A second step could be institutes setting up alliances with other institutes, joint programs drawing on resources beyond what any one institute has on its own

In fact, a program in psychotherapy such as I was suggesting above, might have a better chance to succeed if it were not tied to any one institute. A consortium could draw from a wider pool of faculty and supervisors than exists in any one. And it might stand a better chance of operating free from the internal political pressures that constrain planning and decision-making in particular institutes.

A consortium of institutes might also be able to set up programs focused on continuing professional development, courses that addressed specific clinical problems or new theoretical developments that other therapists want to learn about. It might also be able to draw on a greater concentration of recognized experts and outstanding clinical practitioners than any one institute could offer.

To be sure, in the beginning such consortiums would be seen to be in competition with comparable programs in individual institutes—and, indeed, they would be. Some institutes might be resistant to "throwing in their lot" with them if they think they might be more successful on their own or if they fear being associated with institutes of lesser status. But, in the long run, they would be more viable.

Applied psychoanalysis has been insufficiently explored by institutes, despite the fact that many individual practitioners have had significant success, and there is enormous opportunity

Many executives seek consultation because they know the advantages of having help in seeing their blind spots and understanding more deeply their competitors' thinking. It gives them a significant advantage.

"Coaching," as this is sometimes called, has proliferated to the point that many businesses and other organizations routinely offer it to their top executives. However, this is generally an unregulated and highly varied area, and takes many forms. Although often efforts are made to protect the confidentiality of the coaching relationship, many clients are wary of services offered by their organizations, preferring to hire outside coaches themselves where there is far less danger of information leaking to superiors. On the other hand, organizations are reluctant to pay for help with little control over the form it takes or guarantee of its benefits.

At the highest levels, though, superb advisory services are currently being offered by psychoanalysts and they are being well compensated for it. This help requires not only the ability to understand unconscious motives or to discern obscure intentions, skills psychoanalysts are trained to develop, but also a grasp of organizations and the business dilemmas their leaders face.

Along those lines, institutes could offer training in organizational consultation, helping organizations face the hidden, unconscious obstacles they inevitably encounter. These are just a few of the many opportunities available to the institutes and practitioners who venture out beyond the realm of individual clinical work. Political candidates often use such help to decipher the messages of their opponents and their unconscious appeal; advertising agencies can use help understanding and crafting subliminal communications in the service of their clients. Diplomats can be helped in grasping the psychological profiles of their counterparts, or their vulnerabilities (see Eisold, 2010).

Whatever institutes do, however, whatever programs they offer in psychoanalysis, psychotherapy, or applied psychoanalysis, it is essential that evaluation and review be key components. Faced with a proposal to alter training, it is easy to imagine many of our colleagues will say, "If it ain't broke, don't fix it." I have heard that refrain all too frequently, suggesting how hard it is to see the degree to which our training programs have become ritualistic, impervious to change. But continuous assessment and evaluation does not require an admission of failure as a place to start, just a willingness to improve, and it could be the starting point for creative conversations among those of us interested in education and training. Possibly umbrella organizations such as the International Psychoanalytical Association and the American Psychoanalytic Association could institute annual reports on the state of psychoanalytic education as revealed by annual surveys, reports that could include information on innovations and experiments that some institutes have attempted.

Continuous evaluation has been established as an essential element in today's organizations. We see it reflected in the "learning objectives" we are now required to submit along with our proposals to our professional meetings. However, rather than being annoying formulas with which we are obliged to comply, we could accept it in the spirit of actually wanting to know the impact of what we do.

Some final thoughts

Traditionally, we have been preoccupied by theories of psychic structure and mental processes. We pay attention to the process of change and development in our patients, not so much in ourselves as professionals or in our organizations. It might be time to be broader and more inclusive in our thinking.

My own limited practice in organizational consultation has made me aware of how resistant to change organizations are, in general, as well as ingenious in subverting initiatives that require altering established practices. In this, they are generally worse than individuals. And that is not to take into account the rigidities specific to psychoanalytic institutes.

So, change would have to come slowly and in small increments. But new initiatives would not go unrecognized, especially if they succeeded in attracting candidates. Programs in applied psychoanalysis that meet a need will similarly attract attention.

Change must come, if only the slow change of decline and eventual failure.

References

Ahmed, J. (1994). Meeting of directors of training institutes. *Bulletin of the International Psycho-Analytical Association, 75*: 184–185.

Arlow, J. A. (1972). Some dilemmas in psychoanalytic education. *Journal of the American Psychoanalytic Association, 20*: 556–566.

Arlow, J. A. (1982). Psychoanalytic education: a psychoanalytic perspective. *Annual of Psychoanalysis, 10*: 5–20.

Eckhardt, M. H. (1978). Organizational schisms in American psychoanalysis. In: Q. Carlson (Ed.), *American Psychoanalysis: Origins and Development* (pp. 69–87). New York: Brunner/Mazel.

Eisold, K. (2007). The erosion of our profession. *Psychoanalytic Psychology, 24*: 1–9.

Eisold, K. (2010). *What You Don't Know You Know*. New York: Other Press.

Freud, S. (1919a). Lines of advance in psycho-analytic therapy. *S. E., 17*: 157–168. London: Hogarth.

Frosch, J. (1991). The New York psychoanalytic civil war. *Journal of the American Psychoanalytic Association, 39*(4): 1037–1064.

Gitelson, F. H. (1983). Identity crises: splits or compromises—adaptive or maladaptive. In: E. D. Joseph & D. Widlöcher (Eds.), *The Identity of the Psychoanalyst* (pp. 157–179). New York: International Universities Press.

Grosskurth, P. (1991). *The Secret Ring*. Reading, MA: Addison-Wesley.

Hale, N. G. (1995). *The Rise and Crisis of Psychoanalysis in the United States*. New York: Oxford University Press.

Kächele, H., & Thomä, H. (2000). On the devaluation of the Eitingon–Freud model of psychoanalytic education. *International Journal of Psychoanalysis, 81*: 806–807.

Kernberg, O. F. (1996). Thirty methods to destroy the creativity of psychoanalytic candidates. *International Journal of Psychoanalysis, 77*: 1031–1040.

King, P., & Steiner, R. (Eds.) (1991). *The Freud–Klein Controversies*. London: Routledge.

Masson, J. M. (1985). *The Complete Letters of Sigmund Freud to Wilhelm Fliess, 1887–1904*. Cambridge, MA: Harvard University Press.

Roudinesco, E. (1990). *Jacques Lacan and Co.: A History of Psychoanalysis in France, 1925–1985*. Chicago, IL: University of Chicago Press.

Sachs, H. (1944). *Freud: Master and Friend*. Cambridge, MA: Harvard University Press.

Turkle, S. (1992). *Psychoanalytic Politics* (2nd edn). New York: Guilford Press.

Wallerstein, R. (1993). Between chaos and petrification: a summary of the Fifth IPA Conference on Training. *International Journal of Psychoanalysis, 74*: 165–178.

CHAPTER FOUR

Current aspects and challenges of analytic training

Cláudio Laks Eizirik

This chapter starts by highlighting certain characteristics of contemporary analytic practice, since the ultimate goal of our educational institutions is to experience and address this specific scenario in order to prepare or encourage the training of analysts. Next, I examine aspects of personal analysis, supervision, and psychoanalytic institutions, as well as the challenges I consider most relevant in this endless process of developing and striving to maintain an analytic identity.

Have the patients we treat changed?

From about the 1980s, references began to appear in the literature concerning changes in analytic patients (Ahumada, 1997; Gaddini, 1987) and new descriptions gradually emerged that contrasted with Freud's classic indications of neurotic patients. Kernberg's research on borderline patients is well known, as are studies by Marty on psychosomatic patients (Aisenstein, 2014), new maladies of the soul (Kristeva, 2002) and perversions (McDougall, 1983), a set of clinical conditions in which difficulties with verbal expression and symbolization present specific barriers to analytic work. André Green's psychoanalytic work is based on French theoretical and clinical observations and the contributions of Bion and Winnicott, in which they described, understood, and suggested possible approaches for non-neurotic structures (Green, 2002, 2010; Urribarri, 2013).

All these contributions indicate that contemporary practice includes a new type of patient, while simultaneously raising more questions than answers: are all of these, in fact, new pathologies, or are some merely new versions of the structures described by Freud and his contemporaries? To what extent do cultural changes, which increasingly encourage what has been described as liquid modernity or hypermodernity, contribute to these new versions of pathologies? To what extent has a new vision of the psychoanalytic approach made it necessary to attempt to access more regressive patients, or has a greater ability for analytical listening made us more capable of penetrating areas previously considered inaccessible or invulnerable to analytic methods?

Regardless, a number of possible approaches have identified changes in clinical practice and the types of patients seeking treatment (for example, Eizirik et al., 1999).

To what extent does this occur? In observing my own practice and comparing it with colleagues, I found that neurotics or those with personality disorders continue to predominate, with a relatively small number of patients such as those described by the abovementioned authors; the difference is that we may not previously have accepted them for analysis or would not have had the resources available now to pursue emotional contact with these patients. On the other hand, the presence of elderly patients appears to be a growing trend, both in the literature (Junkers, 2006) and current practice. As I described recently (Eizirik, 2014b), with the notable exception of Little Hans, in the first decades of the past century all analysts and patients were simply adults.

With the advent of contributions by Melanie Klein and other authors, psychoanalysis discovered childhood, and today both this field and that of adolescence are fully developed.

Over the past two decades, it seems we have made a new discovery: old age exists, and the mind and psychological distress of the elderly is a new area of study and psychoanalytic treatment.

Here, it is important to consider another variable, which seems to be largely disregarded: the life cycle of patients and analysts, and to what extent each moment is related to certain types of patients, in relation to whom we are either more or less open to a proper analytic listening. It has been reported that elderly analysts experience greater difficulty (including physical) conducting systematic analysis with children. Or that analysts with more experience, or who have learned more from their therapeutic failures than successes (Baranger, 1993), might be more emotionally available to listen to regressive situations.

Has the setting changed?

Although I am aware that the setting is far more akin to a mental framework within which we work with the patient, it is important to point out that the method and structure developed by Freud as ideal for analysis would invariably undergo changes, adaptations, and modernization.

In and of themselves, formal elements of the setting, such as the contract, payments for sessions, frequency, vacations, using a couch or not, are not the most important aspects of the setting. They are safeguards, beacons, in short, a framework within which we seek to combine the ideal conditions for psychoanalytic treatment aimed at profound and intimate emotional contact with the inner world of both the patient and the analyst. They are part of the scenario in which we establish specific psychoanalytic fields with each patient. In the same way as every analyst's office is unique in one or more aspects, although all of them have at least an armchair and a couch, each analysis is also unique, though all of them involve the search for the unconscious (even though we know there are different versions of this search).

In my view, the risk is the transformation of these elements into a type of fetish and, unfortunately, there is much controversy surrounding the selection of a single element as the focus of dispute and bitter disagreements. The extensive discussion and approval of three analytic training models (Eizirik, 2011) aimed at recognizing the diversity of possible training formats, with frequency consistently highlighted as only one of the elements of recognized models, whose application requires consistence between their objectives and structure.

With respect to current analytic practice, analysts are increasingly seeing fewer patients four or even five times a week, with most cases involving one to two weekly sessions. Several reasons have been put forward for this decline in session frequency, including financial problems, resistance, the large distances in urban centers, analysts' difficulty protecting and defending a setting suited to the method, competition with other methods requiring fewer sessions, the current trend favoring less contact and faster treatment, etc.

The essential question is the following: can treatment consisting of fewer than three weekly sessions be considered analysis? But why three and not four? Or five? Or six, as initially used by Freud? And who decides if this name can be used? The IPA (International Psychoanalytical Association)? Each society? Each analyst? The superego of each analyst?

A convenient alternative would be to apply the term analytic psychotherapy to this smaller number of sessions and think no more about it. However, the subject must be discussed, since it troubles a number of colleagues in the field and causes discomfort, or even a sense of transgression.

It seems insufficient to apply only this indicator to define the treatment being used. It is important to consider whether an analytic process is under way, if there is an established transference neurosis, dream analysis, or an analytic field was established, whether countertransference is being addressed or psychic changes have been observed, if the analyst has a developed and established analytic identity and sufficient experience with the usual method to deal with less frequent sessions; if the answer to these questions is yes, I see no reason not to use the term analysis, regardless of session frequency. After all, this is one of the many themes talked about in the hallways at conferences: patients who came (or come) four times a week with little headway, and others whose sessions are less frequent but analysis progresses. That said, extensive clinical experience has taught me that the analytical method benefits from more frequent sessions, but, at the same time, some patients unable to do so can still be accepted and analyzed.

In regard to other elements of the setting, some patients are unable to use the couch for a period of time, or even never, for a number of reasons (control, paranoid anxiety, etc.); others have such a rigid mental structure that they collapse on the couch in the first session and cannot move beyond this for some time, or the entire time, and there are those who follow a predictable course of spending some time face to face, and then moving on to the couch, satisfactorily completing their analytic treatment.

In relation to establishing a mandatory regime of paying fees for sessions, the time in which patients were solely responsible for maintaining this regime has long passed; today, individual situations are examined to determine resistance and real need so as to pursue a course that is neither rigid nor *laissez faire*, but as analytical as possible. The same is true for vacation time, both on the part of analysts and patients.

There is also the interesting and challenging issue of distance psychoanalysis by phone, Skype, or using other forms of virtual communication. In fact, patients are increasingly communicating with analysts (and *vice versa*) via text message or WhatsApp, rather than the almost obsolete answering machine, and more and more images, videos, iPhone or iPad recordings are being brought into sessions and form part of the modern-day setting. The literature demonstrates the effectiveness of these approaches (Scharff, 2012), but it is important to continue studying the advantages and limitations. In my opinion, it is important, and even indispensable, that analysis involve a period or periods of in-person treatment, which continues to be the manner in which the method was developed and provides the conditions for an optimal setting.

What about the mind of the analyst?

On the one hand, it is increasingly easy to be an analyst in modern times, and, on the other, increasingly difficult.

It is easier because we have the work of Freud, Ferenczi, Abraham, Klein, Bion, Winnicott, Lacan, Erikson, Kohut, Mahler, Laplanche, Green, and Joseph in our wake, alongside our own analysts and supervisors. All this vast experience allows us to navigate paths, depths, and shortcuts with a contemporary clarity unavailable to our predecessors; however, our successors will be even more successful for the same reasons. There has also been a series of innovations in the psychoanalytic community, such as those provided by programs like CAPSA (Analytic Practice and Scientific Activities Committee), which emerged from the pioneering and passionate work of Haydée Faimberg and her "listening to listening" groups, which multiplied into working parties that are perhaps the most stimulating part of every psychoanalytic conference.

However, analysts' work is also more difficult, partly because of the same reasons previously stated: difficulty accompanying so many developments, new contributions, forms of listening and proposals, as well as coping within different institutions with their rivalries, nitpicking, competition, and professional envy, alongside undeniable moments of cooperation and creative work. How does one keep abreast of a world that is constantly changing and challenging us in its complexity and almost endless supply of ideas, books, films, expressions of popular or classic culture of which we are required to have at least minimal knowledge, since they are also part of the world of our patients and their associations.

The mind of the analyst is increasingly considered a vital element of the analytic relationship. In an interesting summary of psychoanalytic work, Levine (2010) suggests the existence of two models. The first is the so-called archaeological model, which is best suited to situations in which psychic elements have achieved representation and are more or less symbolically invested and associatively linked to one another. This model works well in the treatment of neurotics, but is problematic for other analytic patients, for whom Levine suggests the transformational model is more appropriate, since it centers on the functioning of the mind of the analyst as part of the analytic dyad in the creation and reinforcement of psychic elements, rather than, or in addition to, their discovery. He emphasizes that psychoanalysis is a two-person activity that involves the creation of symbols, thoughts, feelings, and the unconscious as opposed to analyzing defenses or uncovering hidden meanings; in short, the analytic process is a double operation: giving a container to the patient's content and content to his container. This echoes the ideas of Green, Ferro, Ogden, and the Barangers.

The contemporary challenge for psychoanalysis is that of switching between the archaeological and transformational models, between states of understanding and not understanding, and of tolerating the inevitable fluctuations in our own mental state, that of the patient and that which we build together.

It is here, perhaps, in addition to all the aspects cited above, that the incomparable fascination of psychoanalysis lies (Eizirik, 2014b).

Construction of the analyst

Are analysts constructed or do they construct themselves? Are they constructed or under construction? As I wrote this paper, I was reminded of a poem: "Construction worker", by Brazilian poet Vinicius de Moraes (1960), in which he describes a construction worker's growing realization of his circumstance. There is a dialogue in which the construction worker, tempted by the manipulative wiles of his boss who failed to bend his will, finally tells him: you cannot give me what is mine! Loosely translated, the poem ends as follows: "And in the still afternoon / Loomed the logic / Of a poor forgotten man / Logic nevertheless that made / A constructed worker / Of the construction worker".

By this, I mean I am not a great believer in the idea of a construction analyst, but, rather, in a dynamic, continuous, and always incomplete process of an analyst under construction. Contrary to the poet's sorrowful conclusion, I feel that our case is not one of a constructed analyst, but, rather, that we experience a fluctuation between mental states in which we feel more or less constructed or under permanent construction (Eizirk, 2012).

Since 1920 and the onset of formal analytical training at the Berlin Policlinic and subsequent developments, it is undeniable that the tripartite system of personal analysis, theoretical and clinical studies, and supervision have been maintained, and that since the IPA finally acknowledged reality and approved the three training models, we are now more easily able to recognize that these aspects have countless variations and nuances that change from one institution to another. Committees in charge of studying what goes on at different institutes carefully examined the situation and found, for example, that despite following the famous tripartite system, the more traditional and prevalent Eitingon model exhibited countless variations. Successive modifications within the IPA under different management have observed and described with increasing realism the different formats used in different institutions to organize psychoanalytic training (Eizirik, 2011; Kernberg & Tyson, 2011; Widlöcher, 2011). Freud likened psychoanalytic technique to chess, in that opening and closing moves can be specified, but there are countless possible variations that occur throughout the game. Similarly, after visiting countless analysts' offices in recent years, I found that all of them had a couch and an armchair, as well as other furniture, but each had a feature that distinguished them from the rest; for example, the relationship between the armchair and the couch varies significantly, with countless positions ranging from the analyst being completely outside the patient's field of view to being almost beside them, so the patients need only shift their head to see them; in short, institutions provide the conditions for analysts to construct, but whether this occurs or not is outside institutional control.

Personal analysis

I feel there is consensus regarding the need to maintain strict training procedures and strive to ensure the internal consistency of the model we adopt, but analysts will develop or not, for reasons that go beyond our best intentions. I have read and heard that, to different degrees, the key element of training is the personal analysis of future analysts and, in general terms, I agree with this statement, but is this always the case? At this point, it is important to underscore the complex web of unconscious fantasies, projections, and dissociations that are established, in almost all cases, between patients and their analysts, supervisors, teachers, colleagues, institutional authority figures, and culture, the tradition of each society and its countless family dramas. All of this combines with the experiences of each future analyst with their family, background, tradition, and fantasies about the future they are building in their mind. Bolognini (2013) carefully examined a series of situations that analysts in training experience, illustrating what he calls their institutional and imaginary family throughout the training process.

In the best cases, personal analysis is a space in which these elements can be examined within the possibilities of each analyst, who also participates in this drama either in fantasy or reality; on many occasions, even when analysis is successful and the analyst is humble enough to recognize his transitional role in the patients' lives, without expecting their eternal gratitude (by mentioning the analyst's name in papers, referring patients, idealization, etc.), this development will occur *a posteriori* through self-analysis, by observing the facts of institutional life, analytic experience, and sharing experiences with colleagues and friends. Several authors emphasize that this type of analysis is necessarily contaminated by all the external factors involved.

In my experience, and I have had the opportunity to hear similar experiences from colleagues, there are roughly two major groups of analytic patients who undergo training. The first consists of patients seeking treatment for their personal needs and emotional suffering, who, at a certain time during treatment, or following years of psychoanalysis, perceive a desire or motivation for analytic training. In general, or in most cases, training is only one period in their analysis, which continues after institutional procedures until formal completion of the analytic process. For these people, training was something incidental that occurred during analysis. The second group comprises people who seek out analysis for the purpose of training, despite recognizing the existence of emotional difficulties. There is often an element of urgency or pressure in this type of analysis, and the patients frequently end it as soon as they achieve the institutional requirements. There are many apparent reasons for this: cost, distances, family demands, etc. It would not be fair to generalize, but my observation demonstrates that the first group contains those analysts who identify more closely with analytic function and identity.

This is where a question emerges that I feel deserves greater attention: why did Freud have the curious idea of recommending re-analysis every five years? Was it because analysis at that time was insufficient or too quick, or because his usual astuteness had perceived the self-limited nature of all analysis, and the powerful presence of resistance to the unconscious that leads to our tiresome tendency to repress, reject, or deny the unpleasant aspects that our analyst(s) spent years trying to show us. Perhaps I am being unfair or misinformed, but I have the impression that re-analysis is not very common among analysts; as a working hypothesis, I suggest that it is difficult to remain sharp and up to date in our field if we do not have the humility to undergo what Freud refers to as periodic psychoanalytic purification.

The psychoanalytic institution

One element that can either stimulate or not the construction of an analytic identity is the institutional climate that predominates in each society or institute, as well as how the trajectory of each future analyst is viewed within each psychoanalytic culture.

To what extent is critical and independent thinking welcomed? To what degree do procedures and rules become a type of fetish that must be obeyed just because? To what extent are analysts in training encouraged to establish and administrate their own candidates' associations? How often are theoretical differences welcome and listened to with respect and interest? To what extent are curricula flexible and do they include optional seminars, allowing each psychoanalysis student to follow their own interests? To what extent does the institutional climate stimulate future analysts to participate in its activities and offer opinions at meetings, or to remain in shy and fearful silence, which will only be broken many years and countless meetings later? To what degree are topics related to analytic training discussed with those who are undergoing the experience? Do institutions revise and modify their curricula, procedures, and manner of understanding analytic training over time, as new national and international ideas on the subject and the learning process itself emerge?

All of these questions, as well as detailed discussion on many of them, have been the subject of successive papers by Kernberg. One of the aspects most highlighted by Kernberg (2000) is the so-called training analysis and the concentration of power to a limited number of training analysts, often resulting in an oppressive and paranoid institutional climate. On my part, I have observed situations in which this does, in fact, occur, and others in which the existence of a growing number of analysts who analyze future analysts offer a form of dilution of power, facilitating dialogue and open, free discussion. Even institutions that adopt the Eitingon model have undergone changes in terms of allowing all full members to analyze candidates. But what is the justification for keeping the analysis of future analysts solely in the hands of those who are training analysts or full members? Aside from the obvious of focusing power among fewer hands, I feel the justification of greater psychoanalytic experience is not enough. I have observed and experienced situations where an analysis with an associate member progresses satisfactorily until the patient decides to undergo analytic training and must then switch to a training analyst. In many cases, this change might ruthlessly interrupt an analytic relationship that was developing well, while in others it might be beneficial. Perhaps we should put more emphasis on the fact that an adequately trained analyst, recognized as such by his society, may be capable of carrying out analyses, regardless of who is being analyzed. After all, a training analysis does not actually exist, since it is not a pedagogical or educational procedure, but, rather, an analysis of a person that might one day become an analyst.

In a recent study, Garcia (2014) discusses several aspects of the institutionalized transmission of psychoanalysis. His central thesis is that of the singularity of each analyst's training, and that the role of institutes should be to offer the best possible conditions for every future analyst to carry out their own training, including the values learned from previous generations with current cultural characteristics, as well as protecting future analysts from institutional resistance to essential freedom and individuality.

Among many possible new ways of promoting progress in the analytic training, and taking into account the most prevalent model of training, the Eitingon model, in my view institutes could consider some aspects of the other two models in order to improve what we have until now. In this sense, the analysis of a candidate (from now on I will call this colleague an analyst in training) could be conducted by any member of the society, mainly in the cases when the patient is already in analysis with one of these members, and not only the so-called training analysts; there should be a limit of analyses of future analysts (in some institutes, there is a limit of three, in others five, but in many there is no limit, which is a real danger, not only of concentrating power, but of confining the analytic practice of senior analysts to a very narrow sample of patients, with the other side effect of dealing with cross transferences and countertransferences); there should be a very strict limit of the number of supervisions per supervisor, for similar reasons; analysts in training should have an active participation in the discussions on curricula and other relevant aspects of training, including their own progress and/or problems with their increased analytic identity; analysts in training should have their progress candidly evaluated, and the papers they write discussed and evaluated by their teachers and peers; there should be a limit of age for receiving new analysts in training, as already exists in some institutes, but is strongly resisted in others; there should be an evaluation of the function of training analyst, from time to time, in order to assess whether these colleagues remain active in the life of their societies and institutes, follow the analytic literature, participate in meetings, write papers, and so on. In short, these procedures would stimulate analytic work and discussion, stress that our instrument, our mind, needs to be challenged and protected from internal and external pressures, and create an atmosphere of collegial joint effort to keep high standards for our senior, as well as our younger, members.

About analytic supervision

There is also extensive literature on analytic supervision and it is well known that its relevance varies according to the model adopted. In any event, it is undeniably an area that significantly affects the training of analysts, since it is a more open relationship than personal analysis, which can be a source of stimulation as well as joint and mutually enriching work, or a space for transmitting a way of thinking or analyzing centered on the figure and authority of the supervisor. It is a delicate relationship in which maintaining a certain distance and asymmetry alongside natural and spontaneous interaction requires constant attention on the part of the supervisor. As with the analytic relationship, this is a naturally ambivalent relationship, but has the potential to stimulate creativity and the establishment of an independent analyst. In my opinion, the most noteworthy among many significant contributions is the recent special issue of *Psychoanalytic Inquiry*, edited by Imre Szecsody and Melvin Bornstein and entitled *Never Ever Stop Learning More About Supervision* (Eizirik, 2014a).

Never Ever Stop Learning More About Supervision is a very adequate title for this gathering of excellent papers on supervision, as well as being a very proper motto for Imre Szecsody's extraordinary and tireless contributions to our current understanding of this complex process that is at the very core of analytic training.

In my view, the papers presented here show the many dilemmas, complexities, and controversies on analytic supervision. On the one side, we see nowadays a consistent search for objectivity and of measurable learning objectives, as the papers from Mega and Cabaniss, and Watkins and Scaturo clearly suggest. For instance, Watkins and Scaturo show how to use the Learning Alliance Building and Maintenance and state that psychoanalytic supervision is a formative, developmental, learning experience and intervention; that it is educational in its mission, process, and product and should be guided by a vision that is founded upon, and grounded in, educational psychology and theories of learning; Mega and Cabaniss present a plea for clearly delineated measurable learning objectives and show how this can be used and its relevance for analytic training.

From another perspective, we can see a qualitative research on two cases of supervision of analytic psychotherapy and follow Stromme's concern on what could characterize a good and a bad supervision process. One of her findings was that the expression of negative views of the supervisee on the supervisor might have a negative impact on the supervisory process. Kahl-Popp criticizes the use of teaching and learning goals from one generation to the next, stresses the importance of freedom in the learning process, illustrates the usefulness of dreams, both from the supervisee and the supervisor, to understand what is going on in the supervisory process, and states that supervision can improve or not the psychoanalyst's clinical competence. The relationship experience in supervision and its influence on the psychoanalyst's identity are studied by Nagell and colleagues in a research conducted with different psychoanalytic institutes in Germany, and they were able to identify four working styles in the supervisors (defensive–controlling; pragmatic; experiential and relationship oriented; facilitating–holding) and in the supervisees ("phobic"–avoidance; open–interested; authentic–researching; reserved–adaptive); these and other findings of this study seem to be extremely useful when one thinks on his/her experience with supervising younger colleagues.

Taking advantage of his long experience in several settings of analytic training, Gabor Szonyii offers us a stimulating discussion on the Budapest model of supervision, inquires about the reason for the silence about it, and shows the possible strong and weak points of it. While reading this paper, what came to my mind was the fact, so often heard in congresses' corridors, or from analytic candidates, that, in fact, from time to time, even the most conservative analyst cannot avoid playing the Budapest model during a session with a candidate in trouble with a difficult case.

So, in my perspective, there is certain tension here between two sets of papers: one group of them stresses the relevance of clear learning objectives, and sees supervision as part of a training in which skills and abilities can be clearly established, pursued, and monitored;

another group relies more on a process of building inner abilities or expanding the mind, or on a sort of emotional learning, following Bion. The emotional relationship between supervisor and supervisee takes the main role here.

These two views seem to be related to cultural factors, economic pressures for showing effectiveness, the presence of competing therapies with their supposed greater effectiveness, and even an overall current trend to idealize the so-called competence. What I mean by this is that I understand and acknowledge the relevance of establishing and trying to use more objective tools for researching and monitoring analytic skills, but, at the same time, I see with some concern the risk of not taking sufficiently into consideration the uniqueness and the peculiar nature of each analytic relation and the process of each analyst acquiring some kind of analytic identity. By the way, in my view, this identity, as Kahl-Popp also stresses, is not something obtained after a number of analytic hours of analysis and supervisions and seminars, but an ongoing process of working through one's own inner world and continuous fluctuations among different mental states. In this process that, in German, is called Bildung and, in English, training or education, while we have in French *formation*, as well as in Spanish *formación*, or in Portuguese *formação*, perhaps we may learn from these apparently minor linguistic differences two basic differences that are clearly reflected in this volume.

I see all these papers as extremely well grounded, and following a clear and well designed methodology, each one of them being able to stimulate the reader to never ever stop learning more about supervision, and I also think that they show the state of the art at this particular moment. As in so many other aspects of analytic activity, diversity is the trade mark of our international community, and, while reading each of these papers, I was reminded of several situations from my own experience as supervisor, supervisee, researcher, or teacher. This might be one of the main riches of this collective effort, under the inspiring leadership of Imre Szecsody: it will certainly stimulate more research along these and other lines, it will increase the interest in seeing supervision as an area full of life and possibilities, and, last but not least, it will help both supervisors and supervisees, as well as analytic institutes in the long and never ending process of helping new colleagues to make their way to becoming part of our shared work in progress.

Becoming and remaining an analyst

And what of this person who will one day tell himself he feels like an analyst?

As in previous areas, there is relevant literature on the complex process of becoming an analyst. Particularly useful are texts in which analysts reflect on their own motivations and personal journey in this complex process of acquiring an analytic identity. At the same time, I feel that the very notion of an analytic identity may contain a threat, in that it prioritizes the idea that analytic identity is obtained or established and is not a work in progress or a process under way. To cite three examples, a good illustration of the vicissitudes of this process can be found in *Un Psychanalyste Engagé* (A committed psychoanalyst) (Green, 1994), about the professional and personal life of André Green, in a special issue of *Psychoanalytic Inquiry* (2005), in which several Latin American analysts reflect on their individual careers, and in the more recent *Comment on devient psychanalyste . . . et comment on le reste* (2010) by Daniel Widlöcher.

These accounts and countless others attest to the fact that each analyst develops based on a series of cultural, conscious, and unconscious motivations, identifications, life experiences, traumatic situations, a wide range of neurotic aspects, the search for reparation, ideals, and so on.

I believe that a central element in becoming an analyst and remaining one in subsequent years is linked to clinical experience and the accumulation of psychoanalytic hours, as well as the possibility of achieving success, failure, and positive results with the patients treated. The ability to share in a patient's psychological changes, the expansion of their mind and ability to love, feel, and work helps strengthen belief (according to Bion) in our method. Tolerating failures teaches us humility in regard to the scope and limitations of this method.

Meltzer (1967) highlights the combination of athletic and artistic activity present in psychoanalytic work, and the importance of simplicity and stability in clinical activity, something I also heard from Bela Grunberger.

It is perhaps even more difficult to remain an analyst than to train one, given the countless temptations to relax in the difficult work of addressing the unconscious within an analytic field that requires constant maintenance and protection. Once the formal steps within an institution are complete, each analyst follows his own path and the inevitable vicissitudes of his personal and professional life cycle, facing not only the difficulties of demanding clinical work, but the circumstances of a culture that challenges the relevance and validity of psychoanalysis. Remaining an analyst means being able to tolerate attacks and challenges that emerge naturally from the work itself through emotional suffering, as well as an often ambivalent external reality. Remaining an analyst means being able to move between tradition and invention without denying the inevitable fluctuations of mental states or the losses and gains of each stage of the life cycle. Since analysts potentially work for longer than other professionals, the aging process deserves special attention, not only because of the limitations it can bring, but also in terms of greater clinical acuity and courage in dealing with close analytic contact with more primitive levels of the mind. Analytic institutions can play an important role in this process, in that they maintain a program that could be referred to as continuous, stimulating psychoanalytic training. Despite the inevitable disappointment of many analysts with their local, national, and international institutions, I still observe that a feeling of "us", a certain sense of belonging and pride in the achievements that can be obtained through joint work, are elements that might have a containing function for different types of anxiety previously mentioned.

Is there a way to characterize how analysts feel about their work, their fluctuations between tradition and invention, and their successive mental states? Between their moments of understanding and non-understanding, as Betty Joseph would say? Between feeling constructed and in construction?

Among so many possibilities, as I wrote this paper I remembered a long-forgotten time when, in the voice of Brazilian actor Paulo Autran, I heard the words of Louis Javet and Jean Louis Barrault, collected by Millôr Fernandes and Flávio Rangel for the play *Liberdade Liberdade* (Liberty, Liberty), staged as a demonstration against the dictatorship in place in Brazil at the time, and perhaps reflecting more astutely than analytic descriptions what it means to identify with a profession: "I am simply a man of the theater. I always was and always will be a man of the theater. Anyone capable of dedicating their entire life to the humanity and passion on these few meters of stage is a man of the theater".

References

Ahumada, J. (1997). Crise da cultura e crise da psicanálise. *Revista de Psicanálise da SPPA, 4*(3): 51–70.

Aisenstein, M. (2014). Abordagem psicodinâmica do paciente psicossomático. In: C. L. Eizirik, R. W. Aguiar, & S. S. Schestatsky (Eds.), *Psicoterapia de orientação analítica: fundamentos teóricos e clínicos* (3rd edn) (pp. 659–667). Porto Alegre: Artmed.

Baranger, M. (1993). The mind of the analyst: from listening to interpretation. *International Journal of Psychoanalysis, 74*: 15–24.

Bolognini, S. (2013). The institutional and fantasy family of the analyst. *Psychoanalyse, 29*(3): 357–372.

Eizirik, C. L. (2011). The IPA administration from 2005 to 2009. In: P. Loewenberg & N. Thompson (Eds.), *100 Years of the IPA: The Centenary History of the International Psychological Association, 1910–2010: Evolution and Change* (pp. 515–524). London: Karnac.

Eizirik, C. L. (2012). O analista em construção. FEBRAPSI Notícias, *XIV, 46*: 2–4.

Eizirik, C. L. (2014a). Discussion: never ever stop learning more about supervision. *Psychoanalytic Inquiry, 34*: 642–643.

Eizirik, C. L. (2014b). Algumas questões sobre a clínica psicanalítica contemporânea. *Psicanalítica, XIV*(1): 9–16.

Fernandes, M., & Rangel, F. (1997). *Liberdade, Liberdade.* Porto Alegre: L & PM Editores.

Gaddini, E. (1987). *Cambios en los pacientes psicoanaliticos hasta nuestros dias.* Monografia número IV. London: Associación Psicoanalitica Internacional.

Garcia, J. (2014). La transmisión institucionalizada del psicoanálisis en los comienzos del siglo XXI. *Revista Uruguaya de Psicoanálisis, 118*: 139–155.

Green, A. (1994). *Un Psychanalyste Engagé.* Paris: Calmann-Levy.

Green, A. (2002). *Idées directrices pour une psychanalyse contemporaine.* Paris: PUF.

Green, A. (2010). *Illusions et disillusions du travail psychanalytique.* Paris: Odile Jacob.

Junkers, G. (Ed.) (2006). *Is It Too Late? Key Papers on Psychoanalysis and Ageing.* London: Karnac.

Kernberg, O. (2000). A concerned critique of psychoanalytic education. *International Journal of Psychoanalysis, 81*(1): 97–120

Kernberg, O., & Tyson, R. (2011). The IPA administration from 1997 to 2001. In: P. Loewenberg & N. Thompson (Eds.), *100 Years of the IPA:*

The Centenary History of the International Psychological Association, 1910–2010: Evolution and Change (pp. 485–502). London: Karnac.

Kristeva, J. (2002). *As novas doenças da alma.* Rio de Janeiro: Rocco.

Levine, H. B. (2010). Creating analysts, creating analytic patients. *International Journal of Psychoanalysis, 91*: 1385–1404.

McDougall, J. (1983). *Em defesa de uma certa anormalidade: teoria e clínica psicanalítica.* Porto Alegre: Artes Médicas.

Meltzer, D. (1967). *The Psychoanalytical Process.* London. Heinemann.

Moraes, V. (1960). *Antologia Poética.* Rio de Janeiro: Editora do Autor.

Scharff, J. S. (2012). Clinical issues in analysis over the telephone and the internet. *International Journal of Psychoanalysis, 93*: 81–95.

Urribarri, F. (2013). *Dialogues avec André Green.* Paris: Itaque.

Widlöcher, D. (2010). *Comment on Devient Psychanalyste . . . et Comment on Le Reste.* Paris: Odile Jacob.

Widlöcher, D. (2011). The IPA administration from 2001 to 2005. In: P. Loewenberg & N. Thompson (Eds.), *100 Years of the IPA: The Centenary History of the International Psychological Association, 1910–2010: Evolution and Change* (pp. 503–513). London: Karnac.

CHAPTER FIVE

Psychoanalytical training in flux

Gigliola Fornari Spoto

My contribution to the current debate about psychoanalytical training is based on the psychoanalytical culture I am familiar with, which is that of the British Psychoanalytical Society and my long involvement with its training, including a recent experience as Chair of its Education Committee. My perspective is unavoidably based on such a culture, its ethos, its history, its institutional dynamics and conflicts, and my identification with it, as well as my personal evolution as a psychoanalyst. So, this chapter contains the limitations that accompany such perspective, although in recent years, thanks to the effort of organizations such as the EPF, we have been able to become more familiar with other training models and less insular in the way we approach issues of training.

The transmission of psychoanalysis is a complex task which combines experiential and formal learning: the different training models which have evolved throughout the years in psychoanalytical societies have tried to address such complexities, developing institutional and organizational structures which deal with the whole process of training, starting from the selection of candidates, the setting of a syllabus, the evaluation during the training, through to the assessment of the competences deemed necessary to qualify as an analyst. Everybody who has been involved in psychoanalytical training is confronted with a fundamental intrinsic dilemma: how can we have a psychoanalytical training which is predicated on the specificity of the psychoanalytical ethos and process, is enabling rather than controlling, promotes freedom of thinking rather than conformity, while maintaining educational standards which ensure transmission of the essence of psychoanalytical thinking and clinical practice, and, at the same time, leading to the acquisition of a professional identity recognizable in the outside world? A training, in other words, which is modeled on the psychoanalytical process rather than one which abandons it in favor of organizational and bureaucratic concerns. In the Eitingon model, which requires the candidate to undergo an analysis with a training analyst, the analytical dyad and its relative freedom have to come to terms with the presence of several thirds: the aim to train as an analyst while being a patient in analysis, the presence of the institution which provides and evaluates the training, the relationship of the training analyst with the training institution, the interaction with one's analyst in an institutional setting, contact with analytical siblings, etc. This is, of course, one of the main reasons why, in the so-called French model, the analysis is kept separate from the training. The complexity of the analytical situation in the Eitingon model of training is also one of the reasons why higher levels of competence in the training analyst are deemed to be necessary.

Sklar (2014), in a recent paper presented to the British Society, sees the tension between developing authenticity and learning technique as central in shaping the identity of the future psychoanalyst and warns about the institutional constraints which can obstruct such a process. Formally learning analytical technique and developing a psychoanalytical identity is not one and the same thing. It takes, on average, in the British Psychoanalytical Society, 4.5 years of training to qualify as a psychoanalyst, that is, to be able to treat patients independently, but it is generally acknowledged that it takes much longer to develop a psychoanalytical identity that feels secure and independent. It also can take longer to develop a substantive clinical practice. As well as the naturally lengthy process of growing as an analyst, it is well known how institutional dynamics can contribute to a climate of prolonged dependence on transferential figures, where the children never fully grow up and never leave home, remaining dependent on the charismatic figures in the Society. It is often said that psychoanalytical institutes operate like families, but not always functional ones. Being a psychoanalyst can be a lonely profession and one depends on colleagues for support and for referrals. Idealization of the work and ideas of senior figures, seen as the parents one never separates from, can lead to a sense of belonging to a well identifiable analytical family which is both comforting and disturbing. This state of affairs can discourage independent thinking and promote powerful dynamics of exclusion. Career progression can be perceived as based on patronage and on being a member of what is seen as the most influential elite in the psychoanalytic society.

Much has been written in recent years about the damage done by institutional psychoanalysis to the development of psychoanalytical trainees (perhaps no more eloquently so than by Kernberg (1986, 1996, 2012)): there is a view that maintains that psychoanalytical training takes place in a hierarchical, authoritarian, antidemocratic atmosphere which promotes conformity with the dominant psychoanalytical ideology and stifles individual creativity. Kernberg and others sharing his position are convinced that the antidemocratic and authoritarian nature of psychoanalytical training, which is then repeated in the way psychoanalytical institutions run themselves, is a major contributing factor to the overall decline of psychoanalysis and its status in the world. His solutions are organizational ones: to separate the analytical functions from the educational and administrative ones, the teaching function from the analyzing function, to abolish training analysts and what he sees as their detrimental privileged status and power, and to adopt a research orientation. The view expressed in this kind of position is that psychoanalytical institutions, animated by unrecognized and repeatedly enacted unconscious group dynamics, tend to subvert, when it comes to training, the very essence of the psychoanalytical experience, its freedom of expression, and its emphasis on unconscious dynamics.

In the trainings which adopt the Eitingon model, the tension between learning and development is already present, before entering the arena of organized training, in the syncretic quality of the training analysis itself, and its dual function: the candidates learn analytical technique (albeit in an experiential way) while learning about themselves and their unconscious processes. Analytical technique is learned in the heat and the complexities of the transference situation. Adam Limentani (1974) recognized the complications of this dual function when he said that "Ambiguity may in fact be a more emotional and accurate word than syncretic to describe this situation" (p. 71).

Psychoanalytical institutions can restrict freedom of thought and creativity if they operate at the level of basic assumptions, but they also have the important function of containing anxiety and conflict and looking after professional identity. Sklar (2014) stresses some of the historical anxieties which have contributed to the progressive transformation of psychoanalytic training from Freud's days to the present. The first anxiety in relation to psychoanalytical training was, and still remains, the anxiety about transmission. Sklar quotes Bernfeld (1962), who thought that the threatened loss of Freud, at the time of the diagnosis of his cancer, made people feel they were responsible for the future of psychoanalysis and its orthodoxy, and pushed various institutes into a competition about who was the holder of the most rigorous training.

The anxiety about loss of power and influence has been central in the present life of psychoanalytical societies worldwide. I do not think it is possible to think of issues of training without acknowledging that training organizations do not only have the task to transmit and protect what is seen as psychoanalytical orthodoxy, but that they are now under increasing pressure to offer something (training and treatment) which will be taken up by members of the public. The concentration on internal transmission has given way to concerns about the relationship with the external world. The internal functioning of psychoanalytical institutions has been challenged by external social and cultural needs.

There are many reasons for our apparent decline and many anxieties generated by it. The recent loss of cultural and clinical power which psychoanalysis has been experiencing means that there are fewer patients who choose analytical treatment and fewer people who apply for psychoanalytical training. This is a worldwide problem that affects most countries where psychoanalysis has a well-established history and all training models and has many causes. I think it is important to stress that it is not so much our different models, but psychoanalysis itself that is going through a crisis and that it is unproductive to focus on one single cause and try to remedy it in isolation, with single solutions. Most of us, who passionately believe in the contemporary relevance of psychoanalysis, have had to come to terms with the fact that analysis does not find favor with legislators and public policy makers, and we, as analysts, and our psychoanalytical institutions, have to deal with the powerful depressive feelings which this produces. In our Society, as, I am sure, in many others, people have been talking about the unavoidable extinction or even the suicide of psychoanalysis, depending on what they saw as the causes of our present decline. Powerful depressive anxieties are also experienced when analysts, especially newly qualified ones, do not have a sufficient number of patients in treatment to sustain a psychoanalytical practice: this leads to a disturbing loss of identity and generativity. We cannot keep our good object alive and our good object, in turn, does not sustain us any more, in some kind of painful vicious circle. In a country such as the UK, where all psychoanalytical treatment is privately funded, it can be very difficult for somebody entering the profession at the present to earn a living working only as an analyst (i.e., doing intensive 4–5 times a week work) and/or to occupy a leading position in the field of mental health.

Our ageing membership (out of a membership of around 400 at the end of 2014, twenty-one members were younger than fifty (5.1%), almost 52% of the membership were aged sixty-five or over, 17.8% were aged seventy-five or over, 29.7% were over seventy) and the average age of our candidates at the time of being accepted for training (about forty) can lead to a tangible anxiety about the Society shrinking into decline. The cost of the training and its length are often quoted as the main reasons that prevent younger people from embarking on a lengthy and expensive course of training. Fewer younger people, who are essential in ensuring generational continuity and in renewing the increasingly ageing membership, join our rank, despite the fact that there is some encouraging evidence, over the past few years, that the interest in psychoanalysis in public mental health (where we have always recruited the majority of our trainees from) is, in fact, on the increase, possibly because of the hegemony of short therapeutic interventions and their limitations, hegemony dictated by financial constraints and by the emphasis on research-backed clinical trials. We are also seeing an increase in applications for training from older people, who are interested in a second career and arrive at our doors in their late forties or early fifties.

These anxieties about decline and extinction can make institutions become even more protective and more controlling of the transmission of psychoanalysis, in the belief that only by maintaining what are seen as the highest possible standards can we keep analysis alive and protect it from the outside financial, social, and cultural attacks to which it has been subjected. However, these anxieties can also mobilize a reparative effort to engage with the new social realities and to re-examine how we do things and how we present ourselves to the outside world. Depressive anxiety, as we know, can also generate persecutory reactions and this can lead to an unhelpful singling out of what is seen as impeding the necessary progress and change: this often takes the shape of the internal "enemy" in the institution, such as the training analysts who want to preserve their power and influence, or a certain committee, such as the Admissions Committee, which is too restrictive in the way it selects candidates for training. The debate can become extremely polarized. Some people feel that analysis has, after all, always been at the margins, has never been fully integrated with other, more established disciplines: to some extent, this is where it derives its strength and its capacity to survive. As long as we keep the passion and the conviction alive, maintain and protect our distinctive identity and our high standards, and engage, with muscular resistance, with the pressure of external forces, we should be able to see this crisis through. The other, as it were, camp believes that the social and financial reality in which analysis operates has considerably affected our position in the world and we need some very substantial changes to our training models and institutional structures in order to survive.

This is very much the debate we have been having in our Society in recent years. As is often the case with psychoanalytical institutions, themes of exclusion–inclusion have been central to it. Some people have voiced a strong concern (Taylor, 2013) that psychoanalysis has been (to its detriment) too focused on transmission and training, excessively valuing the people involved in it, and has not given enough importance to its so-called applications in the wider world and to its wider professional identity, which have received lower status and attention. This could also be seen as another version of the never-ending tension between internal–external reality, which continues to inhabit the psychoanalytical discourse. Many of our members who work in the National Health Service felt that their essential contribution in promoting psychoanalysis has not been sufficiently recognized, as if they were occupying a lower status in the Society.

There have been pressures to move outside the consulting room, and to be less inward looking and insular. Steps have been taken to move psychoanalysis into the wider social and cultural context, to promote its clinical efficacy through research, to be more connected with the world of psychotherapy and allied disciplines, to improve recruitment: all these measures tend to be more successful if taken with a positive, fight-back attitude, rather than a defensive, doom-laden one.

It is undoubtedly true that, as a Society, we have invested a lot in its training and hugely value its rich history and tradition. The British Psychoanalytical Society has been home to many influential and creative psychoanalytical thinkers and continues to be so, and our members can feel a strong and reassuring sense of identification with such figures, past and present.

Just a brief reminder of what the essential aspects of our training comprise. Candidates are expected to be in five times a week analysis for at least a year with a training analyst before starting lectures and seminars and they continue to be in analysis throughout the length of their training. They are assessed throughout the training, with reports written by the different seminar leaders. The need to represent all the theoretical and clinical traditions in our Society is reflected in the way the curriculum is organized: our history continues to affect what we teach. Ensuring pluralism in the teaching owes something to the political compromise post the "Controversial Discussions", but it also leads to a very extensive curriculum where trainees can become familiar with a broad range of psychoanalytical perspectives. The average length of training is about 4.5 years. After the first year of theoretical seminars, the trainees see two patients in five times a week analysis under supervision, the first case for at least two years and the second patient, who can be taken on after a year with the first case, for at least one year. Trainees can recruit analytical patients from their existing private practice, but they usually see patients who have been assessed by the London Clinic of Psychoanalysis. The patients pay a low fee, well below the going rate (a common contribution can be as little as £5), to the Clinic, not to their analysts. The candidates are considered to be part of the Clinic staff.

The existence of the Clinic ensures two very interrelated aims: the first is that patients who would otherwise never have access to an analytical treatment can do so. This has important social implications and, of course, goes back to the aspirations of early psychoanalytical clinics which made analysis accessible beyond the confines of the wealthy classes. Given that the Clinic and its Director are important presences in the training, interesting triangulations can develop between the trainees, their patients, and the Clinic. Sometimes the Clinic can represent a helpful "third", sometimes it can be felt as an intrusive, regulatory one. One could argue that some of the functions of the money and the payment as analytical third are transferred to the Clinic in our system.

The second aim is that candidates can rely on a "supply" of five times a week patients, whom they would have great difficulty in recruiting themselves. The therapeutic tradition of five times a week relies heavily on the existence of a psychoanalytic clinic. Training cases tend to be more disturbed than in the past: long gone are the days where candidates would see one so-called " good" hysteric and one obsessional case. Candidates have to be prepared to analyze very troubled individuals who can act out, break off treatment prematurely, and struggle with the boundaries of the analytic setting. The experience can be a bit like "a baptism of fire", but I think it remains invaluable in establishing the basic parameters of clinical work and contributes in a major way to the internalization of a psychoanalytical identity.

The availability of suitable analytical patients is seen as essential in maintaining a viable training and the Society has invested in the Clinic, which has had, for many years, a salaried Director and administrative staff as well as a physical basis in our headquarters.

Before moving to a more detailed description of the discussions that have taken place in the British Psychoanalytical Society and of the changes which such discussions have promoted, I want to cast a glance over the past. As I said before, institutions can act as containers for anxiety. Institutions are also shaped by their history, and their history shapes the way they deal with, and contain, group processes and the conflicts generated by such processes. Riccardo Steiner, who has scholarly explored with Pearl King the history of the BPAS at the time of the so-called "Controversial Discussions", wrote recently (2014) about "Controversies terminable and interminable", describing some aspects of the present debate as new versions of an old debate about power and hegemony; unfortunately, he thinks, without the passionate exchange of views about scientific differences, which characterized the "Controversial Discussions", and he urges us to revisit our history. At the time of the "Controversial Discussions", the BPAS managed to avoid an acrimonious and damaging split and to remain together as a Society. Pearl King says that the "BPAS managed to compromise and adapt and it maintained a social structure". Elsewhere (1981), she calls this the British experiment. The so-called gentlemen's agreement, which was the compromise that brought to an end a potentially destructive conflict, stipulated that there should be a representation of the so-called three groups in the Society in every committee (in today's description, the Kleinians, the Contemporary Freudians, and the Independents), to prevent a group taking over too much power. A certain ability to recognize, contain, and survive conflict and the capacity for pragmatic compromise have been inscribed, as it were, in the institutional DNA of the Society, since the traumatic experience of the "Controversial Discussions" and its resolution.

What is also part of the "British experiment" is something that has been more generally present in British culture: tolerance of difference, pragmatism, and tradition can be all valued at the same time. The gentlemen's agreement contributed, for many years, to the containment of the conflict about hegemony. With the passing of years, though, it was increasingly felt that the gentlemen's agreement had lost, by then, its containing function, acquiring instead a stifling political quality. People believed it was no longer needed in an atmosphere that had become, over the years, much less divisive and polarized. Perhaps it is worth noting that the gentlemen's agreement came to an end in 2005: this meant that people would be appointed or elected to various committees on the basis of being the "best person for the job", rather than their affiliation to a particular "group". This took place together with a process of democratization about various appointments and elections in the Society, which aimed to be more meritocratic, less patronage based. While there is a shared sense that the politicization of the groups was an unhelpful thing, there is some concern that, paradoxically, the absence of well defined "groups" has contributed to a reduced freedom in scientific exchanges among members: some people miss the very polarized and heated debates which used to happen in scientific meetings and the passion which went with that. Despite their official abolition, the influence of the different groups continues to be an important, subterranean, and possibly not sufficiently recognized influence in the life of the Society.

The new challenges which psychoanalysis has had to face over the last few years have, nevertheless, meant that the preoccupation with the internal conflict about group hegemony has become less relevant, superseded by the need to face such challenges as a united and purposeful organization, with a clear sense of identity which could be presented to the outside world. This process, though, has meant that the Society has had once again to look at itself and at its internal ways of functioning. It is not, perhaps, surprising that, while psychoanalysis as a discipline has had to deal with an increasing sense of being excluded and not sufficiently valued in the clinical domain and more generally in the world at large, the same dynamics of exclusion–inclusion have been at the center of our internal debate, where several people had a painful sense of being excluded and not sufficiently valued. The crisis of the relationship of psychoanalysis with the outside world was mirrored by an increasing sense of internal crisis in the Society. The external crisis manifested itself with lower recruitment of candidates and patients. The second and internal crisis was about an increasing sense of unhappiness and disaffection among some members, especially about issues to do with progression in the Society, particularly about assessment at the threshold of changing status from Member to Fellow and to Training Analyst. (There are two categories of membership, Member, at qualification; and Fellow, which is postgraduate. People become Fellows either by presenting a clinical paper to a large Panel, or via a combination of a postgraduate course, consultations with senior colleagues, and a final clinical presentation to a small Panel.) Being aware of the difficulty of understanding group processes from the inside and that, on the whole, we are better at understanding our patients' unconscious dynamics than our own unconscious institutional ones, the President and the Board decided, after consultation with the membership, to use the expertise of an external institutional consultant, and this has proved to be a most useful exercise. There were many meetings with the whole membership. The organizational consultant sent out questionnaires to all members and had several one-to-one meetings with a large amount of people, participated in the general meetings, and attended all the various committees.

A clear task was identified at the end of this process of consultation: how to find a way to open ourselves to change and development while maintaining the essence of psychoanalysis and our cultural and clinical identity. A corollary to this task was to be able to carry on with the discussion and the suggested changes while trying to avoid defensive splits between those who saw the future of the Society based on preserving tradition and those who thought a future was possible only if there were major changes. I think it is significant that the structure of the training as such was not at the center of recent discussions, as if there was an implicit agreement that our training is, on the whole, good enough and that the Eitingon model, as we understand it, was serving us well. Questions were raised about the role of the training analysts, which I shall address later.

It is difficult to have a clear sense of what the experience of training is like for our trainees. Most of the ones who have responded to questionnaires about their experience of training seem to describe it as a largely positive and enriching experience. People can, of course, also have much less positive experiences. Probably transference dynamics interfere with an objective perception of what people think about their training experiences. Our training is very structured and demanding; you could describe it as very "containing", but also, to some extent, infantilizing. Trainees, though, have a reasonably robust voice. Their representatives sit on the Board and they are involved in the general decision-making, although, perhaps not surprisingly, very few trainees have been attending the recent discussions.

The discussions, as I said, have centered much more on issues of inclusion–exclusion and progression in the Society, on the need to recognize the various different professional identities which people have, avoiding the defensive idealization of the "pure" analyst and the denigration or lack of respect for the colleagues who do less intensive clinical analytical work and are engaged in promoting analytical work in other settings, on the basis of the reductive tribalism of "he is one of us" or "she is not one of us", "he/she is a real analyst".

The consultant put forward a formulation about two different models to explain how the group was operating: the first is the "conservation/warehousing" model, where the aim is to preserve the excellence of the past while keeping it in the present in a relatively unchanged state; the second is the "developmental/horticultural" model of growth, where new ideas might develop and flourish, ideas which might challenge views held in the past and might, therefore, have an impact on the idealization of the past. The tension between these two positions was felt by the consultant to have partly to do with anxiety about how to preserve what is held dear while continuing to develop.

The consultant also identified an anxiety about psychoanalysis being contaminated and becoming something else, an old anxiety that dates back to the concerns about preserving Freud's legacy, as I have highlighted earlier. A good example of this kind of anxiety is exemplified in the debate about the frequency of sessions: is five sessions a week the best way to train a psychoanalyst? Can analytical work take place with a reduced frequency of sessions? The rigor of five times a week analysis has been one of the defining characteristics of psychoanalytical training in the BPAS. It distinguishes our training from many others in almost "brand" defining terms. The long established conviction, so embedded in the British psychoanalytical tradition, that five times a week analysis is considered to be the most appropriate way of training a future analyst, has been nurtured and strengthened in the shared clinical experience of our consulting rooms and in the evaluation of our training. The experiential/clinical dimension has historically been at the core of the training ethos of the BPAS. The experience of the five times a week personal/training analysis continues to be considered by many people in our Society to be the central plank in the development of an analytical identity, although it is the supervisors and the other teachers who determine the speed of progression in the training. Conviction in one's training model is a necessary basis to provide effective training, but it can also generate a narcissistic phantasy of uniqueness and a related phantasy of being the standard bearers of the analytical canon. The culture, albeit one passionately held and confirmed by clinical experience, that five times a week analysis is the best way of training a future analyst can become equated with an unquestioned conviction that it *is* the best way to train future analysts. The formation of a new IPA Society in the UK, the BPA, where the requirement for training is four times a week analysis, has introduced a new "brand" of British psychoanalysis, and has helped us not to be complacent about our training.

The frequency of sessions is, of course, a very distinctive aspect in all our models but, in my opinion, not one that, on its own, can determine or define, in absolute terms, a psychoanalytical approach. The number of sessions is part of an external setting which needs to be supported by an internal one: it is an essential component of the analytical process, as essential as what has been variously described as psychoanalytical attitude and psychoanalytical listening. The frequency of sessions in itself is not a cast iron guarantee of the depth or the quality of the work, and does not necessarily provide exclusive access to the analysand's inner world and unconscious processes. I think, though, and this is a view very much shared in our Society, that something fundamental would be lost if we moved in the direction of reduced number of analytical sessions in the training analysis. It becomes even more important, in an environment where people have to struggle to maintain their identity as psychoanalysts, to be able to have solidly internalized such an identity during the training. Although it is plausible to think that a training which requires lower frequency analysis and training patients might be more attractive to possible applicants, by reducing the cost involved in psychoanalytical training, our evidence in London, where such a psychoanalytical training has existed since 2010, does not confirm it.

I think it is significant that in our discussions there was not much call to reduce the number of sessions in the training. There has been, on the other hand, a debate about bringing four times a week patients to Fellowship Panels. The relative paucity of five times a week patients meant that people who were seeing patients less frequently could not progress to the level of Fellow. It is now possible to present material from a four times a week analysis in a Fellowship Panel, and this represents a small but substantial change.

Role of the training analyst

The function of the training analysis and the role of the training analyst define the Eitingon model in a structural way. In societies which adopt such a model in its various versions, the status and role of the training analyst have been increasingly challenged, partly because of the dissatisfaction with what I described as the duality or "ambiguity" of the training analysis and what is seen by some as its restricting impact on the psychoanalytical process, partly because of an antiauthoritarian stance which has become much more prominent in society at large and in our psychoanalytical culture, contributing, in these times of lower recruitment, to a perception of psychoanalysis as out of step with prevalent values. It is felt by many that the psychoanalytical hierarchy generated by the figure of the training analyst promotes an institutional antidemocratic verticality not in tune with contemporary sensibilities and with the psychoanalytical ethos. The dissatisfaction with a *status quo* in which power is perceived as being unequally distributed can lead to very painful feelings of exclusion. Many of our members have voiced the need to have more democratic participation and more collective involvement in decision-making. Training analysts can be seen as having too much power and influence, but also, more importantly I think, they are seen as the ones who have much easier access to five times a week patients (candidates or people who wish to train) and, thus, can sustain their analytical identity while earning a decent living as well. Although it is often repeated in psychoanalytical societies that adopt the Eitingon model that training analyst is a function and not a lifelong status, becoming a TA is unavoidably seen as the final step in career progression and status is undoubtedly associated with it. The shared perception is that TAs have more status and more influence in the Society; they also do not just train people in an abstract way, they do so through a process akin to filiation. I spoke earlier about the perceived power of the TAs. I think it is perhaps more appropriate to talk about authority rather than power. I believe that the notion of power can be more easily infiltrated by the distortions of phantasy and projection. It is difficult to think about the constitutional position of TAs in our Society without also considering how, as a group, they are represented in the collective unconscious of the BPAS. Despite the fact that the training analysts, as a group, are quite a heterogeneous bunch, they are often perceived as a collective and well-defined entity, the TAs, sometimes in juxtaposition to other sections of our Society, the elite privileged few *vs.* the undervalued majority. Themes of inclusion–exclusion and access to generativity shape these perceptions. I think there are many contrasting narratives about the validity of the figure of the training analyst. I can think of at least two of such narratives. Not surprisingly, since they are about exclusion and inclusion, they both have an oedipal undertone. People who support what could be described as the relative verticality of the present system talk about the reluctance/resistance to accept the (generational) differences in experience, clinical competence, and scientific output, which is required in many other institutions where transmission of knowledge takes place, such as universities. People who favor a more "horizontal" model, where there is not a specific TA role, tend to see the training analyst group as representing an endogamic, oedipal couple who wants to maintain the monopoly of generativity and prevents the children from taking up their proper position in life. People believe that this constellation has contributed to the decline of psychoanalysis. Stefano Bolognini, using the everyday language of family relationships, talks about the difficulty of becoming grandparents, wanting to hold on forever to the role of parents.

Our discussion about the role of the training analyst in this time of change has been aiming to find a pragmatically useful way of defining clearer lines of authority and more democratic ways to include non training analysts in the educational structure of the Society, and to facilitate progression to training analyst level. It has not, on the whole, challenged the structure of the Eitingon model.

What authority and what kind of authority do TAs have? This is, of course, a different question from what responsibilities TAs have. Many training analysts, of course, are uncomfortable with the idea that TAs have a lot of power and prefer to think of their role as TA as one where they are been given the extra responsibility of contributing to the training process.

In the BPAS, TAs analyze, supervise, and teach. A criticism which is sometimes raised, and which I think has implications for the constitutional position of the role of TA, is that TAs, although entrusted with the transmission of psychoanalysis, are not democratically elected by a large base, but are selected, in our present system, by a (relatively small) group of peers, in a process which aims to assess experience and clinical competence. Some people fear that what amounts to being co-opted by peers can be interfered with by patronage or a need for conformity with the prevalent psychoanalytical culture, although the main aim of the Panel is to assess advanced clinical competence. It is generally accepted that we require greater levels of competence at TA level and a great deal of work has been done over the past years to describe what is meant by competence at TA level, what is the difference with competence at Fellowship level, and what criteria are used to assess it. A very comprehensive list has been drawn up of what are the expected competences a future training analyst needs to show in a Panel. The general requirement to apply to become a TA, as they are described in our Handbook, are depth and breadth of clinical experience, an internalized, well formulated, and articulated clinical model, a capacity to encompass the double responsibility of the TA, and a willingness and capacity to take on the wider tasks of the training staff. The Panel which selects the future TA attributes huge importance to clinical competence, and this is in keeping with the whole ethos of our training and our psychoanalytical culture, which remains clinically heavy.

It is, of course, the Society at large, represented by the elected Board, which delegates to the Education Committee the responsibility and the authority to select the people who can train our candidates and to oversee that the selection process for TAs is appropriate, transparent, and fair. The consultation process has led to a much clearer description of the authority relationship between the Board and the Education Committee, strengthening the position of authority of the Board over the Education Committee, but also recognizing that the Education Committee holds the anxiety about the whole system, about standards and career progression, and is just more subject to tensions and projections. It is significant that, whereas in the past, the Chair of the Education Committee was selected by the training analysts, the past two Chairs of the Education Committee have been appointed by a Panel which was formed by the various stakeholders in the Society in a more democratic and transparent manner. Another major symbolic and pragmatic change has been the election, a few years ago, of a president who is not a training analyst: up until then all presidents of the BPAS had been training analysts. Seniority, contributions to psychoanalysis, academic credentials, possessing the necessary quality to run a complex organization, are, of course, not qualities which only training analysts possess, but in the past there had almost been an unhelpful assumption about this.

There has been an effort to include non training analysts in the teaching programme, based on their specific competence in a required area. There has also been a challenge to the idea that TAs can analyze, teach, and supervise equally competently. There have been efforts to introduce more "quality control" over the supervising and teaching functions of the training analyst, given that a good clinician is not automatically a good teacher and a good supervisor.

There have been other important changes. Whereas, in the past, only TAs could sit on the Education Committee's sub-committees, now we have many Fellows who do so. There has been a recognition that what often prevents people from applying to become a TA is the lack of a sufficient number of hours of four and five times a week patients, and measures have been taken to facilitate this progression. It is now possible for a Fellow who has in analysis a patient who is accepted for training to become a training analyst for that patient and to apply, at a later stage to become a training analyst. These are, admittedly, small changes, but psychoanalytic institutions are known for their resistance to major change and introducing small changes is a way of dealing with such resistance. The changes also represent an acknowledgment of the criticism about concentration of power in the hands of the TAs.

Recruitment and professional identity

Increasing recruitment remains the first collective priority and responsibility for our Society. Many measures have been put in place to promote recruitment. The organization as a whole has been strengthened by the appointment of a CEO, somebody experienced in managing educational establishments. The term of office of the president has been extended to guarantee the continuity of the process of change that has been initiated by the recent discussions and will have to continue with future presidents. As in many other Societies, we run Open Evenings, Introductory Lectures, and a pre-training Foundation Course for people who are interested in the training. They are generally well attended and signal that the interest in psychoanalysis continues to be alive, without giving any room for complacency. Recently, following the EPF suggestion, we have been running a successful Summer School, based in one of the London universities, which has attracted younger people. There has also been an emphasis on the need to be generally more encouraging and more open toward people who want to train with us. We have introduced a scheme where experienced psychotherapists can join our ranks by undertaking a modified and reduced version of our undergraduate training. We have also been looking again at how our Admission Committee, entrusted with being the gatekeeper, makes its decisions about accepting people for training. The admission process, as it stands now, is based on a psychoanalytical instrument, the in-depth psychoanalytical character interview, and the resonance that such an interview has with the interviewers and the other members of the Admission Committee. Some people have been questioning the validity of such interviews, which make hypotheses about the suitability of an applicant on the basis of a relatively short interaction, loaded with the transferential interaction between two people. Another criticism of the admission process has been that it tends to favor conformity, to the detriment of creativity and difference, choosing "safe" people. It has also been said (most of our applicants are already in analysis) that when we reject people, we do not, paradoxically, trust enough the transformative power of the analysis and the changes that it will continue to promote.

Our efforts to recruit more trainees will need to continue. However, we have also to be mindful of many other relevant questions related to the issue of recruitment. Perhaps it is important to start by recognizing that the efforts to develop an optimal training structure have tended to prioritize the progressive development of a psychoanalytical identity, which requires several years, while taking for granted the possibility of a professional identity which is also financially secure. The first question for me is what it means to train people as psychoanalysts when the future of the profession is uncertain, and, more specifically, what it means to try to recruit more people to train as analysts when, if things continue to be the way they are now, not very many of our present graduates will be able to earn a living through an analytical practice (i.e., seeing patients four or five times a week), something which was possible for people of my generation. Are we training people toward a self-sustaining and identifiable profession? How does achieving a psychoanalytical identity, considered to be the central task of our training, relate to the achievement of a recognized professional identity? Can a psychoanalytical identity be seen as a transferable skill that can be used across different professional competences? Do we need our trainees to have five times a week analysis and see two five times a week patients during their training, when, in their future practice, they will probably see many of their patients less intensively? Is the financial cost of psychoanalytical training incompatible with the current financial situation? Is the financial cost of psychoanalytical training a worthwhile investment in terms of future earnings, and is training as an analyst an attractive career choice?

These are just some of the many questions that we need to continue to address, and for which I do not have, at the moment, full answers.

Our institutions need to give a central position to psychoanalysis as a profession and to continue to think and facilitate the construction of a professional identity. Paul Stepansky (2009), in his influential *Psychoanalysis at the Margins*, comments about the pluralism which now dominates psychoanalysis and says it has led to ". . . allegiance to one or another psychoanalytic school to sustain a professional identity that is not analytic but *intra-analytic*" (p. 312). Stepansky believes that one of the consequences of what he calls fractionation in the analytic world, is that ". . . it has made analysts identified with part identities and insensitive to the urgent need for self-transformation in socially responsive ways that will command public respect and political attention" (p. 312). Stepansky, who is not an analyst but a historian of ideas and a psychoanalytical editor, believes that analysts have to move out of the consulting room. Psychoanalysis can survive as a self-sustaining profession, not on the basis of how psychoanalysts define their field, but on ". . . how sympathetically the public embraces them as alternative providers in an era of managed care, fiscal restraint, brief cognitive therapy and psychopharmacology" p. 313).

Psychoanalysis cannot exist as a profession without patients who seek it out: important as it is to revive interest in psychoanalysis in the wider social and cultural field, we need to be better and more active in "generating" patients. However, I also think we need to be able to operate both inside and outside the consulting room: rigorously maintaining psychoanalytical values and practice (and, for me, this includes five times a week training analysis), but also being able to actively present distinctive psychoanalytically informed modes of intervention and thinking to the outside world.

References

Bernfeld, S. (1962). On psychoanalytic training. *Psychoanalytic Quarterly*, *31*: 453–482.

Kernberg, O. (1986). Institutional problems of psychanalytic education. *Journal of the American Psychoanalytic Association*, *34*: 799–834.

Kernberg, O. F. (1996). Thirty methods to destroy the creativity of psychoanalytic candidates. *International Journal of Psychoanalysis*, *77*: 1031–1040.

Kernberg, O. F. (2012). Suicide prevention for psychoanalytical institutes and societies. *Journal of the American Psychoanalytic Association, 60*(4): 707–719.

King, P. H. M. (1981). The education of a psychoanalyst: the British experience. In: *La Formation du psychanalyste* (pp. 93–107). IPA monograph No. 3. New York: International Psychological Association, 1982.

Limentani, A. (1974). The training analyst and the difficulties in the training psychoanalytic situation. *International Journal of Psychoanalysis, 55*: 71–77.

Sklar, J. (2014). Analytic training in the modern world. Between learning technique and developing authenticity. *Bulletin of the British Psychoanalytical Society, 50*(3): 17–27.

Steiner, R. (2014). Controversies terminable or interminable? *Bulletin of the British Psychoanalytical Society, 50*(9): 3–21.

Stepansky, P. E. (2009). *Psychoanalysis at the Margins*. New York: Other Press.

Taylor, H. (2013). UK psychoanalysis: mistaking the part for the whole. *Bulletin of the British Psychoanalytical Society, 49*(4): 35–45.

CHAPTER SIX

Psychoanalytic education: between marginalization and irrelevance

Toward a critical organizational and educational reform

César Garza-Guerrero

> There are two ways of making fools of ourselves.
> One is to believe in that which is not certain.
> The other is to refuse to believe in that which is certain.
>
> (Kierkegaard, quoted in Harman, 1991)

Our disconcerting paradox

Although a growing body of evidence attests incrementally to the efficacy of psychodynamic psychotherapy (Huber et al., 2013; Leichsenring & Rabung, 2008, 2009, 2011; Leichsenring et al., 2013; Levy & Ablon, 2009; Shedler, 2010; Watkins, 2011), this in itself has not contributed to stimulate interest in psychoanalytic education (Watkins, 2011).

Moreover, in many clinical university settings these days, the influence of psychoanalysis as an exploratory framework of reference for personality functioning and as a major integrative conceptual perspective to investigate the interphase of psychological, biological, and socio-cultural etiopathogenic factors forms part of everyday practice in mental health and behavioral sciences. For instance, (1) in contemporary diagnostic methodologies which incorporate the psychodynamic exploration of subjective experience and unconscious motivations (e.g., *Operationalized Psychodynamic Diagnostics* (OPD Task Force, 2001); *Psychodynamic Diagnostic Manual: Personality Patterns and Disorders* (PDM Task Force, 2006)); (2) in the importance of knowing psychoanalytically informed levels of personality functioning in order to estimate a prognostic perspective and to plan a treatment strategy (Clarkin et al., 2006; Garza-Guerrero, 2006, 2011, 2012; McWilliams, 2011); (3) in grasping the psychodynamic meaning of interpersonal relatedness, regardless of treatment modalities and types of interventions (Gabbard & Westen, 2003; Garza-Guerrero, 2011); (4) in the application of psychoanalytic concepts to the empirical investigation of psychotherapies and the formulation of treatment manuals, which are already taught in residency programs of university centers (Caligor et al., 2007; Clarkin et al., 2006; Garza-Guerrero, 2006, 2011).

Nevertheless, none of these contributions has stirred enthusiasm for psychoanalytic education at our traditional society/institute of psychoanalysis. Ironically, these advancements have not been integrated for the most part into the traditional teaching programs of conventional institutes of psychoanalysis. In fact, a large number of our colleagues actively teaching at our institutes are not even aware of these developments. Consequently, prospective candidates clearly perceive that the action is somewhere else. Not surprisingly, memberships at our institutions have decreased steadily worldwide during the past thirty-five years. The upward aging trend at our associations, coupled with our failure to attract young members to maintain a stable age profile, has reached an alarming level, as Charles Hanly warned in his farewell message as President of the International Psychoanalytical Association in 2013.

"Are psychiatric residents still interested in psychoanalysis?" ask Cristian Damsa and colleagues (2010), trying to research and determine the impact of psychoanalysts themselves, their beliefs and their attitudes, on their young colleagues in psychiatry. Their answer: psychiatric residents see us as narcissistic, elusive, and secretive; dismissive of research findings and ignorant of other fields; prone to arbitrary righteousness and imposing, rather than listening; overly confident of a faithful response from others in the absence of evidence or convincing and coherent arguments.

From my own experience with psychiatric residents and clinical psychologists considering psychoanalytic education, in a university setting, three considerations reverberate.

1. The part-time and isolated functioning of most societies/institutes of psychoanalysis, divorced from major centers of education and research.
2. Thus, their marginalization from the financial support of academic centers, and with everything against an adequate education and training.
3. Consequently, the immense economical sacrifice for both teachers and candidates, in contrast to conventional clinical postgraduate training in other professions, paid for, and with the full-time commitment of both students and teachers. These three distressing observations recapture Anna Freud's (1971) acerbic reflection many years ago: "The present part-time system seems as out-of-date to me as if church services were still conducted in catacombs since this is where the early Christians were obliged to meet" (p. 230).

Lowder and colleagues (2008) ask why psychoanalysis evokes an iterative excess of myths, misunderstandings, and criticism. Their answers (among others) are listed below.

1. The lack of affiliations of societies/institutes of psychoanalysis with universities.
2. Their ongoing monastical isolation and functioning, extended to the present time.
3. The scant relevance assigned to idiographic and nomothetic research.
4. The idealization of many of their theoreticians and ethnocentrism.
5. The conviction that psychoanalysis provides a special, privileged, and unquestionable perspective.

Although in agreement with all of these observations, I consider them to be merely symptomatic manifestations, but not causological explanations (Garza-Guerrero, 2002a,b, 2006, 2011).

The dismissal of psychoanalysis is often reminiscent of obituaries: "psychoanalysis is dead" is an admonition that I heard when I applied for psychoanalytic training in the 1970s and continues to echo in my mind. Since our usual response from within is that it is "still alive", perhaps the true question to ask is about *its present and future quality of life*. The contemporary response to this disturbing question from two of our most renowned scholars (both ex-Presidents of our International Psychoanalytical Association, and, therefore, knowledgeable about psychoanalysis worldwide) is: still alive, but without radical organizational and educational transformations we are at risk of "... increasing marginalization as a recondite activity ..." (Wallerstein, 2012, p. 397) and, thus, "... becoming irrelevant to a younger generation ..." (Kernberg, 2011, p. 612).

But are we ready to question our overall organization and educational model; not to mention readiness for an all encompassing and fundamental local, regional, and international reorganization?

The spectrum of positions in relation to our traditional educational model ranges from:

1. Do not change anything, "psychoanalysis is alive and well" (Morris, 1992); to
2. "It only requires minor surgery" (Arlow, 1972; Goodman, 1977); and, more recently,
3. From the denunciation of ostensible shortcomings, to the call for urgent innovative changes (Fonagy, 1998; Garza-Guerrero, 2002a,b, 2004, 2006, 2011, 2012; Holzman, 1985; Kächele & Thomä, 2000; Kernberg, 1986, 2004, 2006, 2007, 2010, 2011, 2012; Michels, 2007; Thomä & Kächele, 1999; Tuckett, 2002; Wallerstein, 2007, 2009, 2012).

A review of recent literature on evidence-based psychodynamic psychotherapy and the present status of psychoanalysis leave us with a disconcerting paradox: whereas outside, as an integrative framework for diagnostic and psychotherapeutic treatment modalities with a demonstrated efficacy (Watkins, 2011), psychoanalysis as a science has gained respect and acceptance; inside traditional societies/institutes of psychoanalysis, their educational and organizational structure continues to repel young applicants (Damsa et al., 2010), and is seen more as a quasi-religious movement, with an enigmatic and abstruse aura (Garza-Guerrero, 2002a,b, 2004, 2006, 2011). In Gabbard's and Williams' words (2004), and in the context of violations of professional boundaries, "For too long, we have lacked accountability by hiding behind institutional structures that encourage mystery, obfuscation and infantilization" (p. 2).

From the perspective of its potential to promote psychoanalysis as a science and a professional discipline, our overall organizational and educational systems, both local and international, appear ostensibly dysfunctional. However, with the very same administrative model, it has been highly successful in the worldwide homogamic preservation of psychoanalysis as a "movement" or "cause" (Garza-Guerrero, 2002a,b, 2004, 2006, 2011).

If we are truly to generate passionate interest among psychiatric residents and mental health professionals in training, we need to attest to the effectiveness of psychoanalytic education as Watkins (2011) compellingly writes: "perhaps we need to begin by researching the largely unresearched process of psychoanalytic education and supervision" (p. 290).

In what follows, a brief review of the etiopathogenic, retrogressive interplay of historical determinants and current organizational and educational structure serves as an introduction to a succinct survey of variants of educational models, with their inherit limitations. In turn, the nature of a reorganizational proposal is outlined, as well as the suggestion of a list of immediate changes and survival measures for psychoanalytic education. The demarcation of five of our most critical, long-range challenges for psychoanalysis as a science and a clinical profession concludes this chapter.

The roots of the retrogressive interplay of historical determinants and current organizational structure

In previous works (Garza-Guerrero, 2002a,b, 2004, 2006, 2011), I have suggested that it would be as naïve to try to explain our current organizational and educational dysfunctionality as merely a passive extension, direct and lineal, of past events as it would be to exonerate its historical determinants. The former position would only constitute a rationalization of our present myths and incongruities, whereas the latter would ignore the proclivity to repeat our history.

Incongruities between educational objectives and the monastic nature of the administrative structure of our institutes has been proposed by Kernberg (1986) to explain, at the local level, the institutional problems of psychoanalytic education. Nevertheless, given the inextricable submission of local societies/institutes to regional and international organizational hierarchies, I consider it ineluctable that a diagnosis of our current marginalization and academic irrelevance requires an elucidation of the inconsistencies between objectives, collective leadership, and organizational structure, at both local and regional levels, as well as at an international one (Garza-Guerrero, 2002a,b, 2006, 2011). Our psychoanalytic organization had its origin in, and gradually evolved toward, a congregational network that blends and binds together the prerogatives and functions of a "movement" or "cause" (i.e., quasi-religious, ideological, and sociopolitical), with the prerogatives and functions of sciences and professional disciplines (Bergmann, 1997; Eisold, 1994, 1997; Garza-Guerrero, 2002a,b, 2004, 2011; Kernberg, 1986, 2011, 2012; Steiner, 1994).

This dissociation between educational and scientific objectives and our administrative structure is an educational model that combines the characteristics of a monastery and a technical trade school (Kernberg, 1986, 2000), which generates serious group regressive phenomena. Among others, an idealization of our referential schemes, tasks, and functions, coupled with a depreciative paranoid stance toward the outside (Bergmann, 1997; Eisold, 1994; Garza-Guerrero, 2002a,b, 2004, 2011; Kernberg, 2010, 2011, 2012). The idealization of training analyses, on the other hand, orchestrated in a confined atmosphere that intertwines therapeutic and educational aims, complicates even more the collective regressive phenomena, contributing in turn to a predominantly doctrinaire instruction and a spiral of paranoid anxieties (Garza-Guerrero, 2006, 2011; Kernberg, 1978). Consequently, both primitive idealizations and paranoid manifestations end up reinforcing the quasi-religious and closed nature of the administrative structure of our institutions, thereby closing an auto-perpetuating and self-destructive vicious circle (Garza-Guerrero, 2002a,b, 2006, 2011; Kernberg, 2006, 2007, 2010, 2011, 2012).

I hasten to clarify that any dysfunctional institution immersed in incongruities between goals and its organizing procedures is vulnerable to collective regressive phenomena (Garza-Guerrero, 2006). However, most functional ones have their own self-corrective systems. It is only those with a group-syntonic and ideologically distorting mission that perpetuate transgenerationally their regressive destiny (Bergmann, 1997; Garza-Guerrero, 2002a, 2006, 2011; Miller, 1993).

Over the period of a century, our isolated societies/institutes of psychoanalysis (with scant exceptions) have amalgamated and regenerated the authoritarian syncretism inherent in the psychoanalytic movement at the beginning of the twentieth century. Since our *original* society/institute in Vienna, we have been syncretically superimposing prerogatives and functions that would be absolutely irreconcilable in any other scientific field or clinical profession (Garza-Guerrero, 2002a,b), such as:

1. Educational and those of scientific research (the tasks of universities).
2. The normativity and regulation of the practice of a profession, including its political and ideological aspects (the task of a conventional society of professionals and technicians).
3. "As-if" accreditation, certification, continuing education, and recertification (the tasks of local, external and independent government and civil institutions, as well as of inter-institutional and autonomous collegiate bodies).

The confusion and superimposition of accreditation and certifying prerogatives, educational functions, and of societal, political, and ideological proselytism, together with their handling as if they were all isomorphic dimensions, not only restricts educational objectives and the exploration of ideas in our institutes, but it also multiplies and perpetuates the multi-faceted expressions of our collective regressive phenomena, alongside the entire hierarchy, both local and international, of our dysfunctional organization (Garza-Guerrero, 2002a,b, 2004, 2006, 2011, 2012). According to Miller (1993), only the church preserves such intermingling of functions, but in consistency with their spiritual aims.

Organizational and educational incongruities, locally and internationally feeding back throughout a century, have evolved into a system of "franchises" that grant the authorization for the exclusive "official" training in psychoanalysis worldwide through our basic unit of ecumenical control: our ancestral societies/institutes of psychoanalysis. And it is in this context of an auto-perpetuating interplay of historical determinants and present organizational structure, where administrative rules, prerogatives, and ritualistic procedures become invested with an ideological and quasi-religious fervor, that literally transfigures them into missionary mandates.

I shall briefly outline some of the internal impediments derived from the distortion of these missionary entitlements that are representative of our universal organizational and educational syncretism (Garza-Guerrero, 2002b, 2006, 2011).

Educational monasticism

With very few exceptions, the tripartite system of teaching in our institutes (obligatory personal treatment, seminars on theory, and supervisions) does not integrate exposition into the critical analysis of ideas or into programs of clinical research; much less are there any efforts to explore the scientific evidence of psychoanalytic literature and its correspondence to, or its external coherence with, allied disciplines. Our institutes transmit, recycle, and reaffirm the same ideas, but without questioning or generating new knowledge (Garza-Guerrero, 2011; Kernberg, 2011, 2012). As Cooper (1995) points out, our traditional societies/institutes, preoccupied with the unquestionable transmission of our doctrines and techniques, ignore the results of contemporary research and run the risk of finding themselves in a solitary position, isolated by their respective ideologies and beliefs.

Conceptual fragmentation and the absence of organizing paradigms

At present, we do not possess an epistemological and referential foundation (i.e., a validated theory) on which we can reasonably base our clinical practice. The epistemological strategy of the clinician is, rather, derived from an enumerative inductivism (in contrast to one of an eliminatory nature) and, consequently, is always prone to reconfirming interactive therapeutic patterns that are, in turn, vulnerable to becoming indoctrinating commandments. In Fonagy's words, "We are no longer accumulating knowledge . . . we are all developing the discipline in our own individual direction" (1998). The absence of an organizing paradigm has, he suggests, led us into a "major epistemological problem of conceptual fragmentation" and, consequently, to "the confusing absence of shared assumptions": hence, to our pluralistic sectarianism.

The universal lack of external, local, and independent systems of accreditation, certification, continuing education, and recertification

The worldwide lack of external and independent accreditation and certification systems is living proof of a quasi-religious isolation and of our operation as a homogamous and ecumenical movement rather than a professional and scientific discipline. Dissociated between efforts to preserve the unquestioning transmission of our ideologies and beliefs (psychoanalysis as a "movement"), on the one hand, and our need to participate in the scientific exploration in the field of mental health, on the other (Levinson, 1994), we persist in adhering to a one-hundred-year-old supraordaining system that centrally blesses from abroad (the IPA Board, and the Board of Professional Standards in the USA) the exclusive "recognition of the official training in psychoanalysis".

Our hegemonic system for the exclusivity of franchise control has confused for a century the collective communion in, and loyalty to, our homogamous system, with an acceptance of what would be genuine independent and external systems of accreditation and certification of psychoanalysis as a scientific and professional discipline solely based on the evaluation of theoretical, clinical, and professional competences (Israelstam, 2011; Kernberg, 2010; Körner, 2002; Tuckett, 2005; Tuckett et al., 2008). Quality and standards are confused with membership and affiliation.

*Psychoanalytic training as a potentially regressive professional undifferentiation and a "*sui generis*" re-professionalization*

Any effort at resolving the problems connected to independent accreditation and certification systems would have to start with the questions: What kind of programs should we accredit, and what type of graduates should we certify? If we take into consideration that:

1. More than a hundred years after its foundation, what a psychoanalytic treatment is and how and for whom it works, are very much in doubt, within and outside the discipline (Tuckett, 2000; Tuckett et al., 2008).

2. A qualitative and quantitative exploration of some of our central concepts (e.g., "psychoanalytic process") reveals the inability of ten training analysts from the same institute to reach a consensus (Vaughan & Roose, 1995; Vaughan et al., 1997).
3. We still lack a validated epistemological framework that might permit sifting through our imaginative soliloquies (Olds & Cooper, 1997), and, as a result, our profession does not yet satisfy major canons as a scientific activity (Fonagy et al., 2002).
4. The essential ingredients of "classical psychoanalysis" have not yet been defined in any consensual, or even communicable, way, and, therefore, in teachable fashion (Ellman, 2000; Tuckett, 2000).
5. The disjointed "articles of faith" (in Wallerstein's terms, 1988) of our multiplicity of "schools" are just beginning to divest themselves from their infiltrated myths and fallacies in the light of contemporary advances in neuroscience, psychology, and psychiatry (Fonagy, 2000; Kernberg, 2011, 2012; Panksepp, 2000; Panksepp & Biven, 2012; Wallerstein, 2012),

If we attend to the above considerations, we might well ask whether psychoanalysis today might be defined as an "independent profession", supraordinately accreditable and certifiable, in the complex world of contemporary mental health and behavioral sciences.

At present, with regard to accreditation and certification, at least four frameworks overlap: psychoanalysis as a clinical sub-speciality, an "independent profession", a "special specialty", and a unique re-professionalizing "supra-education". In general, the last three variants find it necessary to remain marginalized from external certifying boards: for these, paying fees to the IPA serves as an "as-if" accreditation and certification (Garza-Guerrero, 2002a,b, 2004, 2006, 2011). The American Psychoanalytic Association (as a regional component system of the IPA) has its own internal Board of Professional Standards (BOPS) to accredit their component institutes and certify their own psychoanalysts—thus reproducing the same syncretism and, consequently, the same political tensions and educational conflicts described within the IPA at large, between local societies/institutes and their BOPS (Garza-Guerrero, 2006, 2011).

Under our present syncretic entanglements, what defining frameworks and genuine systems for evaluating competences (Kernberg, 2010, 2011; Garza-Guerrero, 2002b, 2011; Tuckett et al., 2008) would regulate an external accreditation of our programs and the independent certification of our graduates, in common with any other discipline offering a clinical service to the community?

Our local and international missionary co-dependency

As I have pointed out elsewhere (Garza-Guerrero, 2002a,b, 2004, 2006, 2011), it is time to ask ourselves whether at present we can still justify our homogamous and syncretic organizational model at both local and international levels. It is time to review the regressive impact of the pathologically complementary local and international, organizational and educational incongruities that preserve our adherence to our monastic model (Kernberg, 2000, 2010, 2011, 2012). It is also imperative to evaluate how this monastic model has, in turn, contributed to a consolidation and perpetuation of the very collective and universal dysfunctional structure that brought it about in the first place, and which traps us in a vicious circle (Garza-Guerrero, 2002a,b, 2004, 2006, 2011).

As Thomä concluded, a long time ago, in a systematic review of problems in psychoanalytic training, "Without revolutionary changes in current psychoanalytic education and the structure and function of the International Psychoanalytical Association, stagnation or regression will prevail" (1993, p. 3). To attend to the complications that arise from organizational regressive phenomena at both local and international levels will continue to be the most painful aspect of the task of evaluating our present organizational and educational crisis in psychoanalysis (Garza-Guerrero, 2002a,b, 2004, 2006, 2011).

Homogamous organizational variants of our societies/ institutes: toward a differentiating and integrative proposal

At present, three apparently different archetypes are used in psychoanalytic training: the Eitingon–Freud model, and the French and Uruguayan models. The Eitingon–Freud model, established in 1923, was intended to become a psychoanalytic policlinic, which would provide services to the indigent and integrated research programs. However, nowadays, as Kächele and Thomä (2000) point out, what prevails is a devaluated version of this model, which centers around the tripartite system of treatment, seminars, and supervision, but depreciates research and the critical exploration of clinical practice. The French and Uruguayan models have disseminated to a lesser extent, reaching some psychoanalytic societies outside France and Uruguay.

It must be underscored that, although the French and Uruguayan models emerged, in part, as a critical response to the limitations of the deteriorated version of the Eitingon model, differences between the three have been more philosophical and virtual than structural and substantial. None of them is free of the complications derived from the aforementioned organizational syncretism.

Kernberg (2000) has underlined the universal problems common to psychoanalytic education at large: among others, the infantilization of candidates; scientific isolation and ignorance; irresponsibility regarding candidates' educational experience; authoritarianism, violence, and arbitrariness; the denial of external reality and its effects on psychoanalytic education.

Moreover, insofar as we are organizationally immersed in a local and internationally interactive homogamous and franchising system, it is no surprise that we share worldwide, well-known difficulties, such as:

1. The lack of candidates and patients (Damsa et al., 2010; Watkins, 2011).
2. The absence of research divisions that might prevent indoctrinating processes (Garza-Guerrero, 2011; Kernberg, 2010, 2011, 2012; Kernberg et al., 2012; Wallerstein, 2012).
3. Scant or no scientific productivity of high impact (Kernberg, 2010, 2011, 2012; Wallerstein, 2007, 2012).
4. The urgent need of genuine systems for the evaluation of theoretical, clinical, and attitudinal competences (Garza-Guerrero, 2011; Kernberg, 2011, 2012; Körner, 2002; Tuckett, 2005; Tuckett et al., 2008).
5. A perennial economical uncertainty about the viability of our programs, including the payment of local and international membership fees (Garza-Guerrero, 2004, 2006, 2011).

Although all of these ancestral limitations just mentioned call for immediate changes, the auto-perpetuating nature of the interplay of past inertias and current organizational structure prevents them. And, to complicate matters further, the administrative procedures and rules to form new psychoanalytic groups in our present international association contribute to merely recreating them. Our International New Groups Committee (INGC) obligates that every new group should closely follow the model initially used by their founding predecessors, in their respective countries. Here, we have another gem in our splendid garden of paradoxes. Our committee on "New Groups" alludes to about to be new groups, or newly formed groups, not to new groups which may be evolving and responding innovatively to the contemporary challenges of psychoanalysis (Garza-Guerrero, 2011; Kernberg, 2011; Wallerstein, 2012).

Even though Freud (1926e), insinuated a future university-like conception ("a college of psychoanalysis", p. 206) for psychoanalytic training (Wallerstein, 2009), the Eitingon–Freud model generally evolved away from universities and academic settings in Europe and Latin America (and remained so, until now). In the USA, the original European model (i.e., outside of universities) was followed in New York, Boston, Philadelphia, Baltimore-Washington, and Chicago. Other societies became associated to universities such as: Columbia, Cleveland, Pittsburgh, and Downstate (now, New York University), Colorado, and, more recently, Emory. Cleveland and Pittsburg soon ran into conflicts and were unable to sustain their respective links to universities. David Shakow's plan (1962), a full-time, research-focused proposal for an independent institute in a university setting, never prospered. The Menninger School of Psychiatry and the Topeka Institute for Psychoanalysis (1949–1999), on the other hand, provided a privileged university-like setting for full-time training in both tracks. Unfortunately, without the attendant advantages, which provide a university setting, the program could not go on. They are now integrated with the Department of Psychiatry at Baylor College of Medicine in Houston, Texas, but stripped of their psychoanalytic institute (Wallerstein, 2009).

Besides, some institutions deserve special mention, such as those that have more recently tried to respond with some innovative variations of the Eitingon model and to the limitations in the overall functioning of our societies/institutes (Kernberg, 2011): the Anna Freud Centre in London, a full-time clinical training in child analysis; Philadelphia and San Francisco reorganized their structure to implement a "center model", which does not seem to solve the problem of the isolation from the world of science and academia (Kernberg, 2011); the Psychoanalytic Center of Emory University; the New York University Psychoanalytic Institute; the Psychoanalytic Association of Buenos Aires, which has developed an Institute of Psychology granting a Masters Degree in Clinical Psychology; the German International Psychoanalytic University in Berlin; more recently, the Center for Psychoanalytic Education and Research, in Monterrey, Mexico. All of these very welcome variations have ameliorated, no doubt, the limitations described before.

None of these arrangements, though, entirely resolves the problem of the truly full-time commitment of both students and teachers, or provides the stable human resources and financial support for adequate clinical training and research found within the conventional structure of university settings with strong links to medicine, to the behavioral sciences, and to the humanities. In Wallerstein's terms (2012), "The ultimate redemption of psychoanalysis . . . will only come when full academic-university placement is achieved" (p. 393). Without it, we will remain condemned to increasing marginalization and irrelevance (Wallerstein, 2012, p. 397).

There is, at present, no ideal model for psychoanalytic education, but any reorganizing effort will have to distance itself from our prevailing syncretism in search of a congruity between objectives and our overall administrative structure, both local and international. With these premises in mind, I have outlined the nature of a long-range proposal in previous works (Garza-Guerrero, 2002a,b, 2004, 2006, 2011).

1. A radical reversal of our retardant organizing inertias (a homogamous legacy of psychoanalysis as a movement of the early twentieth century), local and internationally interwoven, that syncretically amalgamates incompatible prerogatives and functions (educational and scientific, societal, and political, and "as-if" accreditation and certification) through our basic control unit represented by our local societies/institutes of psychoanalysis.
2. Toward an educational university model, within or outside conventional universities, devoid of societal–political prerogatives and exclusively geared toward the critical exploration of ideas and the generation of knowledge.

3. Finally, a reorganization of our entire membership into an international federation of psychoanalysis, which agglutinates the common collective interests of genuinely autonomous component societies of psychoanalysis, and with privileges strictly limited to functions of membership, promotion, and scientific diffusion without any supraordaining influence over educational, accrediting, and certifying prerogatives that functionally should correspond to local, national, or regional independent arbitration: that is, European, Latin American, and North American, like any other scientific discipline.

Any new proposal aimed at changing the *status quo* of our psychoanalytic organization is destined to be baptized as utopian and unrealistic at best, or irrational at worst. And although a whole array of reasons and arguments are raised, the most powerful opposition has an ideological origin. Elsewhere (Garza-Guerrero, 2006), I have outlined the pros and cons of different reorganizational variations, including psychoanalysis as a clinical sub-specialty in departments of psychiatry or psychology divisions in university structures (to me, the most readily possible), both entirely viable and implementable, if it were not for ideological impediments.

Immediate changes and survival measures

In what follows, I outline eight of our most pressing survival measures and educational changes. Again, all of these changes could be entirely workable if collective group regressive phenomena and ideological obstacles at our traditional societies/institutes were overcome.

Relationship to universities

Academic institutions do not need psychoanalysis to survive and implement their functions. On the contrary, it is highly questionable whether in the long run psychoanalytic societies-institutes could survive without a link to them (Auchincloss & Michels, 2003; Garza-Guerrero, 2004, 2006, 2011; Kernberg, 2011; Michels, 2007; Wallerstein, 2012). Psychoanalytic institutes are in urgent need of joint collaborations with universities for their teaching and research programs, as well as for the legitimization of the congruity of their educational objectives. Without a mutually enriching and reciprocal collaboration, or, even better, their own insertion in universities, further isolation and exclusion will prevail (Kernberg, 2011; Wallerstein, 2007, 2009, 2012). A relationship of psychoanalytic institutes to universities is of such significance that Kernberg (2012) ironically considered it necessary to "establish a lifeline with local universities" as a top priority in his list of "suicide prevention guidelines" for psychoanalytic institutes and societies (p. 22).

Any practicable and productive relationship with universities would have to be a clearly educational two-way street, in contrast to the unilateral proselytizing efforts of traditional institutes solely to seek the enrolment of candidates (Garza-Guerrero, 2006, 2011). It also needs to be acknowledged that although most psychoanalysts away from universities would not be able to compete with the level of competences and expectations demanded by contemporary teaching and research positions in academic settings, they still should furnish valuable contributions to universities, particularly to the humanities.

Finally, it should be reminded that a *university setting* might not be synonym of a *university model*. What matters is an organizing system aimed at genuinely generating knowledge.

Theoretical seminars

Primitive idealizations and paranoid processes are fertile ground for the "phenomenon of not learning" (Riesenberg Malcom, 1990) and indoctrination (Garza-Guerrero, 2004, 2006, 2011). And the danger of indoctrination is rooted precisely in not realizing how we indoctrinate (Steiner, 1994). Our pluralism of explanatory metaphors (our multiplicity of "schools") obligates us to remember that none of our present theoretical systems could serve as a "general unifying theory", and neither do they cover the current needs of a general scientific structure (Garza-Guerrero, 2006; Wallerstein, 1990). Each one of these general theories needs to be explored, though, in terms of what they might offer to our conception of a basic psychoanalytic model "or common ground" (Wallerstein, 1990, 1992). And, while every conceptual theme should depart from Freud's contributions (when ordered), it would only be as a starting point (in contrast to its eternal exegesis) toward the exploration of where we stand today with those same ideas in the context of contemporary idiographic and nomothetic research. Besides, our theoretical pluralism and the growth of knowledge in neighboring disciplines call for a curriculum design that encourages the development of epistemological perspectives that serve as guiding frameworks to help candidates and teachers to think critically about what is proposed as psychoanalytic knowledge (Glucksman, 2006; Rees, 2007).

Supervisions

Supervisors should have demonstrated their competency in individual supervisions, as well as in continuous case seminars and collective supervisory situations; to be a training analyst, *per se*, does not guarantee anything. They should be willing to expose their own clinical material, thus preventing our conventional stultifying expectation that candidates learn only from other candidates (Garza-Guerrero, 2004, 2006, 2011; Kernberg, 2007, 2011), and be readily available to co-participate with seminar leaders in the ongoing evaluation of candidates. The task of evaluating candidates is too important to be left to any monolithic system (e.g., training analysts, in the Eitingon model, or supervisors, in the French model). Nowadays, the supervisory tasks need the support of an objective system to evaluate a candidate's competences (Israelstam, 2011; Tuckett et al., 2008).

The ability to supervise calls for: (a) experience in integrating the three communicative channels represented by verbal narration, the non-verbal aspects of communication and countertransference (Clarkin et al., 2006; Watkins, 2013), as well as for the identification of parallel phenomena (Gediman & Wolkenfeld, 1980); (b) humility to avoid the authoritarianism and pseudo-sapience derived from the adherence to one single mechanism of therapeutic change ("my own"), instead of a multi-systemic conception of multiple and varying mechanisms of psycho-structural changes (Gabbard & Westen, 2003; Tuckett et al., 2008; Watkins, 2013); and (c) demonstrated aptitude to listen, from the perspectives of others and, thus, the ability to contrast the comparable and incomparable in one's own and the other's framework of reference (Tuckett et al., 2008)—hence, contrary to the sneering arrogance of the: "that is not so".

Training analysis system and "educational committees"

The primitive idealization of the training analysis leads to the splitting revealed in submissive behavior toward the institute authorities in charge of a candidate's progress, on the one hand, and a displaced opposition to other systems of the institute or other "schools" (Garza-Guerrero, 2011; Kernberg, 2010). The idealization of the training analyst has also led to a two-level hierarchy, with the nonsensical expectation that psychoanalytic candidates should receive better psychoanalysis than ordinary patients in our communities (Kernberg, 2010).

The training analysis system should be abolished (Kernberg, 2010, 2013), as well as the concentration of power in "educational committees" formed exclusively with training analysts: our maximal expression of our homogamous syncretistic proclivities and authoritarianism (Garza-Guerrero, 2002a,b, 2006, 2011). And the problem with intellectual incest is that it accentuates the worst of our organizational defects. To replace both (i.e., the training analysis system and pseudo-educational committes), there exists the imperative need to develop a genuine and independent system of certification, continuing education, and recertification, in terms of demonstrated competences, theoretical, clinical, and attitudinal, away from our present conformism to our "bean counting" approach (solely based on the accumulation of minimal criteria) to the selection of training analysts (Kernberg, 2010, 2013; Körner, 2002; Mullen & Rieder, 2002; Tuckett, 2005; Tuckett et al., 2008). Societal and political prerogatives, decided by democratic consensus, should be strictly delimited of educational and scientific matters, resolved by functional criteria, and open to any genuinely certified member.

The teaching and training of psychoanalytically informed psychotherapies

Primitive idealizations and paranoidizing processes, added to the transgenerational institutionalization of emotional counter-reactions with respect to the defense of a presumptive psychoanalytic "identity" continue to self-destructively reduce psychoanalytic training to a treatment modality, indicated and justified only in less than 1% of the epidemiologically potentially available referrals in the area of mental health (Garza-Guerrero 2002a,b, 2006, 2011; Jiménez, 2000; Kernberg, 2011, 2012). Contrary to parochial positions, the exposition of candidates to the teaching and training of psychotherapies does not dilute, but, rather, consolidates, psychoanalytic identity and enhances professional skills (Garza-Guerrero, 2011; Kernberg, 2012; Wallerstein, 1986).

Within the present context of contemporary research in psychotherapies, as Gabbard and Westen (2003) poignantly state, we need to ". . . avoid single-cause theories of therapeutic change" (p. 837). Therapeutic changes occur through multiple mechanisms. Nowadays, we could not refer to psychoanalysis and psychotherapy as "first- or second-rate treatment", but as modalities of intervention, with areas of convergences and divergences, dimensional and categorically definable, derived from the same framework, but with specific strategic, technical, and tactical variations, and with different indications and justifications for distinct clinical situations and circumstances (Garza-Guerrero, 2006, 2011; Kernberg, 2010, 2011, 2012; Ticho, 1970; Wallerstein, 1988).

We urgently need to integrate our traditional programs to the full exposition of the teaching, training, and research of psychotherapies, not merely as an introduction, or as parallel complementary seminars, but throughout the entire duration of professional training (Garza-Guerrero, 2011; Kernberg, 2012).

Research

Without research, our traditional educational model will remain doomed to rejection and marginalization (Kernberg, 2011, 2012; Michels, 2007; Stepansky, 2009; Wallerstein, 2009, 2012). Contrary to the presupposition that psychoanalysis is a unique intersubjective experience and an incomparable field of knowledge, it is self-destructive not to integrate research divisions with our educational programs, either autonomous or affiliated with universities (Kernberg, 2012; Garza-Guerrero, 2011; Wallerstein, 2012). The problem with treating psychoanalysis as an unquestionable relic is that it invalidates it as a science, and the only way of paying due respect to psychoanalysis as a scientific activity is to stop its veneration.

The integration of information from both idiographic (including conceptual and hermeneutic perspectives) and nomothetic research (even if implemented by outside institutions and neighboring sciences) to our curricular plans and clinical practices is mandatory, not only to maintain congruity with educational objectives, but, even more importantly, to counteract the indoctrinating processes and habitual innocence of our claustral ambience regarding advances in the contemporary broad horizon of mental health (Garza-Guerrero, 2011; Kernberg, 2012).

International "New Groups" Committee (INGC)

Our present INGC guarantees that "new psychoanalytic groups" preserve, follow, and closely adhere to administrative procedures, rules, and standards of training that homogamously reproduce their loyalty to psychoanalysis as a "movement". This is to say, usually, the imposition of the Eitingon model or the French or Uruguayan variations. Nevertheless, the strict adherence to rules and procedures prevents any deviations that might attempt to correct or respond to existing challenges of psychoanalysis in the complex field of contemporary behavioral sciences. Our INGC safeguards continuity and divulgation to "new places", but prevents innovation and creative transformations (Garza-Guerrero, 2004, 2006, 2011).

The overall functioning of our present INGC is: (a) overly bureaucratic, dysfunctional, and excessively expensive (three colleagues from three different and distant countries, visiting "new groups" two to three times annually). They usually arrive without any real experience in administration, education, or research (with nothing more than their conventional training); (b) insufferably slow (there is a lapse of eight to sixteen years for "new groups" to become "autonomous" societies); (c) they are exclusively concerned with the blind adherence to homogenizing mandates, "politics of the moment", or what is "ideologically correct" (e.g., most of them are dismissive of research, the integration of outside interdisciplinarity, and the joint teaching of psychotherapies).

Our present educational needs call imploringly for: (a) an international, truly facilitating and innovative committee for psychoanalytic training and research, jointly working with local institutes toward their respective badly needed transformations; (b) an integration of colleagues with genuine trajectories and experience in education, research, and administration; (c) with the professional and moral integrity to extricate themselves from societal and political undercurrents or hidden agendas from within or from abroad; (d) the ability to distinguish between societal psycho-cloning ruptures and genuinely transformative separations. Under our present rules and procedures, during societal schisms, the group that splits off and tries an innovative reorganization is forced to repeat the very same administrative structure that they tried to leave behind—another of our paradoxical and perplexing inconsistencies.

Moreover, in a context of the transgenerational transmission of primitively idealized rituals and mandates, it is imperative for our colleagues working in our INGC to become familiar with contemporary criteria to evaluate genuine theoretical and clinical competences (Birksted-Breen, 2008; Israelstam, 2011; Tuckett et al., 2008), sufficiently to at least be able to distinguish between subservient obedience to the anachronistic inertias of psychoanalysis as a "movement" and the present demands of psychoanalysis as a science and professional discipline.

Regarding psychoanalysis as a movement, it is worth mentioning the functions of the recently created European Institute of Psychoanalysis, and the Latin American Institute of Psychoanalysis (under the umbrella of the INGC), aimed at the dissemination of our traditional models of psychoanalytic education to places where there are no societies/institutes of psychoanalysis. If, under conventional conditions, the overall functions of our institutes leave too much to be desired as to their capacity to further the advancement of psychoanalysis as a science and a professional discipline, under the much less than average resources and the highly constraining procedures of the EIP and the LAIP (e.g., concentrated training analyses, Skype, and telephone supervisions, online seminars, concentrated seminars in hotel lobbies during psychoanalytic meetings, etc.), our inadequacies merely increase.

The EIP and the LAIP might doubtless accomplish their proselytizing mission of spreading our psychoanalytic "gospel" to "new places", but with their present resources and structure they are not in a position to contribute to the real development of psychoanalysis as a science and a publicly accountable professional discipline.

Ironically, although many of these "new communities" could really benefit from the most workable integration of the teaching and research of psychoanalytically informed psychotherapies with clinical divisions of psychology and psychiatry in university settlings, these projects are perfunctorily dismissed as "non-analytic activities".

In a future federation of psychoanalysis, constituted with truly autonomous psychoanalytic societies, the present administrative structure of our International New Groups Committees, along with their intermingling of ostensible syncretistic and dysfunctional activities, should disappear entirely.

Psychoanalytic congresses and our institutionalized writing and publishing "epistemophobia"

Nothing confronts us more with our real level of knowledge, or ignorance, than the responsibility of writing and publishing on the nature of our teaching, research, and clinical practices. However, ". . . the collective 'epistemophobia' of writing and publishing would seem to be a universal symptom" in our traditional institutes (Ramón Ganzarain, 1995, personal communication).

The majority of societies/institutes do not have an indexed journal that integrates an authentic committee of arbitration. Moreover, most of our institutes have not published in an indexed journal in the last twenty-five to thirty-five years; some, not ever since their foundation. Nevertheless, all of them usually celebrate annual congresses where hundreds of papers are submitted. Yet, less than 1% of those presented may have the quality of argumentation and standards of writing necessary to reach the level of an indexed publication. With very honorable exceptions, most works presented at congresses (i.e., local, regional, and international) seem to serve as a testimony to our faith in our beliefs and ideologies, but do not generate knowledge. As Fonagy (1998; Fonagy et al., 2002) sharply cautions us, the epistemological strategy of most psychoanalysts is derived from an enumerative inductivism that fosters the proliferation of theories, pseudo-explanatory metaphors, and progressive conceptual fragmentation.

It is critical for psychoanalytic institutes today to develop and stimulate a culture of scientific writing and publishing of high impact in indexed journals, for both faculty and students. Candidates should be supported at all levels of training and throughout their entire program. If a candidate does not learn to write and publish a paper during his or her years of training, they most likely will not do it during their lifetimes (Garza-Guerrero, 2002a,b, 2006, 2011).

Long-range challenges

If we were able to reorient psychoanalytic education along the lines of the immediate changes aforementioned, that itself would place us in a position to aspire, reach out, and move toward, not utopian, but more realistic and normative challenges for any contemporary professional discipline pretending to offer an educational and clinical service in our communities. Elsewhere, I have outlined these challenges as follows (Garza-Guerrero, 2002b, 2006, 2011).

An educational university model

An autonomous educational system, independent of societal–political prerogatives and proselytizing admonitions, guided by functional criteria embodying university objectives (i.e., not just transmitting, but also investigating and generating knowledge), rather than our prevailing monasticism and political eclecticism, at the service of reaffirming our internal beliefs and rituals (Garza-Guerrero, 2004, 2006, 2011; Kernberg, 2004, 2007, 2010, 2011, 2012).

Epistemological foundation

The consolidation of an epistemic foundation, idiographic (i.e., integrating conceptual research and an hermeneutic perspective) and nomothetically sustained, consistent not only with our intrinsic methodology, but also with that of neighboring disciplines, would lead to a deductive and inductive exploratory referential framework on which our professional, educational, and research activities could be based (Fonagy, 1999). A well-founded conceptual framework might help to filter our cumulative inductivism, a seedbed of fragmented schools and sectarianism, as well as our cross-sterilization (i.e., outwards, with others, and inwards, among ourselves) and our international pseudo-ecumenism (Garza-Guerrero, 2002, 2006, 2011; Paniagua, 1995).

Accreditation, certification, continuing education, and recertification

External and independent local, state, and/or national sanctioned organisms, with accrediting and certifying functions, divorced from affiliation and membership privileges, and solely based on the evaluation of competences: theoretical, clinical, and attitudinal (Garza-Guerrero, 2006, 2011; Israelstam, 2011; Kernberg, 2010, 2011, 2012; Körner, 2002; Tuckett, 2005; Tuckett et al., 2008).

Authentic autonomous accreditation and certification systems should not only prevent confusing quality and standards with membership and affiliation, as mentioned before, but should also avoid our present psycho-cloning and undifferentiating syncretism, as well as our, by now, reproachable and indefensible franchise control for the only "official" psychoanalytic training.

Social relevance

An external, interactive, and critical reorientation of our psychoanalytic societies, toward their integration with programs of genuine social relevance, might provide a life of their own and a transcending sense of direction beyond the circumscribed idealization of the activities related to the training of candidates, and the perpetuation of psychoanalysis as a movement. Without proving evidence of our potentialities for academic and social relevance, it will not be possible to secure the financial support for our programs.

Creative interdependence

The creative local and international reorganization of genuinely autonomous psychoanalytic societies toward an international federation of psychoanalysis, with the conventional functions of membership, promotion, and divulgation, but without any supraordaining prerogatives over matters of accreditation and certification, which should consistently belong to a local and independent national or regional arbitration just like any other scientific and professional discipline on the planet.

Our unavoidable dilemma and final considerations

Even though numerous corrective measures for our organizational and educational problems begin to glimmer, the inclination is to deny the urgency of immediate implementation (Garza-Guerrero, 2002).

The central argument is that centrifugal "tendencies" (i.e., a decentralized organization) might weaken the IPA "central administrative structures" at a time of external "challenges" and "attacks" (e.g., Widlöcher, 2001, p. 1427).

Nevertheless, from the perspective of the central thesis of this study that points toward the internal origin of our specifically organizational and educational crisis, which is derived from the incongruities between our explicit objectives (psychoanalysis as an open scientific system and a publicly accountable clinical profession) and our implicit international and local administrative structure (characteristic of psychoanalysis as a closed, homogeneous movement), our present situation leaves us faced with an unavoidable dilemma: (a) either we continue with an international, central, homogamous control, syncretically coalescing incompatible functions and prerogatives in one unique ecumenical system (our traditional societies/institutes of psychoanalysis), or (b) we would rather reorganize toward more congruous paths for sciences and professions in general.

With regard to the suggestion of delaying changes until "times are better" for psychoanalysis, would we not continue to blame the outside for our internal ailments, as we have done for a century? Would we not be confusing symptoms (the perennial queries to our professional and scientific practices) with causes (our own internal disarticulation between objectives and administrative organization)? Would it not be more dangerous to continue to retreat in the same organizational structure responsible for the same challenges attributed to the outside (Garza-Guerrero, 2006, 2011)?

The future of psychoanalysis as a science and profession must be nothing less than that of its continuing evolution and transformation. The survival of our local traditional psychoanalytic societies/institutes of psychoanalysis and our overall regional and international organizations is what is being questioned (i.e., psychoanalysis as a "movement" or "cause").

Facing the second century of psychoanalysis, I consider that the harmonization between scientific and educational objectives and organizational structure, local, regional, and international, is essential if we are to loosen the bonds of primitive idealizations that keep us tied to our past and, thus, today, we continue to struggle with marginalization and irrelevance.

References

Arlow, J. A. (1972). Some dilemmas in psychoanalytic education. *Journal of the American Psychoanalytic Association, 20*: 556–566.

Auchincloss, E. L., & Michels, R. (2003). A reassessment of psychoanalytic education: controversies and changes. *International Journal of Psychoanalysis, 84*: 387–403.

Bergmann, M. S. (1997). The historical roots of psychoanalytic orthodoxy. *International Journal of Psychoanalysis, 78*: 69–86.

Caligor, E., Kernberg, O. F., & Clarkin, J. F. (2007). *Handbook of Dynamic Psychotherapy for Higher Level Personality Pathology*. Washington DC: American Psychiatric Publishing.

Clarkin, J. F., Yeomans, F., & Kernberg, O. F. (2006). *Psychotherapy for Borderline Personality: Focusing on Object Relations*. Washington, DC: American Psychiatric Publishing.

Cooper, A. M. (1995). Discussion: on empirical research. In: T. Shapiro & R. N. Emde (Eds.), *Research in Psychoanalysis: Process, Development, Outcome* (pp. 381–391). Madison, CT: International Universities Press.

Damsa, C., Bryois, C., Morelli, D., Cailhol, L., Adam, E., Coman, A., Stamatoiu, D., Lazignac, C., & Freymann, J. (2010). Are psychiatric residents still interested in psychoanalysis? A brief report. *American Journal of Psychoanalysis, 70*: 386–391.

Eisold, K. (1994). The intolerance of diversity in psychoanalytic institutes. *International Journal of Psychoanalysis, 75*: 785–800.

Eisold, K. (1997). Freud as leader: the early years of the Viennese Society. *International Journal of Psychoanalysis, 78*: 87–104.

Ellman, J. P. (2000). Panel: The mechanism of action of psychoanalytic treatment. *American Psychoanalytic Association, 48*: 919–927.

Fonagy, P. (1998). What can we do to further psychoanalytic knowledge? Inter-congress meeting of the International Psychoanalytical Association, London.

Fonagy, P. (1999). An open door review of outcome studies in psychoanalysis. Report prepared by the Research Committee of the International Psychoanalytical Association. Editor and Chair: Peter Fonagy.

Fonagy, P. (2000). On the relationship of experimental psychology and psychoanalysis commentary. *Neuro-psychoanalysis, 2*(2): 222–232.

Fonagy, P., Jones, E., Kächele, H., Krause, R., Clarkin, J. F., Perron, R., Gerber, A., & Allison, E. (2002). *An Open Door Review of Outcome Studies in Psychoanalysis* (2nd revised edn). London: International Psychoanalytical Association.

Freud, A. (1971). The ideal psychoanalytic institute: a utopia. *Bulletin of the Menninger Clinic, 35*: 225–239.

Freud, S. (1926e). The question of lay analysis. *S. E., 20*: 177–258. London: Hogarth.

Gabbard, G., & Westen, D. (2003). Rethinking therapeutic action. *International Journal of Psychoanalysis, 84*: 823–841.

Gabbard, G. O., & Williams, P. (2004). Editorial, *International Journal of Psychoanalysis, 85*: 1–2.

Ganzarain, R. (1995). Personal communication.

Garza-Guerrero, C. (2002a). "The crisis in psychoanalysis". What crisis are we talking about? *International Journal of Psychoanalysis, 83*: 57–83.

Garza-Guerrero, C. (2002b). Organizational and educational internal impediments of psychoanalysis: contemporary challenges. *International Journal of Psychoanalysis, 83*: 1407–1433.

Garza-Guerrero, C. (2004). Reorganizational and educational demands of psychoanalysis training today: Our long and marasmic night of one century. *International Journal of Psychoanalysis, 85*: 3–25

Garza-Guerrero, C. (2006). *Crisis organizacional y educacional del psicoanálisis: desafíos contemporáneos*. Mexico City: Editores de Textos Mexicanos.

Garza-Guerrero, C. (2011). *Psicoanálisis ¿Requiescat in pace? Una crítica desde adentro y una propuesta impostergable*. Mexico City: Editores de Textos Mexicanos.

Garza-Guerrero, C. (2012). Desregulación afecto-cognoscitiva en organización limítrofe de la personalidad y sobremedicación: iatrogenia, ignorancia y seudoprofesionalismo. *Medicina Universitaria, 14*(55): 99–112.

Gediman, H. K., & Wolkenfeld, F. (1980). The parallelism phenomenon in psychoanalysis and supervision: its reconstruction as a triadic system. *Psychoanalytic Quarterly, 49*: 234–255.

Glucksman, M. L. (2006). Psychoanalytic and psychodynamic education in the 21st century. *Journal of the American Academy of Psychoanalysis and Dynamic Psychiatry*: *34*(1): 215–222.

Goodman, S. (Ed.) (1977). *Psychoanalytic Education and Research: The Current Situation and Future Possibilities*. New York: International Universities Press.

Hanly, C. (2013). My last letter to you as your President. Available at: http://www.ipa.world/IPA/en/Newsletters/From_the_President_July.aspx.

Holzman, P. S. (1985). Psychoanalysis: is the therapy destroying the science? *Journal of the American Psychoanalytic Association, 33*: 725–770.

Huber, D., Henrich, G., Clarkin, J., & Klug, G. (2013). Psychoanalytic versus psychodynamic therapy for depression: a three years follow-up study. *Psychotherapy, 76*(2): 132–149.

Israelstam, K. (2011). The interactive category schema of candidate competence: an Australian experience. *International Journal of Psychoanalysis, 92*: 1289–1313.

Jiménez, J. P. (2000). El método clínico, los psicoanalistas y la institución. *Aperturas Psicoanalíticas, 4*: 1–19.

Kächele, H., & Thomä, H. (2000). On the devaluation of the Eitingon–Freud model of psychoanalytic education. *International Journal of Psychoanalysis, 81*: 806–807.

Kernberg, O. F. (1978). Leadership and organizational functioning: Organizational regression. *International Journal of Group Psychotherapy, 28*: 38–25.

Kernberg, O. F. (1986). Institutional problems of psychoanalytic education. *Journal of the American Psychoanalytic Association, 34*: 799–834.

Kernberg. O. F. (2000). A concerned critique of psychoanalytic education. *International Journal of Psychoanalysis, 81*: 97–120.

Kernberg, O. F. (2004). Resistances to research in psychoanalysis. In: *Contemporary Controversies in Psychoanalytic Theory, Techniques, and their Applications* (pp. 86–93). New Haven, CT: Yale University Press.

Kernberg. O. F. (2006). The coming changes in psychoanalytic education: Part I. *International Journal of Psychoanalysis, 87*: 1649–1673.

Kernberg, O. F. (2007). The coming changes in psychoanalytic education. Part II. *International Journal of Psychoanalysis, 88*: 183–202.

Kernberg, O. F. (2010). A new organization of psychoanalytic education. *Psychoanalytic Review, 97*: 997–1018.

Kernberg, O. F. (2011). Psychoanalysis and the university: a difficult relationship. *International Journal of Psychoanalysis, 92*: 609–622.

Kernberg, O. F. (2012). Suicide prevention for psychoanalytic institutes and societies. *Journal of the American Psychoanalytic Association, 60*(4): 707–719.

Kernberg, O. F. (2013). The twilight of the training analysis system. Plenary address of the annual Conference of the American Psychoanalytic Association.

Kernberg, O. F., Canannis, D., Auchincloss, E., Glick, R. A., & Roose, S. P. (2012). Three problematic assumptions about psychoanalytic education. *Journal of the American Psychoanalytic Association, 60*(1): 97–102.

Körner, J. (2002). The didactics of psychoanalytic education. *International Journal of Psychoanalysis, 83*: 1395–1405.

Leichsenring, F., & Rabung, S. (2008). Effectiveness of long-term psychodynamic psychotherapy: a meta-analysis. *Journal of the American Medical Association, 300*(13): 1551–1565.

Leichsenring, F., & Rabung, S. (2009). Author's reply. *Journal of the American Medical Association, 301*: 932–933.

Leichsenring, F. & Rabung, S. (2011). Long-term psychodynamic psychotherapy in complex mental disorders: Update of a meta-analysis. *British Journal of Psychiatry*, 1999, 15–22.

Leichsenring, F., Abbass, A., Luyten, P., Hilsenrot, M., & Rabung, S. (2013). The emerging evidence for long-term psychodynamic therapy. *Psychodynamic Psychiatry, 41*(3): 361–384.

Levinson, H. (1994). The changing psychoanalytic organization and its influence on the ego ideal of psychoanalysis. *Psychoanalytic Psychology, 11*(2): 233–249.

Levy, R. A., & Ablon, S. (Eds.) (2009). *Handbook of Evidence-Based Psychodynamic Psychotherapy*. New York: Springer.

Lowder, G., Hansell, J., & McWilliam, J. (2008). A free-use PowerPoint presentation (www.apsa.org/powerpointresearch). Psychoanalysis (Division 39) of the American Psychological Association.

McWilliams, N. (2011). *Psychoanalytic Diagnosis: Understanding Personality* (2nd edn). New York: Guilford Press.

Michels, R. (2007). Optimal education requires an academic context: commentary on Wallerstein. *Journal of the American Psychoanalytic Association, 55*(3): 985–989.

Miller, E. J. (1993). *From Dependency to Autonomy: Studies in Organization and Change*. London: Free Association Books.

Morris, J. (1992). Psychoanalytic training today. *Journal of the American Psychoanalytic Association, 40*: 1185–1210.

Mullen, L. S., & Rieder, R. O. (2002). The psychodynamic competency test. Unpublished manuscript.

Olds, D., & Cooper, A. M. (1997). Dialogue with other sciences: opportunities for mutual gain. *International Journal of Psychoanalysis, 78*: 215–225.

OPD Task Force (Eds). (2001). *Operationalized Psychodynamic Diagnostics*. Göttingen: Hogrefe & Huber.

Paniagua, C. (1995). Common ground, uncommon methods. *International Journal of Psychoanalysis, 76*: 357–371.

Panksepp, J. (2000). On preventing another century of misunderstanding: towards a psychoethology of human experience and a psychoneurology of affect. *Neuro-psychoanalysis*, 2: 240–255.

Panksepp, J., & Biven, L. (2012). *The Archaeology of Mind—Neuroevolutionary Origins of Human Emotions*. New York: W. W. Norton.

PDM Task Force (2006). *Psychodynamic Diagnostic Manual: Personality Patterns and Disorders*. Silver Spring, MD: Alliance of Psychoanalytic Organizations.

Rees, E. (2007). Thinking about psychoanalytic curricula: an epistemological perspective. *Psychoanalytic Quarterly, 76*(3): 891–942.

Riesenberg Malcom, R. (1990). As if: the phenomenon of not learning. *International Journal of Psychoanalysis, 71*: 385–392.

Shakow, D. (1962). Psychoanalytic education of behavioral and social scientists for research. In: J. H. Masserman (Ed.), *Science and Psychoanalysis* (pp. 146–161). New York: Basic Books.

Shedler, J. (2010). The efficacy of psychodynamic psychotherapy. *American Psychologist, 65*: 98–109.

Steiner, R. (1994). The tower of Babel or after Babel in contemporary psychoanalysis. *International Journal of Psychoanalysis, 75*: 883–901.

Stepansky, P. E. (2009). *Psychoanalysis at the Margins*. New York: Other Press.

Thomä, H. (1993). Training analysis and psychoanalytic education: proposals for reform. *Annual of Psychoanalysis, 21*: 3–75.

Thomä, H., & Kächele, H. (1999). Memorandum on a reform of psychoanalytic education. *International Journal of Psychoanalysis, 8*: 33–35.

Ticho, E. A. (1970). The differences between psychoanalysis and psychotherapy. *Bulletin of the Menninger Clinic, 34*(3): 128–138.

Tuckett, D. (2000). Theoretical pluralism and the construction of psychoanalytic knowledge. In: J. Sandler, R. Michels, & P. Fonagy (Eds.), *Changing Ideas in a Changing World: The Revolution in Psychoanalysis. Essays in Honor of Arnold Cooper* (pp. 237–246). New York: Karnac.

Tuckett, D. (2002). The new style conference and developing a peer culture in European psychoanalysis: Presidential Address, Prague. *European Psychoanalytical Federation Bulletin, 56*.

Tuckett, D. (2005). Does anything go? Towards a framework for the more transparent assessment of psychoanalytic competence. *International Journal of Psychoanalysis, 86*: 31–49.

Tuckett, D., Basile, R., Birksted-Breen, D., Bohm, T., Denis, P., Ferro, A., Hinz, H., Jemstedt, A., Mariotti, P., & Schubert, J. (2008). *Psychoanalysis Comparable & Incomparable. The Evolution of a Method to Describe and Compare Psychoanalytic Approach*. New York: Routledge.

Vaughan, S. C., & Roose, S. P. (1995). The analytic process. Clinical and research definitions. *International Journal of Psychoanalysis, 78*: 343–356.

Vaughan, S. C., Spitzer, R., Davies, M., & Roose, S. (1997). The definition and assessment of analytic process. Can analysts agree? *International Journal of Psychoanalysis, 78*: 959–973.

Wallerstein, R. S. (1986). *Forty two Lives in Treatment. A Study of Psychoanalysis and Psychotherapy*. New York: Guilford Press.

Wallerstein, R. S. (1988). Psychoanalysis and psychotherapy: relationship roles reconsidered. *Annual of Psychoanalysis, 16*: 129–151.

Wallerstein, R. S. (1990). Psychoanalysis: the common ground. *International Journal of Psychoanalysis, 71*: 3–20.

Wallerstein, R. S. (1992). Psychoanalytic pluralism: the resolution of the issue? In: *The Common Ground of Psychoanalysis* (pp. 269–302). Northvale, NJ: Jason Aronson.

Wallerstein, R. S. (2007). The optimal structure for psychoanalytic education today: a feasible proposal? *Journal of the American Psychoanalytic Association, 55*: 953–984.

Wallerstein, R. S. (2009). Psychoanalysis in the university: a full time vision. *International Journal of Psychoanalysis, 90*: 1107–1121.

Wallerstein, R. S. (2012). Will psychoanalysis fulfill its promise? *International Journal of Psychoanalysis, 93*(2): 377–399.

Watkins, C. E. (2011). Is psychoanalytic education effective? Comment on Damsa (2010). *American Journal of Psychoanalysis, 71*: 290–292.

Watkins, C. E. (2013). The contemporary practice of effective psychoanalytic supervision. *Psychoanalytic Psychology, 30*(2): 300–328.

Widlöcher, D. (2001). The IPA and regional structures. *IPA Newsletter, 10*(2): 9.

CHAPTER SEVEN

Thoughts on the present and future of psychoanalytic education*

Otto F. Kernberg and Robert Michels

Introduction

This chapter originated in a series of dialogues between the authors over a period of approximately one year, focused on present problems (and possible solutions) in psychoanalytic education, internationally but particularly in the USA. Both authors have been involved in psychoanalytic education and governance over many years and share a concern with where psychoanalysis presently stands and where it is going. They share the experience of being part of what today is a significant minority of psychoanalysts involved in academic pursuits, thus being situated at the boundary between psychoanalysis and university-based psychiatry as professions. Having been involved in the leadership of both psychoanalytic and psychiatric organizations, they share an interest in organizational theory, an additional joint interest influencing their approach to institutional

* Otto F. Kernberg & Robert Michels, Thoughts on the present and future of psychoanalytic education. *Journal of the American Psychoanalytic Association*, 64(3): 477–493, copyright © 2016 by the American Psychoanalytic Association. Reprinted by permission of SAGE Publications, Inc.

aspects of psychoanalysis. Despite these commonalities, however, they have been identified as having differently shaded positions and views within psychoanalytic politics: Robert Michels as relatively conservative regarding controversial issues in psychoanalytic institutional functioning and governance, and Otto Kernberg as inclined toward rapid change regarding these issues (Auchincloss & Michels, 2003; Kernberg, 2014). This difference determined a dynamic of particular interest in their dialogue: the extent to which mutual respect, yet differing viewpoints, might issue in an analysis and joint recommendations that might be of interest to the field. In what follows, their achievement in that direction is spelled out in some detail.

Psychoanalysis has played a significant role in the development of twentieth-century Western culture, an influence that extends to the present. It is also a major scientific enterprise dealing with fundamental issues in psychology, particularly the influence of unconscious processes on psychological functioning. In addition, it is a mental health profession with membership organizations in Europe, North and South America, Asia, South Africa, and Australia. Its contribution to the humanities has been universally recognized. In recent years, however, its scientific status has been questioned and its professional organizations have taken diminished interest in its scientific and intellectual foundations.

Today, the psychoanalytic community is engaged in limited academic pursuits, and has limited scientific, educational, and interdisciplinary interactions with the academic world. The impact of the field's cultural contributions is significantly restricted by its lack of activity in these areas.

As a profession, psychoanalysis suffers at present from declining prestige, minimal research on its effectiveness, and competition with alternative treatments, particularly psychopharmacological and cognitive–behavioral approaches that are often viewed as more effective for the conditions psychoanalysts have traditionally treated. In addition, the field suffers as a profession from its neglect of derivative treatments, as seen in its lack of psychotherapy training and psychotherapy research, and of any "marketing" of psychoanalytic psychotherapy. The profession suffers also from the low level of involvement by psychoanalytic societies in the professional development of members, and from the lack of prestige these societies command in the academic and university environment. This lack of active, enthusiastic community involvement by psychoanalytic societies stands in sharp contrast to their preoccupation with internal conflicts, particularly surrounding the dynamics of the relationship between psychoanalytic institutes and societies (Berman, 2004; Garza-Guerrero, 2004; Kernberg, 2011; Michels, 2007; Reeder, 2004; Wallerstein, 2010).

The scientific activities of psychoanalysis are virtually paralyzed by its lack of systematic research and research training. There is an urgent need for empirical research dealing with alternative theories and technical approaches that, under the present circumstances, are "ecumenically tolerated" as parallel developments with unresolved questions. This grave neglect of research interest and training in psychoanalytic institutes and the related lack of initiatives to obtain financial support for psychoanalytic research are powerful negative influences on psychoanalysis as a science. The lack of scientifically trained psychoanalytic professionals who would consider academic careers and university professorships as major goals is a consequence of the implicit, or even active, discouragement of such careers by psychoanalytic educational institutions and by some leaders of the profession. Perhaps most disturbing, an increasing number of analysts seem to have little interest in empirical research, and believe that it offers nothing to their work. This attitude persists side by side with their claim for public support and health care funding, as if others should accept their conviction of its value without further evidence and despite the many health care professionals who are equally convinced that it is worthless. This is a classic situation that can be resolved only by systematic research, but the profession remains strangely disinterested. In short, we believe that while the contributions of psychoanalysis to the humanities will continue to be appreciated in their historical context, psychoanalysis, as a science and as a science-based profession, faces severe problems.

The dominant conflicts of psychoanalytic societies and institutes

Both small psychoanalytic societies and larger organizations, such as national associations, experience similar problems and conflicts. Most societies have weak or non-existent relations with local universities. These are institutions that would seem, given their common professional and cultural interests, to be natural collaborators. The impact of psychoanalytic societies on other cultural institutions in their environment is minimal. The membership of psychoanalytic societies generally consists of graduates and candidates of their associated institutes, among whom interest in society activities tends to dwindle once training is completed. And, once again, there is practically no interest in the development of research in psychoanalysis and/or related fields.

A major internal source of the malaise affecting the psychoanalytic community is the conflict between psychoanalytic societies and psychoanalytic institutes and an associated withdrawal from the challenges posed by external reality. This is intimately connected with shortcomings in psychoanalytic education: the lack of research, a failure to orient candidates and graduates to academic careers, and a stultifying conservatism regarding educational methodology. This educational stagnation limits the development of psychoanalytic knowledge, its basic theory of mind, and its relation to adjacent disciplines. This problematic situation relates to the nature and functions of the training analyst system at the core of the psychoanalytic educational endeavor (Kernberg, 2006; Meyer, 2003; Roustang, 1982).

Both of us agree that these problems stem from the combination of a lack of accepted standards of professional competence and the training analyst system (TAS) that evolved as a result, but disagree on the relative importance of these two features. RM believes that the lack of standards of professional competence, reflected in the evaluation of every graduate psychoanalyst, is a fundamental cause of the persistence of the TAS, and that the system will wither away with the development of true and accepted standards to be applied in the certification of analysts.

The real problem is not so much the training analyst system as the "non-training analyst" system, the institute graduates who are viewed as not quite good enough to analyze candidates. This leads to a two-tier profession, hurt feelings, internal conflict, and understandable challenges to the procedures for selecting training analysts. With appropriate criteria for graduating from an institute and becoming an analyst, every analyst would be a training analyst. This is, for now, the view of RM (Auchincloss & Michels, 2003; Michels, 2007).

For OFK, the basic problem is the distortion of the educational system's functioning, the authoritarian absorption of all decision making by training analysts as a self-perpetuating dominant group, and the mystification of the process of training analyst selection as a political tool. The TAS is opposed to research seeking to establish objective, reliable, and transparent professional standards. In practice, OFK believes, the TAS has been the major obstacle to renovation in psychoanalytic education (Kernberg, 2014; Wallerstein 2010).

Both of us agree, however, that a major innovative effort to develop a realistic, functional conceptualization of the standards of competence for the profession of psychoanalysis is urgently needed, and that when this has been accomplished the training analysis system will come to an end. While RM thinks that under such circumstances it will fade away, OFK believes that the natural defensive reaction of an authoritarian elite will be to resist its demise and that its termination might, therefore, have to be actively implemented. We agree, however, on the need to be alert to this dynamic. We agree that were our proposal to be adopted there would be but one category, of certified graduate analysts: that is, all analysts would be "training analysts." Practically, we agree, given the length of time it will probably take to achieve this task, the TAS should be maintained in the transitional period, as long as an active, intensive, undisturbed process of establishing such standards is not interfered with politically by the present organizational structure of psychoanalytic institutions. A new, fail-safe mechanism for elaborating the standards of professional competence is required.

Within this context of a basic agreement regarding what needs to be done, we have each started from differently nuanced assessments of the group processes affecting members of the psychoanalytic community who are not educationally active, the "non-academic" majority. RM believes that most analysts, once they have graduated, become progressively uninterested in any further educational programs of a formal nature, and are skeptical regarding the need for, or advantage of, the profession's continued concern with standards: "They want to be left in peace." OFK, by contrast, believes that many of those members are quite concerned with maintaining and developing high professional standards, precisely because of the academically isolated nature of the profession, and are critical of the authoritarian atmosphere of psychoanalytic institutes that often seems to discourage such standards.

The training analyst system evolved as an elite of highly skilled psychoanalysts charged with maintaining professional standards and transmitting them to future generations, the psychoanalytic counterpart of the peer review and evaluation involved in appointment, promotion, and tenure decisions regarding faculty in university-based professions. Psychoanalysis developed a private educational system outside the academic world that succeeded in preserving the new profession and protecting it from external attacks. However, the system has evolved in the direction of a hierarchical "three-tier system" within psychoanalytic educational institutions: training analysts, graduates aspiring to become training analysts, and candidates. The dynamics of this institutional development have been analyzed extensively in work sufficiently well known as not to require review. On the side of its positive consequences, the training analyst system in the USA has been effective in developing a high level of clinical psychoanalytic education that has been maintained in many institutes. At the international level, the education committees of the various psychoanalytic institutes have, in general, also been able to assure a uniformly acceptable level of training throughout the three major regions. These positive features of the training analyst system were essential in the early years of psychoanalytic education, while its predominately negative features have only emerged over time. These long-range negative effects, we believe, have been a combination of conservatism, an institutionalized unrealistic idealization of the training analyst, infantilization of candidates, a phobic fearfulness regarding external influences that might affect the theoretical belief system of an institute, and an institutional reluctance to carry out research. The organization of training analysts as an intellectual elite dominating psychoanalytic institutes committed to an ideology of preserving present structures as necessary for maintaining high standards of practice has clashed with a growing dissatisfaction among the societies' members, constituted by a majority of non-training analysts, with critical and resentful reaction against what they perceive as an attitude of superiority and authoritarian institutional control by the training analyst elite.

We both agree that the present educational system has serious faults. It has contributed to producing an atmosphere of intellectual stagnation, conservatism, and a phobic attitude toward any questioning of basic theory and technique by candidates, along with a distrust of any interest in outside academic engagements. The system's demand that candidates be in analysis with training analysts, together with the unquestioned assumption that the training analyst represents the ideal of the profession, limits the possibility of analyzing the transference implications of candidates' idealization of their analyst. An atmosphere of widespread submission and implicitly fostered idealization is the flip side of paranoid fearfulness and rebelliousness, the mostly ignored, but quite prevalent, consequences of this situation (Cabaniss et al., 2003; Roose, 2003). Thus far we agree, and we agree also that it is essential that this atmosphere change. It is detrimental to the scientific development of psychoanalysis, to the education of candidates, and, above all, to an open spirit of inquiry.

At this point, our viewpoints diverge. RM sees behind this reality and the corresponding critique of the training analyst system a characteristic of professions generally, replayed typically, for example, at the level of the American Psychiatric Association. There, the general membership, chafing at certification and recertification requirements, was demanding a lowering of standards, while the profession's educational elite, represented, for example, by the American Board of Psychiatry and Neurology, was trying to maintain and upgrade them. RM sees the conflict between the Board on Professional Standards of the American Psychoanalytic Association (BOPS), representing the training analyst elite, on the one hand, and the membership of the American Psychoanalytic Association, represented by the Executive Council, on the other, as a typical illustration of a conflict in which a minority elite is trying to maintain and raise standards, acting without conscious disdain of the non-privileged majority, while that majority is resentful, envious, and enraged at the elite, whose authority it perceives as inappropriate and illegitimate. In essence, in RM's view this is a dynamic unavoidable in large professional organizations that include a specialized body responsible for setting and maintaining standards, on the one hand, and, on the other, a resentful majority that experiences this as an unjustified bureaucratic intrusion on the exercise of its professional functions. OFK, for his part, considers the TAS's intrinsic pathology the essential dynamic of the internal crisis currently plaguing psychoanalysis, with the institutional conflict between BOPS and the Executive Council as a derivative dynamic.

Given these different perspectives, which together we accept as posing a dialectic that needs to be taken into consideration in the search for solutions, we have reached the following understanding after lengthy discussions and formulated a proposal that may be relevant for the specific situation of the American Psychoanalytic Association and, with appropriate modifications, useful to the international psychoanalytic community as well. We both agree that the basic educational psychoanalytic system needs to be changed, and that the membership's resentment of educational standards and controls must be taken into account, even while protecting the standards and requirements of certification from dilution as a consequence of political pressure.

A proposal for change

We started from the hypothesis, a joint basic assumption, that psychoanalysis is a developing discipline, and that the clinical application of psychoanalytic theory and technique for the treatment of patients can be defined, taught, and evaluated. In other words, we believe it is possible to develop reliable, transparent criteria for assessing standards that would justify the certification of a psychoanalyst as a competent member of the profession. The development of such standards would require a definition of the expertise of the clinical psychoanalyst in terms of (1) knowledge, (2) technical ability, and (3) "psychoanalytic attitude," including a readiness to search for, and recognize, the unconscious aspects of the psychoanalytic encounter (Körner, 2002). We believe that it is possible to define minimally expected knowledge (assessed by instruments) and that a broad spectrum of technical capacities can be achieved and evaluated, as has been demonstrated for other medical specialties using clinical examinations that test knowledge and technical ability. Examinations focused on alternative clinical interventions and videotaped material can serve this purpose, as already demonstrated in pioneering research on evaluating competence in psychoanalytic psychotherapy. The complex subjective and attitudinal aspects that constitute the "psychoanalytic attitude" require direct discussion of clinical material, a subjective element that is unavoidable and must be included in any comprehensive evaluative process. Under the conditions of theoretical and technical pluralism currently prevailing in the psychoanalytic community, we believe this clinical evaluation could be achieved by a process that includes examiners both sharing and not sharing the theoretical and technical approaches of the person being examined. Certification should be encouraged by psychoanalytic institutes to strengthen the identification of their candidates with the profession.

Present methods of selecting training analysts often include such a clinical evaluation; one that, in the context of a clear definition of expected knowledge, technical skills, and attitude, may lead, with the help of instruments developed to assess those features, to an examination and certification process that assures psychoanalytic competence. We propose that evaluation under such conditions, conducted several years after graduation—permitting the psychoanalytic graduate to acquire broader clinical experience—is an adequate basis for specialty certification.

We propose that any analyst thus certified would be assumed to have the competence to analyze psychoanalytic candidates. Certified psychoanalysts would not automatically become members of the faculty of psychoanalytic institutes; each institute would add its specific criteria for faculty selection. Some of these criteria are spelled out below.

We propose that two administrative bodies be developed with specific and independent functions. One is a committee on education, with the mission of proposing innovative educational methods and new curriculum content, both designed to achieve psychoanalytic competence. This committee would also be charged with developing criteria for determining such competence. The committee's mission, in short, would be to explore new and creative educational objectives and methodology. Its members should be enthusiastic educators willing to experiment with new ideas. The second independent body would be a board charged with organizing the process of certification, devising an objective, fair, reliable, and transparent system of certification, with appropriate mechanisms for redress of grievances. It would have the final authority regarding criteria for certification, the certification process, and the application of these criteria. The mission of this committee would be to assure a stable, consistent, faithful application of the psychoanalytic institution's educational objectives and criteria of competence to the certification of members and the accreditation of institutes. For large organizations, such as the American Psychoanalytic Association, the directors of psychoanalytic institutes might constitute a third entity of professional interest with input into the certifying process.

We propose that the dialectic of authoritarian decision making regarding standards, on the one hand, and group psychology opposed to bureaucratic controls, on the other, may be resolved by a process in which new initiatives are generated by the education committee and proposed to the leadership of the institute faculty. In case of disagreement, the education committee proposal would be decided by a vote of the entire faculty.

In the American Psychoanalytic Association, this would mean replacing the Board on Professional Standards by a small committee for psychoanalytic education, on the one hand, and an organization of directors of psychoanalytic institutes, on the other. Once a decision regarding educational innovation has been made, this decision may be translated into concrete criteria that determine the operation of the certifying board. That board would be completely independent in its decision making, within criteria and standards that have been approved.

Elimination of the training analyst system should contribute significantly to reducing the organizationally fostered idealization of the candidates' analysts and disconnect completely the personal analysis of the candidate from all other educational pursuits, including the acquisition of knowledge, technical skills, and the psychoanalytic attitude by means of seminars and individual and group supervision. The certifying board should include representatives of the institute directors, have a staggered system of replacing members to assure continuity and preserve institutional memory, and work with the clear understanding that it applies organizationally approved criteria of professional standards but has no authority to modify them. Its decisions could be appealed only on the grounds of faulty application of approved certifying principles.

An additional key function of psychoanalytic education should be the development of interest in research as an essential aspect of psychoanalytic inquiry. Institute faculty should include experts in conveying knowledge, experts in conveying the nature and management of clinical situations, and experts in personal supervision, in addition to experts in the methodology and teaching of psychoanalytic research. The selection of faculty is a complex process that necessarily must evolve differently in small and large institutes, and should, for the most part, be based on participation in group discussions and group supervisions, participation in scientific meetings and conferences, and the presentation and publication of clinical and theoretical material. Because we are largely in agreement regarding the selection of teachers, supervisors, and research experts, we have concentrated mostly on the following practical issues.

Practical recommendations

We strongly believe that teachers must be rotated, that no monopolies of teaching regarding theory, technique, or applications be accepted, while certain seminars require a continuity of teaching with certain instructors who require an extended period of time for a full deployment of their contribution. This means that the mechanical "chopping up" of seminars on technique should be eschewed, so that candidates will be able to identify a particular approach by a particular instructor. Theoretical courses need to be integrated, so that candidates are not subjected to unnecessary repetition of the same material, or exposed to significant disruption in the continuity of related subjects. If an institute does not have instructors for certain subjects, that should be recognized and outside teachers invited to compensate for the deficit. A principal mission of psychoanalytic institutes is the development of a comprehensive and integrated curriculum that differentiates between essential and optional subjects. We are critical of the mechanical review of traditional material and of participation by some faculty members in an educational program they are not aware of in its totality: all faculty should be aware of the context within which their particular contribution is made.

Institute faculty should include supervisors, seminar leaders, and researchers, and should be advised by a representative group chosen by and from the candidates. Ideally, the institute's director would be selected by the faculty, or by academic authorities where the institute is affiliated with a university.

A basic understanding that guided us in crafting this proposal is the risk of a petrified, orthodox institute leadership, on the one hand, and an antiauthoritarian, rebellious organizational membership on the other, a situation in which educational principles and methods would be subordinate to political ends.

We propose a functional reorganization and selection of faculty as the body empowered to decide educational matters. Routine matters would be handled by ongoing dialogue between the education committee and the institute leadership. If conflicts emerge, these would be referred to the institute faculty as a whole, which would have the final say.

Psychoanalysis and the university

The present situation: psychoanalysis as an independent profession

The scientific leadership of medical and psychological professions is embedded in university departments that support progress in science and set the standards for competence within the profession.

Psychoanalysis, by contrast, operates as an independent profession. Early on, when it was a completely new and highly controversial profession, this permitted the field to develop freely. This status as a profession largely unaffiliated with universities—a status unique among the learned professions—has continued into the present. It has served the clinical mission of the profession reasonably well but has been less successful regarding advocacy and public outreach (though in recent years activity in these areas has increased). Although the profession has created an extensive network of training institutes, their work has been hampered by the political problems we have seen between institute faculty and the general membership of the societies. A particularly serious problem arises from the institutes' general lack of university affiliations, as a result of which the field's scientific development has been truncated. Thus, psychoanalysis has become a relatively static intellectual discipline, valorizing tradition rather than progress, and tolerating dialogue without requiring new knowledge. The barrier between psychoanalysis and the university, perhaps necessary in earlier years, might well have become the greatest threat to its survival. While we are aware that pioneering efforts are under way to improve this situation, and have reviewed these efforts in an earlier publication, the basic lack of university representation for psychoanalysis is still a major problem (Kernberg, 2011). Further, many of the affiliations between psychoanalytic groups and universities that do exist involve administrative ties and educational activities, but little participation in the core activity of universities—research and the creation of new knowledge—or the participation of psychoanalysts as full-time university faculty.

We recognize that psychoanalysis is more than a science. It obviously has other dimensions—hermeneutic and artistic, among others. However, we strongly believe that it encompasses important assertions about reality—facts, data. These can be formulated, tested, and accepted or rejected based on the results of these tests. These assertions involve the effect of interventions on the clinical process, the effect of the process on the patient's life, early development and its impact on latter development, and the relationship between subjective experience and bodily functions. Systematic research in these areas will enhance the field. If we have no interest in such research, the non-psychoanalytic world will dismiss us as a cult. The development of such research, and (perhaps even more important) of enthusiasm and support for it within the profession, requires repairing our relationship with universities.

The ultimate success of the reintegration of psychoanalysis and the university will require the development of academic career tracks for psychoanalysts. As part of the academic community, they would do clinical work, teach, and conduct research, each activity supporting the others and being respected by the psychoanalytic profession at large.

Today, some psychoanalytic communities foster a dedication to conducting psychoanalytic treatment as an exclusive activity, anything else being regarded as an inferior alternative, while, in fact, many members are more likely to be engaged also in other activities, psychiatric or psychological, or in university settings. Thus, the majority of psychoanalytic practitioners might have more relations with the external environment—including the university and neighboring mental health professions—than have core institute faculty members dedicated to clinical and educational activities exclusively within the psychoanalytic domain. This situation highlights the need to better integrate psychoanalysis with the university, and raises a basic question: Is the analyst active exclusively in the psychoanalytic realm the true representative of the profession, with the highest "identity" as a psychoanalyst, or is the psychoanalytic professional also engaged in other activities more truly representative of the profession in a world of cultural, professional, and intellectual challenges?

We believe that both types of professionals enrich the profession. Given our present reality, an important task is the expansion of psychoanalysis to include its application in a wide range of clinical situations. In this regard, we believe that psychoanalytic institutes should encourage faculty and candidates to participate in a range of professional endeavors, and to apply psychoanalytic theory in multiple fields. The basic institute curriculum should present knowledge about fields contiguous to psychoanalysis, with faculty representing the social sciences, neuroscience, and the humanities.

The role of the leadership of the psychoanalytic profession is to coordinate the professional, clinical, educational, and scientific activities of the psychoanalytic community, with primary responsibility for educational activities delegated to the psychoanalytic institute, which is responsible for selecting candidates and faculty, organizing the curriculum, and supervising the conduct of research.

Specific functions of psychoanalytic institutes

Selection of candidates

Selection requires evaluation of two aspects of a candidate: (1) personal qualities and (2) professional background and training. Regarding the first, there should be evidence of the candidate's ethical integrity and intelligence. We believe that the predictions that traditionally have been made on the basis of past traumas in an applicant's life, or particular aspects of his or her psychopathology (other than antisocial behavior), have seldom been substantiated and that the capacity for psychological insight may be much more difficult to predict than was once assumed (Kappelle, 1996).

Regarding the second point, however, we agree that applicants should have a solid background in clinical psychiatry, including long-term internships or fellowships in psychiatric institutions where they have learned about psychopathology, differential diagnosis, and alternative psychiatric treatments, or, if applicants come from professions that have not provided such a background, that they must acquire that experience early in their training.

We propose that a parallel track be available for applicants interested in psychoanalytic psychotherapies. This proposal reflects our conviction regarding the importance of psychoanalytic psychotherapy, a point to which we shall return. We should regard candidates with ideological biases for or against particular treatment methods, such as an "anti-medication" ideology, negatively. Our proposal favors broad and open selection, followed by objective and responsible quality control on a step-by-step basis throughout progression.

Seminars

Overall educational objectives should determine the content of the curriculum. In the case of national psychoanalytic organizations, commonly agreed on educational objectives should determine the common core curriculum and be tested in the process of certification. Evaluation and monitoring of seminar teaching is an essential aspect of curriculum assessment. Non-psychoanalytic faculty should be engaged to teach subjects at the boundaries of psychoanalysis. Alternative psychoanalytic theories should be taught, and candidates exposed to active discussion among the proponents of alternative views. The research implications of theoretical assumptions should be explored, and candidates should be encouraged to reach their own tentative synthesis in areas where our knowledge does not yet permit a definitive conclusion. We are critical of a comforting "ecumenical" acceptance of all divergent theories, and prefer to stress the need to accept present uncertainties and, whenever possible, to conduct empirical research to resolve conflicting views.

Technique

The present-day technical alternatives (e.g., ego psychological, Kleinian, British object relations, self psychological, relational, and French approaches) should be presented, along with discussions among their proponents. However, we both agree that beginning candidates are best trained in one, locally prevalent, mode of technical approach, in order to avoid confusion or a superficial eclecticism, and should only later be encouraged to explore alternative views.

Supervision

The purpose of psychoanalytic supervision is providing knowledge and support to the candidate, rather than assuming responsibility for the treatment. Supervisors should help the candidate expand his or her own views, and not simply convey their own. Supervisors should be evaluated in terms of their ability to formulate clinical experience, their possession of knowledge, and their skill in communicating it. Group supervision as a potential tool for the selection of supervisors can be helpful. Supervision should cut across the barrier of graduation, so that candidates have the opportunity to participate in supervision at postgraduate levels as well as supervision as part of their basic educational program. Candidates inclined to follow a particular theoretical school should have supervisors sharing that approach, and at least one supervisor from a different approach. At the point of certification, ideally the certifying committee should include members who share the candidate's approach and at least one member from another approach. A minimum of three members is recommended. We are critical of supervisors not sharing honestly with candidates any critical assessment of their work.

Progression assessment

Progression assessment should be carried out step by step at the end of each year of training, in terms of the educational objectives set for that particular time, and the corresponding criteria and methods for assessing them (Cabaniss et al., 2003; Roose, 2003). We are sharply critical of over-strict selection procedures employing questionable criteria; they run the risk of missing potentially creative and unusual candidates. We also reject the idea of a single, final assessment made after many years of training during which no clear assessment of progression was carried out. Candidates unable to meet realistic expectations need career counseling and guidance. We emphasize the essential tasks of defining criteria for psychoanalytic competence, specifying the educational achievements required to achieve that competence, and developing methods to evaluate them.

Psychoanalytic psychotherapy

The further development of psychoanalytic psychotherapies is an essential task of psychoanalysis. In addition to the traditional individual psychodynamic psychotherapy, a variety of specific dynamic psychotherapies have demonstrated clinical and empirical evidence of their effectiveness (Kernberg, 1999). These modalities have the potential to provide psychoanalytically based treatments to a much larger population than can be treated with standard psychoanalysis. Today, graduate analysts practice psychoanalytic psychotherapy with various degrees of competence. High-quality psychoanalytic psychotherapy training is vital for the survival of the psychoanalytic profession. It should be conducted by experts in this field.

Psychoanalytic research

As we have noted, the development of psychoanalytic research is essential for the survival and development of psychoanalysis as a profession. One of the troublesome consequences of the present training analyst system is the fostering of the training analyst position as the single major professional ideal. Adding other career tracks to this single ideal of psychoanalytic excellence, encouraging candidates aspiring to academic positions, stimulating and facilitating their development and rise within university hierarchies, and encouraging and rewarding candidates conducting psychoanalytic research would broaden the range of psychoanalytic careers. Not every psychoanalyst should become a researcher, and not every psychoanalytic institute is geared to becoming a research institution. However, the fostering of research should be a major goal of psychoanalytic education. Research ensures the questioning of traditionally transmitted assumptions that might no longer be viable.

One requirement for such a development is the availability of expertise in research methodology. A major psychoanalytic institution should develop a research department that includes expertise in research design.

Research on outcome of psychoanalysis, and on the relationship between process and outcome, is particularly important.

Graduation

A concerted effort to define the basic nature of psychoanalytic competence, the criteria by which it can be evaluated, and the educational methods that lead to its achievement is crucial to the development of the entire professional enterprise. The results of such an effort may show up most concretely at the point when candidates graduate. We believe that development of a definition of competence, and of the methodology for achieving it and testing its achievement, is a crucial task for education committees focused on innovations in psychoanalytic education, completely separate from the day-to-day administrative activities of psychoanalytic institutes.

Graduation should be based on the assessment of knowledge, technical skills, and analytic attitude.

As stated earlier, graduation from a psychoanalytic institute should lead to membership in the corresponding psychoanalytic society. This fits with what we have earlier proposed, which is that intimate participation in society activities by graduating candidates should be encouraged as part of eliminating the barriers between institute and society functioning. Society membership should not require certification. The function of certification should be the general recognition of the competence of the certified analyst who has met a national standard. It may be considered equivalent to specialty certification in medicine.

Conclusion

We trust we have developed a model of a structure for creativity, responsibility, and authority in fostering innovation, as well as quality control of education, that might powerfully support the changes in psychoanalytic education that we consider urgent and indispensable for the future of psychoanalysis.

References

Auchincloss, E. L., & Michels, R. (2003). A reassessment of psychoanalytic education: Controversies and changes. *International Journal of Psychoanalysis, 84*: 387–403.

Berman, E. (2004). *Impossible Training: A Relational View of Psychoanalytic Education*. New York: Analytic Press.

Cabaniss, D. L., Schein, J. W., Rosen, P., & Roose, S. P. (2003). Candidate progression in psychoanalytic institutes: A multicenter study. *International Journal of Psychoanalysis, 84*: 77–94.

Garza-Guerrero, C. (2004). Reorganisational and educational demands of psychoanalytic training today: Our long and marasmic night of one century. *International Journal of Psychoanalysis, 85*: 3–13.

Kappelle, W. (1996). How useful is selection? *International Journal of Psychoanalysis, 77*: 1213–1232.

Kernberg, O. F. (1999). Psychoanalysis, psychoanalytical psychotherapy and supportive psychotherapy: Contemporary controversies. *International Journal of Psychoanalysis*. *80*: 1075–1091.

Kernberg, O. F. (2006). The coming changes in psychoanalytic education: Part I. *International Journal of Psychoanalysis*, *87*: 1649–1673.

Kernberg, O. F. (2011). Psychoanalysis and the university: A difficult relationship. *International Journal of Psychoanalysis*, *92*: 609–622.

Kernberg, O. F. (2014). The twilight of the training analysis system. *Psychoanalytic Review*, *101*: 151–174.

Körner, J. (2002). The didactics of psychoanalytic education. *International Journal of Psychoanalysis*, *83*: 1395–1405.

Meyer, L. (2003). Subservient analysis. *International Journal of Psychoanalysis*, *84*: 1241–1262.

Michels, R. (2007). Optimal education requires an academic context: Commentary on Wallerstein. *Journal of the American Psychoanalytic Association*, *55*: 985–989.

Reeder, J. (2004). *Hate and Love in Psychoanalytic Institutions: The Dilemmas of a Profession*. New York: Other Press.

Roose, S. P. (2003). Candidate progression in psychoanalytic institutes: A multicenter study. *International Journal of Psychoanalysis*, *84*: 77–94.

Roustang, F. (1982). *Dire Mastery: Discipleship from Freud to Lacan*. Baltimore, MD: Johns Hopkins University Press.

Wallerstein, R. S. (2010). The training analysis: Psychoanalysis' perennial problem. *Psychoanalytic Review*, *97*: 903–936.

CHAPTER EIGHT

The training analysis: still a roadblock in psychoanalytic education

Douglas Kirsner

The science and therapy that Freud created over a century ago is a significant part of the *zeitgeist*, language, therapy, and conversation of the contemporary globalized world. Despite this success, however, psychoanalysis has become marginalized in academia, psychiatry, and psychology. The external challenges to psychoanalysis and psychodynamic approaches include competing therapies, especially cognitive–behavioral therapy (CBT), psychopharmacology, economic issues of expense from patients, insurance companies, and governments, increasing social demands for quick fixes, scientific critiques of lack of empirical research in psychodynamic therapies, cultural critiques of elitism and increasing anti-individualistic views. Despite some degree of interdisciplinary research in the neurosciences and social and behavioral sciences, there are significant threats within both the professions of psychology and psychiatry, together with ever-decreasing interest in universities in psychoanalysis across the board, even including humanities departments. In this situation, psychoanalysis as a therapy attracts a small number of patients, and institutes attract only a small number of candidates. With such marginalization in scholarship, research, and clinical practice, there is a real question as about the continued viability of the organized profession, which remains at the heart of the field in terms of providing a viable future (e.g., Procci 2013). The future of the field and profession depends on the effectiveness of organized psychoanalytic institutions in driving the transmission, stimulation and development of psychoanalysis. Although the field includes a wide range of organizations with a psychodynamic and psychoanalytic focus, the IPA and its societies must continue to play a central, though certainly not an exclusive role, in order for the discipline to have a future. This is especially true when viewed within the contexts of accelerated social and technological change, globalization and the development of alternative treatment modalities. A vital part of the future of psychoanalysis is to consider these new realities and where appropriate to utilize and adapt to them. Reshaping psychoanalytic educational systems and their objectives so as to align with contemporary realities is central to the future of the field.

The task of examining the roadblocks and requirements of the educational system is crucial for helping the field to become less marginal and to become relevant and dynamic again. External challenges should not divert those working within the field from confronting and resolving longstanding serious internal issues. In his 1952 Presidential Address to the American Psychoanalytic Association, Robert Knight lamented the typical themes of difficulty in psychoanalytic institutes:

> The spectacle of a national association of physicians and scientists feuding with each other over training standards and practices, and calling each other orthodox and conservative or deviant and dissident, is not an attractive one, to say the least. Such terms belong to religions, or to fanatical political movements and not to science and medicine. Psychoanalysis should be neither a "doctrine" nor a "party line". (1953, p. 210)

In Knight's view at the time, "the most pressing issue and the one charged with the greatest emotion has always been that of training" (Knight, 1953, pp. 211–212). Sadly, these problems remain, despite increasing numbers of significant critiques and warnings, and an atmosphere of greater pluralism and tolerance for different approaches.

The many trenchant critiques since the 1930s have increasingly pointed beyond particular individuals or local problems to basic faults in the system itself. Anna Freud declared at a conference in 1976,

> The heart of the matter is that the problem doesn't really seem to have changed much in the last forty-five years! But in listening to you here, I also got the impression that my colleagues who first advocated the introduction of training analysis . . . if they had known of all the dangers, of the positive and negative transferences, and splits, and hates, etc. would probably never have advocated it! They would have said, "Let them be as they are!" (A. Freud, 1983, p. 259)

Classic discussions such as Balint (1948), Bernfeld (1962), and Kernberg (1986) made significant contributions to understanding basic flaws and indicating ways to improve the system and how the system should work optimally. Although many have followed such discussions in similar vein (see Schachter et al., 2014; Thomä, 1993), the problems have persisted and the hierarchical syncretistic system has remained in place. Although training analyst status is one important part of the training system, there are other names or related roles that apply even when the literal term "training analyst" does not exist in the system. Or where all analysts with five years post-graduation experience are included but authorities decide which analysts are selected, the decision is, nonetheless, made by authorities. A caveat: although this chapter directly concerns institutes and societies affiliated to the IPA and their history of the training analysis system, such issues are scarcely restricted to IPA groups. Similar dynamics also apply to a wide variety of institutes around the world not affiliated with the IPA, whatever the professional backgrounds or theories. They are relevant whether they be Jungian, relational, or Lacanian, whether they are constituted by psychologists, social workers, or eclectic, or whether they be in Europe, the USA, or Asia. The central issue in all concerns the right to train and the culture and mind-sets surrounding it.

In the present day, organized psychoanalysis has fallen to the point where the problem is no longer "decline" and "crisis" but the dangers of the lack of a future with imminent death. The critiques have reached a crescendo with the culmination of Kernberg's ongoing critiques of psychoanalytic education. Kernberg's incisively crafted critiques of the system focus on internal systemic root causes of stymying and destruction of creativity and growth in psychoanalysis. Kernberg (1986) posits four models for psychoanalytic institutes: a seminary, a university, a trade school, and an art academy. He suggests that, ideally, psychoanalytic training should take place somewhere between the models of an art school and a university, whereas they have been mainly a combination of seminary and trade school. Recently, Kernberg has sounded severe warnings about imminent professional and scientific death. Kernberg's "suicide prevention" guidelines (Kernberg, 2012) are followed by his 2013 Plenary Address to the American Psychoanalytic Association, tellingly titled, "The twilight of the training analyst system" (Kernberg, 2014). The lecture highlights the necessity of abandoning the dysfunctional training analysis system that has created so many obstacles in its wake. There, Kernberg states,

> I believe it is fair to state that, while psychoanalysis has assured its place as a major contribution to the culture in the twentieth century, its future as a profession and a science in the twenty-first century cannot be assumed. (Kernberg, 2014, pp. 152–153)

Before the 1920s, formal psychoanalytic training did not exist. Psychoanalytic societies were scientific clubs with no accredited schools or curricula. In Europe, for the first twenty years of psychoanalysis, there were no training institutes and no mandatory training analysis. Originally, analysis played a subsidiary role in psychoanalytic education. The analyst-in-training was analyzed so as to iron out blind spots and get a sense of what psychoanalysis was like. It was also short and dealt with symptoms, small and large. A much longer time elapsed before there were "training analysts". The 1925 Bad Homburg IPA Congress unanimously established the International Training Board, chaired by Max Eitingon, to set uniform standards for psychoanalytic training around the world. The Congress resolved that the Board was to be "the central organ of the International Psycho-Analytical Association for all questions connected with psycho-analytical training". Modeled on the Berlin Psychoanalytic Institute, established in 1920, the Board would set the standards for those emigrating from Europe to the USA and beyond.

The early teaching approach for the small groups of students was student-centered and individually oriented. Even as late as 1937, Freud asserts that the simple aims of the training analysis are that the student gains

> a firm conviction of the existence of the unconscious, if it enables him, when repressed material emerges, to perceive in himself things which would otherwise be incredible to him, and if it shows him a first

> sample of the technique which has proved to be the only effective one in analytic work. (Freud, 1937c, p. 248)

For Freud, the analysis would be quite rudimentary and short, but it would continue to stimulate the analyst afterwards. The actual analysis was the necessary setting for the rest of the student's studies to become an analyst.

The short didactic psychoanalysis had educational objectives that were part of a broader educational context and was not an end in itself. It mutated to occupy center-stage—the secondary role became primary in the system. Anna Freud recalls that, for the generation of the 1930s, the major quality for selection of candidates was "a burning curiosity as to how human beings function, what makes them function normally or makes them suffer abnormal conditions, and what makes them develop from children into adults" (A. Freud, 1983, p. 260). This suggests philosophical excitement and inspiration lasting well beyond the training years (see A. Freud, 1983, p. 261). This spirit in psychoanalytic education was lost when the training analysis came to dominate the educational system as the primary identifying shibboleth. So long as the movement was small and Freud was its clear and active leader, many major decisions could be made by him as final arbiter or by some of his trusted colleagues. As the psychoanalytic movement increased in size and spread, the perceived need for organizational decision-making changed. As psychoanalytic education became more formalized, the role of the training analysis grew larger. Considerably different from Freud's own position (Freud ironically referred to "the authorities" (Bernfeld, 1962, p. 462)), the training analysis developed into something quite different—a far longer and mutative regimen, that is, one sufficiently "deep" that the personality of the analysand was to be changed, idealized as a psychoanalytic utopia of "complete psychoanalysis" as a "supertherapy" (Balint, 1954, p. 158).

However, the analysis should not need to be completed in one fell swoop, once and for all during training, any more than an academic needs to write the perfect PhD before being appointed to a university faculty position—the PhD is the beginning not the end of an independent research life for an academic. In the case of the student in psychoanalysis, the analysis during training is often filled with too many expectations. The analyst can undergo analysis again subsequently, whenever needed. Instead of having such intrinsic major importance as the main event, it could be seen as a beginning, one step along the way of, perhaps, a number of analyses over the analytic life cycle as part of life-long learning. Perhaps the adage, "The first analysis is for the institute, the second for yourself", might influence constructive change after all. If the first analysis were downsized to an introduction to the procedure and field, it could be viewed as an internship in the life of the mind, which would inspire further experiences. Just as Freud described it in "Analysis terminable and interminable" (1937c), the analysis during training could be treated as a part of an ongoing process that served certain educative functions, and not as a finished distinct product loaded with unrealistic expectations and irresolvable transferences. Unfortunately, such a downsizing proposal would elicit furious opposition, as it would reduce and question the position and power of training analysts. Yet again, this demonstrates the malignant logic of the structure of the system itself, which cannot be repaired but needs to be abolished *in toto*. Although many options have been tried over the decades, the same intrinsic problems have declared themselves.

In any case, such a short ongoing process is not the way it eventuated. In 1938, Fenichel could assert that the training analysis and the therapeutic analysis are, in fact, "to a high degree the same thing. There is but one analysis, and the candidate has to learn to face and to overcome his unconscious conflicts in the same way as any neurotic" (Fenichel et al., 1980, p. 24). According to Fenichel, the training analysis is especially crucial for the analyst because it is his or her "working instrument". This meant, for Fenichel, that the analysis should go beyond the simple aims that Freud adumbrated, but a problem emerges. Fenichel asserts,

> Whereas Freud taught us that the handling of the transference makes it necessary that between analyst and analysand there exist no other relationship than the analytic one, it cannot be denied that *the training analyst is actually a decisive person in the life of the candidate.* (Fenichel et al., 1980, p. 25, original italics)

This was an issue, then, even in those pre-war days when the training analysis was not yet large, formalized, reified, and rigidified.

The didactic analysis evolved from being ancillary to achieve an independent powerful status in its own right with the aura of being the ritual carrier of esoteric knowledge, more anthropology. Psychoanalytic candidates increasingly came to be seen, and saw themselves, as children who knew little, lying on the couches of those who knew. Psychoanalytic education travelled further away from being a collective voyage of discovery. The appointment of experienced psychoanalysts to fill a training or educational role eventually became transformed into an additional accreditation. It became a powerful position, occupying a status with the allure of a higher caste, a sinecure, rather than performing a specific function within the educational system.

As the psychoanalytic movement rapidly grew and spread, psychoanalytic training became formalized, with the training analysis as its pre-eminent feature. There was an intrinsic syncretism in the roles, such as student and voluntary analysand (Lewin & Ross, 1960), and the power relations involved with the analyst as gatekeeper, educator, judge, guide, leader, and power broker. These intrinsic contradictions made a training analysis more complex and confused, as well as potentially less therapeutic than an ordinary analysis. Psychoanalysis, which studied the role of transferences in everyday life, institutionalized it in its training, thus transmitting and amplifying a basic fault-line across the generations. Noting the symptoms of inhibited dogmatic thinking about psychoanalytic training, Balint (1948) suggests an anthropological explanation.

> The whole atmosphere is strongly reminiscent of the primitive initiation ceremonies. On the part of the initiators—the training committee and the training analysts—we observe secretiveness about our esoteric knowledge, dogmatic announcements of our demands and the use of authoritative techniques. On the part of the candidates, i.e. those to be initiated, we observe the willing acceptance of the exoteric fables, submissiveness to dogmatic and authoritative treatment without much protest and too respectful behaviour. We know that the general aim of all initiation rites is to force the candidate to identify himself with his initiator, to introject the initiator and his ideals, and to build up from these identifications a strong super-ego which will influence him all his life. This is a surprising discovery indeed. What we consciously intend to achieve with our candidates, is that they should develop a strong critical ego, capable of bearing considerable strains, free from any unnecessary identification, and from any automatic transference or thinking patterns. Contrary to the conscious aim our

> own behaviour as well as the working of the training system have several features leading necessarily to a weakening of these ego functions and to the formation and strengthening of a special kind of super-ego. (Balint, 1948, p. 167)

Balint (1948, 1954) and Lewin and Ross (1960) were followed by Bernfeld's (1962) beautiful and regularly cited paper contrasting the flexible, student-centered, informal and wide-ranging training of Freud's time with the modern day when training analysts became king and education became training. Siegfried Bernfeld makes a radical proposal: the dismantling of the whole system of psychoanalytic education which became so bureaucratized as to have lost the spirit and passion of psychoanalysis which belonged to the early pioneers. The formal system would be replaced by an informal one, which would be student centered. There would be no formal requirements about previous training. All the committees on admission, education, and students would be abolished, as would the category of "training analyst". When an analyst spotted somebody who was committed, talented, and passionately interested in analysis, he or she would be brought to meetings and seminars, meet other analysts, receive supervision, and maybe present a paper to the Society. The student would most likely be eager to undertake an analysis through interest and passion. After a while, the student would have met and mingled with the members of the Society, who could decide whether or not to accept the student as analyst (Bernfeld, 1962).

In a significant critical review of the literature on training analysis in 1964, New York analyst David Kairys highlights the inherent contradictions in the training analysis and expands on the basic contradiction that Anna Freud pointed out in 1938. For Anna Freud, the resolution of the patient's identification with the analyst in a therapeutic analysis comes through the interpretation of the infantile roots of the identification. Kairys explains,

> The analysand is thus brought to recognize the unreal character of the identification and can turn his energies to his own life interests. In the training analysis this cannot happen since identification with the analyst takes place in reality and the infantile and real determinants of the identification become fused. The patient in therapeutic analysis ends by becoming independent of the analyst and separating his fate from that of the analyst, while the candidate at the end of training

> connects his future with that of the analyst by becoming his colleague and sometimes his collaborator. This fact must affect the success of any training analysis and sometimes has produced cliques and factions within analytic groups. (Kairys, 1964, p. 501)

In 1964, Kairys thought it was "time to ask ourselves some hard questions" about the training analysis. He asks if it was justified to make students invest a great deal of time, effort, and money in an analysis which is flawed from the start—was it right to ask training analysts to conduct analyses with "so many built-in hazards"? Kairys finally asks if the profession is being served "by continuing a system of training which, we believe, leaves many students unsuccessfully analyzed and in need of further analysis after graduation". Despite the number of technical suggestions to improve the situation, Kairys suggests that "we have an obligation to seek answers that go beyond mere tinkering with the details of the present system" (1964, p. 508).

Training analyses became the master instead of an important servant of psychoanalytic education. During the heyday of psychoanalysis, training analyses could afford a very good living in addition to the analyst being able to practice their art. The tail came to wag the dog. The training analysis came to play a special independent and dominant role in psychoanalytic education. However, it makes more sense for the educational system to have it play a different role, a role that serves as a function, a means to an end serving the general aims of psychoanalytic education, closely connected with the intellectual discipline and practice.

I conclude, from my studies on the internal political histories of psychoanalytic institutes in *Unfree Associations* (Kirsner, 2009), that major conflicts most often surround the issue around the right to train, who appoints whom, and who is a training analyst. I describe the process of "anointment" of training analysts, which is akin to the Biblical laying on of hands. I chronicle the pivotal role played by anointment in the political histories of psychoanalytic institutes in the USA. The idea of an esoteric pipeline to knowledge, special to psychoanalysis, has been intrinsic to all psychoanalytic schools, which train their candidates to the level of their alleged "standards", as though there were some kind of objective reality to these standards. Variations in orthodoxies occur because of regional histories. In the hothouse atmospheres of institutes, followers have often clustered around local leaders directing the local mainstream. Despite some local differences in theory, these events usually concern who possesses the right to train and who does not. As Arlow observes,

> It is disturbing but true that most of the conflicts have originated over who shall have the right to train, that is, who shall be training analyst. The tensions emanating from the division of colleagues into two categories of psychoanalysts, training analysts and just plain psychoanalysts, intrude themselves into the organizational and scientific life of the institutes. This is an ever-present problem, and its impact is accentuated by the aura of special status which surrounds the position of training analyst, a position endowed with charismatic implications. The training analyst is regarded as possessing the psychoanalytic equivalent of omniscience. It is from the training analyst that candidates claim their descent. In many places the professional career of an individual may be determined by who his training analyst was. Greenacre referred to some of this in her study of the so-called "convoy" phenomenon, that is, the situation of the psychoanalytic candidate who is safely guided through his professional training under the protection of some influential training analyst. (Arlow, 1972, p. 559)

The training analysis carries with it a quasi-mystical, symbolic, and unique magical role well beyond an explicit putative or assigned function. The training analysis and the role of training analyst came to acquire a high status and aura that occupies a central role in the identity of being a psychoanalyst.

The training analysis system depends on the idea that there are those who know, despite the lack of evidence that training analysis is superior to an ordinary analysis. Joseph Schachter recently interviewed and submitted questionnaires, receiving responses by eighty-two analysts in institutes of the American Psychoanalytic Association. He finds no evidence that analysis by a training analyst is superior to non-training analysts in terms of patient satisfaction or in terms of therapeutic effectiveness. Schachter and his colleagues confirm the findings of two other studies, and there are no others with a different outcome (Schachter et al., 2014). Neither is there evidence that training analysts are better qualified in other educational functions, such as teaching, research, and supervision (see Kernberg, 2000).

It is as though some "x factor" beyond any evidence makes training analysts special. Such idealization might reflect a wish that there is a revealed truth instead of the reality that there are contested claims to truth. Although a science aims at truth, it requires an environment that encourages freedom of inquiry, which does not take for granted an established truth. There are no settled paradigms. The training analyst imago is like that of a priest with a special status conferred beyond functional criteria. The idealization of the perfect analyst might derive from the transferences of the analyst's own training, including unrecognized institutional transferences. Does it provide a false sense of identity with the image of psychoanalytic leaders with perfect training (real or imagined)? In a phrase Leo Rangell was fond of citing, Otto Fenichel writes, "The subject matter not the method of psychoanalysis is irrational" (Fenichel, 1946, p. 5). Berman (2000) points to the utopian fantasy of a New Person in psychoanalytic training that leads to a false and rigid analytic persona that stifles, rather than enhances, creativity and development. The over-reach appears to have the stamp or trademark of authenticity. Perhaps the relentlessly subjective and deconstructive nature of the psychoanalytic enterprise, with its attendant uncertainty, makes the claim to knowledge more difficult to sustain.

When psychoanalytic education changed from being student centered to institute centered, training analysis moved to center stage as a shibboleth (Kirsner, 2010). Instead of creating a trustworthy system that produces and increases trust and confidence, a spiraling paranoiagenic system was created, reinforcing issues such as idealization, splitting, adherence, identification, and denigration. That is, the system itself then produces, reproduces, and increases the level of suspicion and mistrust if the causes are insufficiently recognized and systemically ignored. Such a system undermines trust and shifts focus away from its educational and work tasks. As Kernberg notes, "It is an open secret that the appointment of training analysts is politically motivated, that the actual qualifications of the training analyst may be less important than his or her reliability with regard to local politics" (1986, p. 805).

Is the division between two kinds of analysts legitimate, or even helpful? As Bernfeld observes,

> We possess no way by which we can rationally rank the membership into Good, Very Good and The Best psychoanalysts. Yet strangely, that is exactly what has taken place. The membership of all our groups

> is divided into members who are good enough for the simple paying patient and into really good ones who take care of our future membership. (1962, p. 481)

Training analyst is not a role but became a status, even though there is no specific or intrinsic difference between how candidates and ordinary patients are analyzed. Nonetheless, there are two classes of psychoanalysts. Functions and roles became castes. The selection of the "really good ones", today as ever, does not necessarily relate to psychoanalytic ability. Kernberg highlights the observation of François Roustang, that

> the purpose of psychoanalysis is the resolution of the transference, while the purpose of the training analysis includes the identification with one's training analyst that is a radical contradiction that raises serious questions about the very nature of training analysis that was not seriously explored at that time. (Kernberg, 2014, p. 158)

This tension in the system is a dynamic contradiction that creates a cycle of systemic counterproductive outcomes. Furthermore, according to Kernberg,

> the increase in the number of training analysts that replicated, at international conferences, the division between analysts and training analysts in specialized meetings reserved for the latter, made painfully clear the existence of two levels of competence fostered by the training analysis system. Can we imagine in another profession, say, in cardiology, the existence of two levels of cardiologists, the regular ones, and the training cardiologists, with the understanding that the training cardiologists would be reserving their clinical work to treat ill cardiologists while the general population would have to make do with the ordinary cardiologists. In other words, many cardiologists would never be able to reach the highest level of their profession, they would not be eligible to become training cardiologists because the election of training cardiologists would depend on subjective criteria in the hands of those making the decisions, without any objective criteria for what it would take to ascend to a training cardiologist. And would the educated public, once it was informed of this stratification, seek out the—second string cardiologists? (Kernberg 2014, pp. 158–159)

This artificial distinction erodes trust in the system as delivering credible outcomes and provides still further evidence as to how severely broken the system is which breeds closed-mindedness and authoritarianism and not authority.

The training analysis system can be seen to be a prime illustration of what Elliott Jaques terms a "paranoiagenic" institution, a system that, of its very nature, breeds suspicion and mistrust. Jaques' idea derives from his work with Melanie Klein. Paranoiagenic institutions have structures and processes that stir any deeper-lying suspicion and mistrust, and intensify selfishness, greed, destructive competitiveness, scapegoating, mistrust, and bad working relationships. This does not mean that individual people are paranoid, but that an environment of paranoia, suspicion, and mistrust is produced institutionally. Thus, removing an internal syncretism by itself would have constructive consequences. That then allows members of the institution to exercise their creative energies and ability to learn, supervise, and research without the constraints and obstacles that are working against them in the organization. Paranoiagenic institutions are the opposite of trustworthy ones. For an institution to function effectively, members do not need to like one another, but do need to be able to have grounds to trust one another. That is, the organization would not, of itself, militate against constructive behavior. Another level beyond this is what Jaques terms philogenic institutions, which are trust inducing. As against paranoiagenic processes, such philogenic processes contribute to the possibilities of individuals functioning in relation to each other on the basis of trust and confidence, enhancing trust and confidence in their working relationships (Jaques, 2002). Kernberg quotes an apposite Roman proverb in relation to psychoanalytic institutions: *Senatores boni viri, senatus mala bestia,* which translates as "Senators are good men, but the Senate is a nasty beast" (Kernberg, 2014, p. 166). Structures have consequences that cannot be overcome by individual goodwill alone. This characterizes a paranoiagenic system that militates against its members, even where everyone is doing their best. Art academies and universities are founded on the creativity of their members and, at least in theory, work individually in a bottom-up direction, the reverse of the international structures that sanction training in particular countries. The challenge for psychoanalysis has been to reach out beyond the prevalent closed, internally focused cliques toward an open system where creativity, critique, and diversity are valued.

This involves an emphasis on the priority of local institutes, the "local" not being "authorized" by higher levels any more than universities are. They need to be marketplaces of ideas, institutions in particular cities, countries, and cultures deriving much from their indigenous surroundings and needs rather than being just imported from organizations in other countries and, thereby, receiving a stamp of authenticity. This is the wrong way around. People need to develop their own ways that are sensitive and responsive to their cultures and histories. Others can coach, advise, recommend, but not command and decide (see Kirsner, 2012).

Freud supported the Berlin Institute's research program and the idea of the *Lehranalyse*, the didactic analysis, to "refine the future analyst's mental capacities" or "enrich the personality". As Reeder contends, it is "clear that at least during the first ten years of the Berlin Institute the view of training analysis did not conform with what today would be regarded as 'psychoanalysis proper'" (Reeder, 2004, p. 96). Moreover, as Kächele and Thomä maintain, the Eitingon Berlin model was that of a 'minor university' with a Trinity of teaching, treatment and research which, they claim, 'degenerated into a tripartite training model, in which the pseudo-private personal analysis is at the concealed center of everything' (Kächele & Thomä, 2000, p. 806). Training became a pale shadow of the spirit and direction of the promise of a university model of the Berlin Institute, which, of course, was destroyed with the advent of Nazism. It did not thereafter become a feature of mainstream psychoanalytic education (see Balint, 1948). According to Kächele and Thomä, students can be evaluated solely on the basis of supervision and clinical courses, and it is particularly unethical

> to administer and to request a candidate to undergo a "supertherapy" (Balint) as a prerequisite for his or her profession. The dilemma of the training analysis derives from a confusion between therapeutic goals and professional qualifications. It cannot be the business of educational institutions to make qualifications dependent upon the diagnosis of the person. (p. 807)

Without adopting the university model either inside or outside its institutions, psychoanalysis came to be directed by cliques of insiders against outsiders who were not content to be working within a new field of inquiry but, instead, wanted to be part of a particular set of schools within this field. The insiders' authority was based on no further evidence than that they were anointed by previous insiders. Arbitrariness and subjectivity reigned.

The special type of training involving a training analysis increasingly marked the territory of the uniqueness of the psychoanalytic approach from more general educational methods. Training took place within the established paradigms of the school, and the training analysis evolved into the special path to knowledge and experience that set analysts apart. Students tend to follow their analyst's positions—or sometimes rebel against them. Somehow, the position of training analyst was separated from the rest of the educational endeavor and became reified. The shibboleth of the training analysis demonstrated an esoteric quasi-religious line to knowledge not subject to the normal academic protocols of university-based disciplines, which are generally fields that often include orthodoxies but normally go somewhat beyond them.

As what became the shibboleth of psychoanalytic education, the training analysis helped to entrench particular schools and conformity. Education needs to be organically connected with critique and research, and the training analysis seen as a means to an end of furthering the attitude of what it takes to have a critical and inquiring mind. It involves promoting the virtues of scientific humility, dependent on observation and outcomes instead of faith, belief, and subservience (see Meyer, 2003). This depends upon a facilitating and opening structure instead of one built upon a shibboleth.

The early one or two orthodoxies developed into a plurality of orthodoxies. As Arnold Cooper observes,

> Unfortunately, plurality in itself does not assure an open competition of ideas. In fact, what we have is a growing plurality of orthodoxies that are responsive to authority rather than to data. Kleinians, Kohutians, Bionians, Sullivanians, Lacanians, relationalists, even Freudians—each group sheltered under its own guru, tending to be self-enclosed, self-satisfied, and fighting off all the others. Thought collectives can be amazingly powerful. (Cooper, 2008, p. 250)

There can be a plurality of groups within a psychoanalytic association that are internally structured in the same orthodox way as, for example, a national association. That larger group may be an amalgam of these groupings from the British Psychoanalytic Society to the

IPA, which also has Freudian, Kleinian, and independent groupings constituting it. Even clustering around many different leaders ensures the same foundational organization through the evocation of an esoteric pipeline of anointment. Different *dramatis personae* but the same *modus operandi.*

It is vital for the educational and research system to be respectful and tolerant of different approaches at all levels. In a field without mandatory theories and approaches but with the recognition and respect for difference, even robust differences, a clearing, a mental space is established.

The abolition of the training analyst system would remove a significant roadblock to reshaping and reorienting the culture and ethos of psychoanalytic education. The orthodoxy of the training analyst system has fostered conformity, constraint, and inhibition for decades. Its ending would contribute to creating more open and trust-inducing institutes. These, in turn, would foster creativity by rekindling some of the early spirit of psychoanalytic education prior to the training analyst system. Such a reform would contribute greatly to the capacity of psychoanalytic institutions to effectively address the considerable challenges psychoanalysis faces today.

References

Arlow, J. (1972). Some dilemmas in psychoanalytic education. *Journal of the American Psychoanalytic Association, 20*: 556–566.

Balint, M. (1948). On the psycho-analytic training system. *International Journal of Psychoanalysis, 29*: 163–173.

Balint, M. (1954). Analytic training and training analysis. *International Journal of Psychoanalysis, 35*: 157–162.

Berman, E. (2000). The utopian fantasy of a new person and the danger of a false analytic self. *Psychoanalytic Psychology, 17*: 38–60.

Bernfeld, S. (1962). On psychoanalytic training. *Psychoanalytic Quarterly, 31*: 453–482.

Cooper, A., (2008). American psychoanalysis today: a plurality of orthodoxies. *Journal of the American Academy of Psychoanalysis and Dynamic Psychiatry, 36*(2): 235–253.

Fenichel, O. (1946). *The Psychoanalytic Theory of Neurosis.* London: Routledge and Kegan Paul.

Fenichel, O., Gill, M. M., & Fleming, J. (1980). Theoretical implications of the didactic analysis. *Annual of Psychoanalysis, 8*: 21–35.

Freud, A. (1983). Some observations. In: E. D. Joseph & D. Widlöcher (Eds.), *The Identity of the Psychoanalyst* (pp. 257–263), Monograph 2, IPA. New York: International Universities Press.

Freud, S. (1937c). Analysis terminable and interminable. *S. E., 23*: 209–254. London: Hogarth.

Jaques, E. (2002). *The Life and Behavior of Living Organisms*. Westport, CT: Praeger.

Kächele, H., & Thomä, H. (2000). On the devaluation of the Eitingon–Freud model of psychoanalytic education. *International Journal of Psychoanalysis, 81*: 806–808.

Kairys, D. (1964). The training analysis—a critical review of the literature and a controversial proposal. *Psychoanalytic Quarterly, 33*: 485–512.

Kernberg, O. (1986). Institutional problems of psychoanalytic education. *Journal of the American Psychoanalytic Association, 34*: 799–834.

Kernberg, O. (2000). A concerned critique of psychoanalytic education. *International Journal of Psychoanalysis, 81*: 97–120.

Kernberg, O. (2012). Suicide prevention for psychoanalytic institutes and societies. *Journal of the American Psychoanalytic Association, 60*: 707–719.

Kernberg, O. (2014). The twilight of the training analysis system. *Psychoanalytic Review, 101*: 151–174.

Kirsner, D. (2009). *Unfree Associations: Inside Psychoanalytic Institutes*. New York: Rowman and Littlefield.

Kirsner, D. (2012). All psychoanalysis is local. *Psychotherapy and Politics International, 10*: 146–156.

Knight, R. (1952). The present status of organized psychoanalysis in the United States. *Journal of the American Psychoanalytic Association, 1*: 197–221.

Lewin, B., & Ross, H. (1960). *Psychoanalytic Education in the United States*. New York: Norton.

Meyer, L. (2003). Subservient analysis. *International Journal of Psychoanalysis, 84*: 1241–1262.

Procci, W. (2013). Psychoanalysis and APsaA in the twenty-first century: their fates may be different. *Journal of the American Psychoanalytic Association, 61*: 879–896.

Reeder, J. (2004). *Hate and Love in Psychoanalytic Institutions: The Dilemma of a Profession*. New York: Alton Press.

Schachter, J., Gorman, B., Pfäfflin, F., & Kächele, H. (2014). A questionnaire/interview comparison of satisfaction with training analysis to satisfaction with analysis by a nontraining analyst: implications for training analysis. *Psychoanalytic Psychology, 31*(3): 357–374.

Thomä, H. (1993). Training analysis and psychoanalytic education. *Annual of Psychoanalysis, 21*: 3–75.

CHAPTER NINE

Rethinking psychoanalytic education: some critical points for reflection

Elias Mallet da Rocha Barros

I do not intend to review extensively what happens in the diverse institutes worldwide, but to discuss the question of psychoanalytic education from the perspective of a concerned critique (Kernberg, 1998) and to focus on reflections regarding the different controversies related to the question of transmitting the psychoanalytic way of thinking.

I consider that we are mature enough to think critically about Eitingon's tripartite model that has been adopted by nearly all institutes. This is neither an invitation to discard nor to reaffirm our adherence to this model, but to deepen our understanding of the theory and of the ideology underlying this model, and to invite the psychoanalytic community to reflect on how we are educating the future generations of psychoanalysts.

Nevertheless, while examining the Eitingon's model, we should keep in mind an important remark made by Jacqueline Amati-Mehler (1999) when she said that

> The core issue is not the tripartite side of it (Eitingon's model), but rather how these three legs of the training combine, interact and are interwoven with each other to configure a certain system and the

weight that each of these three variables has, according to different conceptualizations that underlie the training.

All the IPA approved models (Uruguayan, French, and Eitingon's) at present are tripartite, and what varies between them is mainly how these variables interrelate.

Much of what we do is a product of tradition, but perhaps, as a profession, we are now sufficiently mature to be able to examine the basis of the theory we have been using in our educational practices up to now. Considering the amount of critical literature in relation to the classical model, we are surprised to find that no important changes in our basic model have been put into practice. This point merits special study to enable us to understand why resistance to innovation seems to be quite high in this area. I consider that the area of rethinking psychoanalytic education involves throwing light on all the paradoxes it entails. In this way, we can create a collective effort for the renovation of this very special type of education.

When Freud introduced psychoanalysis, his ideas were a complete novelty. He was creating a new field of knowledge, proposing a method of investigation and a therapeutic practice. At that time, psychoanalysis had to be presented as a practice exercised with tremendous rigor, in order to make it acceptable, even more so because it was "learned" outside the university. This rigor was expressed in the creation of training institutes, in Eitingon's proposal, and especially in the guarantee that every analyst had previously been analyzed by a more experienced member approved by the institution.

Today, after over a hundred years of clinical and theoretical practice, psychoanalysis is now part of the shared heritage of human culture. In view of criticism from supporters of the neurosciences and from some epistemologists, as well as from a natural consequence of our own development, we are led to think that we need again to introduce a new rigor in the training process. However, it is quite probable that this ought to be different from the way it has been done so far. Because psychoanalysis is the shared heritage of human knowledge, having entered the academic world and being used by scholars in other areas of knowledge, we who participate in this complex task of training psychoanalysts in our institutes now have a further obligation: to define the specificity of psychoanalytic practice and thinking in relation to other forms of psychological approaches.

For this reason, part of the job of the psychoanalyst engaged in educating our candidates should have an academic character, as we are helping future psychoanalysts to participate in the debates taking place in our social environment and in the university. However, we also have to balance the academic approach with the training and establishment of the specific and special psychoanalytic kind of listening in the therapeutic setting. Thus, a large part of our training function consists in helping to develop and preserve this "analytic ear".

The psychoanalysis taught in universities aims not to train analysts, but particularly to assist the academic community in learning a method and a theory on the constitution of the human mind. I consider that the task of the institutes is to continue to struggle to define the specificity and singularity of the fact of becoming an analyst. Just as we need to deal with the crisis in the cultural and social environment that psychoanalysis is facing, we also need to help future analysts to differentiate between the psychotherapeutic aspect of psychoanalysis and its essentially psychoanalytic aspect.

In view of the demands of contemporary society, what is the function of the institutes? How can we preserve the essence of psychoanalytic attitude and practice and, thereby, also preserve the possibility to continue to investigate the functioning of the human mind more deeply without diluting it in a psychotherapeutic practice whose objective is immediate efficiency? Or, in other words, how can we preserve the psychoanalytic essence of our instrument of investigation of the functioning of the human mind while neither ignoring social demands nor yielding to the pressures of the market?

When we teach psychoanalysis, we are conveying its entire history from Freud onwards, but we are also communicating a very specific kind of attitude and *listening* and, at the same time, an ideal that makes psychoanalysis continue to exist as such. We convey psychoanalytic thinking, difficult to define, but easily recognizable when it is missing.

Our objective as educators is to promote concomitantly the competence and creativity of our candidates.

If we wish to guarantee the survival of psychoanalysis, as a field of knowledge, we certainly cannot consider our preoccupations concerning the quality of the candidates or any training regulation as a necessarily authoritarian exercise. Are there any ways to control quality that can be done democratically, respecting the singularity of analytic practice?

Our preoccupation should be how to avoid authoritarianism, stimulated by the dominant structure of political power in the societies, both formal and informal, so that we can preserve the high quality of psychoanalytic training and the purity of the psychoanalytic method and of clinical practice, while promoting a totally innovative development.

The Association Française de Psychanalyse, for example, when it answered a question from the Committee for Psychoanalytic Education of the IPA (COMPSED) on the organization of its psychoanalytic training, commented: "Our Institute created a system of professional training in which neither the Institution nor any of its members can exert an act of power that is not justified by a theory that governs our system of psychoanalytic training". In this context, *all exercise of power is limited to a process of constant reflection on its meaning* and the power would seem to be exercised without the evils of authoritarianism.

This requires constant reflection in regard to the theory of psychoanalytic training and creates the ideal conditions for psychoanalytic education to be based on something different from simple tradition.

When Freud refers both to training analysis and the model for educating new analysts, he sometimes uses the term *Lehranalyse,* which derives from the words *lehren* and *lernen,* whose meaning is "to teach", while, at other times, he refers to *Ausbildung,* whose semantics field comprises "to construct", "to form".

The diverse connotations given the term that names the process of educating new analysts have also been reflected in the different emphases placed on each of the aspects of the tripartite model (training analysis, supervision, and theoretical seminars) suggested by Max Eitingon in 1922.

Psychoanalysis is a process of subjectivation and, therefore, is opposed to any practice of "teaching". Consequently, it would be much more appropriate to think of it in terms of "psychoanalytic training". Renato Mezan (1991, p. 277) says in this regard,

> Of all the formulas, it seems to me that "training"—as long as it is interpreted on the basis of its origin—concentrates the greatest wealth of connotations, in extension and intensity: it encompasses the pedagogic dimension, the strategic and normative aspect, the question of inheritance and, especially, the profoundly conflictive nature of becoming an analyst. (Translated for this edition)

The author also asks us to give attention to the critique, originating among French psychoanalysts, that shows the paradoxical aspects of psychoanalytic training: "the same procedures destined to ensure that the training of psychoanalysts is good, have the capacity to harm or distort them seriously".

Later, I will discuss in more detail this question of the possibility of distorting the ideology underlying the use of the model of mothering, totally inadequate in my view, as a model for psychoanalytic education based on the same model (misleading, too, I believe) for the psychoanalytic session. The institutions that imperceptibly assimilated this model seem to represent the world as constituted by ill-cared-for children, lacking in attention from their mothers, misunderstood and defenseless. This model is extremely attractive because, with this type of clientele (abandoned children), there is practically no way to be wrong in what is offered. Thus, psychoanalytic work is simple, creates no conflict, and produces no great anxiety. The main objective is to produce immediate relief instead of facing the tensions inherent to any process of transformation, meaning that it tallies with the demands of consumer society. Actually, in the short term, effective analysis tends to provoke a feeling of discomfort because it interferes with a fragile and defensive equilibrium that is well maintained. Relief is the product of slow and progressive integration, the result of long analytic work.

The model, based on mothering, is simplistic. Practice is dissociated from theory, which might even be disqualified as being unnecessary. In this context, certain concepts tend to be trivialized or simplified. Examples of that are the concepts of "containing" and "holding", which lose their heuristic value when they are removed from all their rich complexity. These concepts become synonymous with "patience" and "reassurance" and lose, in this simplistic context, their core meaning associated with the promotion of transformations by means of enabling critical thinking. Psychoanalytic education following this simplistic model is then carried out by simple identifications with the great master and the more fashionable training analysts of the institute who are rarely questioned. Up to this point, the model, in the short term, looks attractive because of the simple fact that it does not provoke anxiety. However, I should say, it also does not produce a passionate relationship with psychoanalysis, the revolutionary approach to the mind created by Freud.

The exploration of transference in the psychoanalytical setting, over the hundred years of psychoanalytic practice, has allowed us to understand much better how our experiences are internalized and how our reason is educated and developed by a process of learning with experience. Emotions underlie our sensibility and reason. The process of our education cannot be dissociated from our sensibility.

I use the term sensibility in two senses: (1) the skill for perceiving and feeling and (2) mental responsiveness, including the capacity to respond to esthetic stimuli.

Susan Langer (1980, p. 27) comments that only people who have skill for artistic discernment are capable of being enthused by the perception of forms. These persons possess a kind of intuitive awareness to grasp the fact that feelings are inherent to each imaginary form. The development of the skill for artistic discernment mentioned by Langer is intimately linked to increased sensibility in relation to the meaning of emotional experiences as well.

I consider that this characteristic, which Langer called "intuitive awareness", is also important in the process of selection of candidates for psychoanalytic training.

We know quite well that it is not enough to go through experiences for a person to change; it is also necessary to understand them. This means that the transforming element that leads to a broadening of sensibility, to an education of sensibility, is the fusion of the experience with its emotional meaning, a process that makes it thinkable. This process is necessarily conflicted because it forces a standoff between the conservative tendencies—which resist any alteration of subjectivity—and the new elements appropriated by the self that transform the essence of being.

The process of acquisition of knowledge is relational and deeply marked by the meaning acquired by the emotional experience associated with the process of knowing that defies the *status quo*. Knowing cannot be reduced to the process of acquisition of information. Above all, it is an activity that modifies the person's way of being, because it places the individual in the position of facing the new, in an attempt to make it something of his/her own. The feelings must be processed as thoughts if sensibility is to be broadened. To *construct* oneself as an analyst is not the outcome of a process of harmonic development. It consists, above all else, in accepting a great challenge: to confront the new, to be face to face with otherness, to access the unknown—all of which create conflict with the more conservative forces of our personalities. The tendency to maintain the *status quo* is recurrent in our personalities. In the position of psychoanalysts–educators (be it as supervisors, faculty members, or just as analysts), we are constantly called to exert the function of containers of these conflicts, for which we should always be on the alert.

I owe Dr. Miguel De La Puente (1993, p. 343) a reflection, which I consider illustrative, on the etymology of the word "knowledge". Dr. De La Puente says,

> To know is a word that derives from Latin, from the word cognoscere, which in turn took its meaning from the Greek verb (which exists only in the present tense of the indicative mode) konnein, which means to know. More exactly, konneo has a meaning composed by the word koinós (kon) "common" and the adverbial (koinê) "in common", and by noein (nein which means "to understand". Therefore, to know means to understand with someone, in common. It is a communicative act that involves noetic aspects (from noein) and affective aspects (kon originated the Latin preposition cum).

In this way, human knowledge is seen as something that is generated, not eternal and in itself, and is done with someone. *Human knowledge is not; it becomes*. From this derives the meaning of learning.

The process of psychoanalytic education involves a great transformation of the candidate's emotional structure. This transformation is not only an objective to be achieved; it is the very condition for an individual to become an analyst.

Neuroscientists suggest that the brain's neurochemical system always reacts to the new. When new information reaches the brain, its cells release a mechanism in the memory files for a search of the correlative registers that have been obtained during the individual's lifetime. If the person has not had this type of meaningful experience registered on the different temporal levels of memory, from the most recent to the oldest, there is emotional impoverishment. If meaningful experiences are not found, the person no longer feels sadness or joy and his or her experience of life is marked by a void, a lack of meaning. Of all the mental functions, memory contributes the most to giving meaning to the present. The wealth of memory is what keeps the past alive. These discoveries are in the same line as the ideas of Bion, who suggested that the most important opposition in mental life is not between opposed feelings (such as love and hate, for example), but between emotion and opposition to emotion.

These discoveries suggest that psychoanalysis is correct when it underscores that experiences must be associated to meanings if they are to be assimilated and produce mental growth.

Psychoanalytic education demands a great variety of life experiences. It is said in London that Anna Freud answered a girl who asked her how she could become an analyst by saying that she should read the great works of universal literature, watch the best films, the exhibitions of humanity's greatest artists, go to the theatre, travel a lot, and meet people.

The unconscious fantasies interpreted by the psychoanalyst in the session are expressions of unconscious ways of shaping the relational world according to certain patterns in the internal world, organized around meaningful nuclei of emotional experience.

The interpretation is a way to introduce analysands to themselves and to create the conditions for them to recover lost aspects of their experiences and mental functions, and, thus, become persons able to observe themselves. Interpretations are not true or false. They are relevant or irrelevant, plausible or not, effective or ineffective. Validating an interpretation ultimately depends on the patient, on how he listens to it, and how he reacts on the unconscious level. What the supervisor can offer to the analyst in training is to listen to how he hears the patient's response to the candidate's interpretation. By proceeding in this manner, the supervisor is evaluating the plausibility and coherence of the candidate's listening. It is from this perspective that, in our opinion, supervision becomes an activity to contain analytic experiences on the symbolic level.

Through successive insights, analysands experience a varied spectrum of emotional states and become familiar with the different aspects of their personalities, becoming more tolerant of psychic states that they had been avoiding up to that time. This experience leads them to greater integration. In this perspective, to know one's self is to change. We could add that this change takes place through a process of education of the sensibility that broadens the spectrum of emotions so that we are able to perceive and differentiate meaning. The understanding of the meaning of emotional experiences acts as a key that opens new affective networks. The education of sensibility in this context has nothing to do with pedagogical processes. It is an agogic activity, based only on the fact of guiding and showing, in contexts in which experiences acquire meaning for the analysand. In this way, a pedagogy inspired by psychoanalysis would have an agogic character directed less to information and much more to the meaning of the experience in the process of its acquisition.

Noam Chomsky refers to the recursive function of language, meaning the capacity to understand words never heard before. I think that a successful analysis, and also a good enough educational process, establishes what we could call, in metaphoric terms, a recursive function of the psyche, or the capacity to understand the meaning of new experiences while experiencing them, which saves us from disorganization of our systems of representation.

To be educated in psychoanalytic terms, in the perspective described above, depends, in the first place, on the existence of a life rich in emotional experiences that are broadened by association with their meanings on the domain of thought. This process constantly broadens sensibility, an essential instrument for both analytic practice and the development of creative thinking.

As I have said at the beginning of this chapter, our present dissatisfaction with the way we are educating the new generations of psychoanalysts stems, in part, from the fact that, since its establishment in 1920 (with the introduction of training analysis), the model of psychoanalytic education has not been modified, while the world around us has changed almost to the point of being unrecognizable for someone who might emigrate directly from 1920 to our day.

This model was inspired by the teaching of medicine, which dissociated the learning of theory from the learning of clinical work. One part of what was taught was given in the amphitheatres with the structure of a formal lecture (theories) and another part was given in the wards, in contact with the patients (clinical practice), under the guidance of an experienced professor who diagnosed with his "clinical eye", a product of a mixture of former experience, intuition, and theoretical knowledge about the human body and its pathologies.

I believe that we can say that, even in this twenty-first century, theory and practice have a tendency to be split in the teaching of both medicine and psychoanalysis.

The emphasis on clinical psychoanalytic training has very positive aspects, but it has encouraged the "trade" side of psychoanalytic practice. What I mean is that psychoanalysis has become a liberal profession, and the psychoanalyst, a self-employed professional offering services to the public. In this environment, interest in critical reflection and investigative work decreased notably. An analyst, in my perspective, is always in the state of becoming.

Herrmann (1996, p. 39) answered the following question: "Are we still Freudian?" by saying,

> The real problem is becoming Freudian in the strong sense of the word, which means being able to produce psychoanalysis with the freedom and scope with which Freud produced it. Above all, it is a goal, not a point of departure. It is a place I wish to attain, not a place where I choose to stay. It is an objective to become Freudian. (Translated for this edition)

André Green (1991), at the Training Congress in Buenos Aires, commented that it is not only a question of training future analysts what they must know in order to be able to face new situations based on general principles (the basis of theoretical teaching), in order to be able to become analysts, but, above all, it is fundamental to stimulate them so that they are always reflecting on "the analysis of analytic theory" (p. 3).

To recover the inspiration and passion that colored the beginnings of psychoanalysis, in my view, will be possible only if we develop an investigative mentality that feeds reflection and promotes the development of the psychoanalytic model. The great enemy of this attitude is a kind of benevolent acceptance of the differences, a type of conceptual indifference that does not enrich thought and keeps us in a state of intellectual somnolence. We have a tendency to base ourselves on authors we adopt, even our own selves, without subjecting our thinking to critical examination.

Rethinking the theory of psychoanalytic education implies finding ways to promote an investigative mentality that challenges, that relates to the theories, *stressing their divergent aspects* and their insertion in the history of psychoanalysis and in the history of culture. I believe that the acritical acceptance of pluralism without ever arguing about what we agree with and what we disagree with fosters a state of theoretical sleepiness.

Bhaskar (1978, p. 3) suggests that there are generating structures that will be known rather by inference based on their effects than from the sum of observations performed, considering that this description is the one which best characterizes the mode of accumulation and validation of knowledge in psychoanalysis.

Psychoanalysis, as a theoretic–practical construct, is based on the idea that there are structures (conceived as generating by Bhaskar) underlying consciousness, dynamically "hidden" (existing in the form of states of mind expressing object relations) from the latter, which generate effects on the way of perceiving and feeling in our patients' world of relations. These structures produce effects in the form of feelings, perceptions, and modes of thinking. Without this conception of the existence of hidden structures, we would have little to offer our patients besides sympathy and comments based on common sense.

Kernberg (1986) considers that psychoanalytic education combines practices that include the model of academic teaching, the type of learning found in the trades, and that of a young artist in an *atelier* with a master artist and, also, the learning given in a religious seminar. The author, in this text and recently in a highly productive and broadly encompassing article (Kernberg, 1998), emphasizes the academic character of psychoanalytic knowledge, marked by critical examination, thirsting for innovation and colored by an artistic type of inspiration.

Because psychoanalysis is essentially conveyed through personal analysis, a fertile ground represented by the transference is established for indoctrination, based on affiliations and hierarchical structures of descendants in relation to founders. In this context, psychoanalysis simultaneously combines a great exposure of the self in the diverse contexts where it is conveyed—personal analysis, supervision—with the need for systematization controlled by an institution whose objective is to protect the individual in training from this exposure and also his or her future patients from an intervention in the subject's individuality that can either positively reconstruct or destroy them.

Michael Rustin (1991, p. 90) comments on this matter,

> The psychoanalytic organizations, as well as two-person psychoanalytic relationships, have to combine these opposed characteristics of highly personal and idiosyncratic modes of work-each analysis being different from every other-with the need to maintain a permanent predictable institutional form.

John Stuart Mill (1991[1859]) believed that whatever restrictions were placed on the individual in the form of normative regulations, or even in the form of laws or opinions, were justifiable only if they were based, formally or informally, on *a principle* rather than preferences or prejudices of sectors of the reigning power. The control of individual behavior, exercised by an institution, was only justifiable if it served to "prevent damage to another" or to avoid a person provoking ill to another. This ideology had a significant impact on the shaping of modern democratic societies.

Within this context, the psychoanalytic institutions have oscillated historically between a perspective that placed emphasis on the need for institutional control and another that accentuated the importance of intuition, originality, creativity, freedom from regulatory intervention, which they consider kills creativity. After attending several meetings on models of psychoanalytic education in recent years, I have often been surprised to find that the discussions were limited to a possible opposition between a so-called democratic organization of psychoanalytic training and another considered authoritarian. The first model is based on a minimum of regulations. This model of training is supposed to omit any kind of evaluation of quality. To my mind, it often leads to a loose structure that is a source of confusion for candidates. The other system is described as being highly regulated, based on constant preoccupation with the quality of the analysts being trained and viewed, in this context, as antidemocratic and authoritarian.

At first, in view of this polarization, it is easy to understand that due to the dominant political ideology of our modern societies, the sytem defined as democratic would be the one to have most supporters.

Nonetheless, it seems to me that the training problems we are facing are far more complex than those contemplated by this simple opposition.

Actually, the option for the democratic system and for the absence of quality control is a response to the authoritarian atmosphere, which is thought to infantilize and inhibits the development of new knowledge. The solution, on the other hand, seems to me too simplistic, both in its diagnosis of the situation of crisis in respect to our conception of psychoanalytic education as well as the solution proposed.

I think that some of the questions we have to face today are:

1. How can we create regulations that only set norms in order to safeguard the training process without making it rigid?
2. How can we avoid the destructive effects of authoritarianism and indoctrination, aspects that are enemies of creative thinking, and, at the same time, maintain the high quality of psychoanalytic education?

This dilemma has no simple solution.

In 1991, at the Fifth Conference of Training Analysts, the theme debated was "Between Chaos and Petrification", which is still an expression of the dilemmas we are facing.

I consider that the themes discussed in our Conferences of Training Analysts since its beginnings seem to be a nearly inevitable consequence of our dissatisfaction with the tripartite model adopted in 1922, following Max Eitingon's proposal.

However, to this day we have not found a substitute model, although our dissatisfaction with the way of preparing future generations of psychoanalysts has grown. The IPA's recognition of the existence of two other educational models besides Eitingon's represents, in my view, a step forward and against old ways of thinking, but it has not solved the problem of the quality of the psychoanalytic training of new generations.

Today's epistemological crisis in psychoanalysis will have a fortunate outcome, meaning that it will result in the deepening of the psychoanalytic model, only if we make radical changes in the way we educate future generations of psychoanalysts.

Kernberg (1998) insists on the need to create the conditions to make psychoanalysis more attractive so that the most brilliant intellectuals of our generation will be encouraged to join our training institutes.

Widlöcher (1997) comments that the university students with whom he works even have some liking for psychoanalysis, but that this positive attitude is not enough to persuade them that it is worth the effort to seek a deepening of their experience through a psychoanalytic experience. People, even those in the academic world, feel familiar enough with psychoanalytic concepts to recognize that they can contribute something new besides a simplistic explanation of the ways human beings feel.

Could it be that the analysts, especially we who are involved in the training of new generations, are partly responsible for this loss of interest? Could it be that we ourselves have lost sight of the singularity and specificity of the analytic experience? Do we continue to believe that the analytic experience is unique and surprising? Do we still have the conviction that the feeling that accompanies an important insight has the quality of something new and unique?

Perhaps part of the responsibility for the impoverishment of psychoanalytic reflection and the conception of psychoanalytic education can be attributed to a certain deformed and restricted interpretation of the theories of object relations. This has encouraged a vision of psychoanalysis based on mothering, as I have previously mentioned, instead of using psychoanalysis to understand mothering itself.

Another deleterious aspect of the unconscious model of education unconsciously based on the exercise of mothering makes the need to investigate, to reflect critically, and understand the modes of functioning and manifestation of the unconscious, disappear. How often do we hear, in the most contrasting psychoanalytic institutions, in order to justify criticism of candidates or to soothe them when they doubt their talent, that neither intelligence nor knowledge of theory is necessary for being a mother? In this case, the idea is that it is enough to have intuition and sensibility. This example is paradigmatic to understand how the model of mothering invaded the conception of what it is to be a psychoanalyst. Our field has been so deeply marked by this idea that today it even sounds disagreeable to say that to be a psychoanalyst it is not enough to be intuitive and sensitive, but also to be intelligent, to know the theory well, and to have theoretical questions in order to constantly question psychoanalytic practice.

The model of what a psychoanalytic session is, as well as what psychoanalytic training is, had become simplistically based on the model of the mother–infant relationship, as I suggested at the beginning of this chapter, as if this is the single necessary condition to establishing the possibility of analysis of the oedipal situation. Without being aware of the consequences, we abandoned the model of the session based on the concept of formation of the unconscious, constituted similarly to dream work. The interpretation stopped existing, as such, and was replaced by a kind of maternal benevolence that operates in some parts of the world under the name of a pseudo-Bionian term that explains and justifies everything: "containment".

If the situation had not acquired such proportions, it would be unnecessary to stress that the Bionian concept of containment has nothing to do with this type of conception. For Bion, containing is not a synonym of accepting, good intentions, soothing, or patience; containing is transforming meanings whose model is the operation of the unconscious that, at first, transforms drive pressure into mental representation.

I consider that the key idea, on the basis of which we can think about the question of contemporary clinical work and psychoanalytic education, is related to the conditions of establishment of the analytic situation. Therefore, it is not a question of reforming just the formal aspects of psychoanalytic training, but the entire conception of what training is. It is important for us to spend time on the basic concepts we convey, explaining their complexities.

Rethinking psychoanalytic education implies reflecting again on the whole scientific life of a society. In 1998, in a panel discussion coordinated by Pulver, at a meeting of the American Psychoanalytic Association, entitled "The system of training analysis: Asset or liability?", nearly all those present spoke out in favor of a complete and radical review of our current system of psychoanalytic training (Masur, 1997).

Luiz Meyer (2003) suggests at several meetings of the Brazilian Society of Psychoanalysis of São Paulo and elsewhere that the training analysis is a fetish, and that the training analysis is a form of ideological indoctrination, producing deep emotional splits and intellectual immobilization among analysts. I think that when Dr. Meyer calls our attention to the danger of ideological indoctrination via training analysis, he has a point that deserves our deep reflection. However, Robert Michels and Elizabeth Auchincloss (1999) have argued, in the discussion of their presentation at the Nice Conference, that the elimination of the position of training analyst does not eliminate power and authority but *only redistributes* them. Excessive authoritarianism, in psychoanalytic education arises not from the existence of hierarchical structures such as those of the centralized curriculum committee or the training analyst position, but primarily from (1) the complete condensation of all important functions into the single position of the training analyst and (2) the lack of an agreed upon methodology for determining the validity of our theoretical propositions.

> It is true that we have no agreed upon strategy for deciding who possesses knowledge in our Institutes where a single professional role

> (training analyst) is so venerated, ambitious students are socialized to imagine that they can close the gap between their relative ignorance and the omniscience of the training analyst not by inquiring into the nature of mental life but by striving to become training analysts themselves. As scientific curiosity collapses into professional ambition, the "authority" of the training analyst position is further exalted and the intellectual life of our Societies and Institutes becomes impoverished. (Auchincloss & Michels, 2003, p. 397)

It seems to me that the solution to these problems does not lie in attempts to obliterate all gaps in expertise and status by doing away with hierarchical structures altogether, whether in curriculum planning, in the training analyst system, or in overall governance. There is no reason to believe that the denial of differences in knowledge and ability can reinvigorate the intellectual life of our field.

I am in agreement again with Michels and Auchincloss (2003, p. 398) when they said at the Nice Conference of Training analysts that we must direct our energies not toward eliminating all gaps "but toward situating our experience of a gap in the area where it most belongs: between what we psychoanalysts and psychoanalytic students feel we already know and understand about mental life and what we do not yet know." I want to suggest that what is important is to keep alive, in all the procedures that constitute training, an investigative mentality. Only curiosity will keep alive a passionate relationship with psychoanalysis.

Agreeing with this point of view suggests an invitation to work at our clinics with a research-oriented attitude, not in the positivistic sense, but in the sense of action-research (Lakatos, 1978, pp. 128–200): for instance concerning the clinical material of the session, trying to collect data in such a way as to allow them to be compared, and to submit them to the shared observation test.

Meanwhile, in view of the push for innovation, we must be extremely careful not to submit to market pressures and to the demands of consumer society. If we do submit, our training system will be directed and guided by the market, even though its medium may be an institute of psychoanalysis.

Creativity in psychoanalysis must not be interpreted as simply a synonym of innovation, of creating something that leads it away from its foundations. There is a dialectic relation between the new and what grounds psychoanalytic knowledge. The positive crisis that can occur is one that demands a constant return to the foundations of psychoanalysis, just as Laplanche proposes.

I want to believe that the current crisis in our system of psychoanalytic education is positive and will lead us to re-examine the set of theoretical bases that inspire the setting in which education takes place.

The formal aspects of the analytic situation (number of sessions, the use or not of the couch, etc.) are what Pierre Fédida (1992, p. 77) elegantly called "our theoretical materiality". This phrase is quite useful because it sums up a large field of reflection by indicating that our clinical practice (our materiality) is the metapsychological expression of a model (the theoretical expression) of the psyche that continues to highlight the dialectic relation between theory and practice.

In my opinion, we must effect a rigorous and profound examination of the theoretical, philosophical, and ideological bases of the setting adopted in the process of training psychoanalysts. Paul Israel (1994, p. 34) considers that we must find, in each institute, what he refers to as "the most invisible thread that connects the theoretical consistency of our work both to clinical practice as well as to our training system".

I would like to emphasize that when I invite our community to reflect on the bases of psychoanalytic education, I am not suggesting that any particular model is better than another and, above all, it is not an invitation to stretch the old models.

The adoption of a radical viewpoint at this historical moment has been easily mistaken for the choice of an attitude of *laissez faire, laissez passer*.

Innovation that is not submitted to rigorous examination of the bases of psychoanalysis will involve the risk of paralyzing the positive crisis that characterizes our field of knowledge. Being revolutionary in psychoanalysis means setting out to examine radically what grounds it, with the awareness that psychoanalysis is not technical knowledge that can be adapted to consumer demands, but is knowledge concerning the essence of the human being.

References

Amati-Mehler, J. (1999). Verbal intervention at the Nice Training Conference.

Auchincloss, E., & Michels, R. (2003). A reassessment of psychoanalytic education: controversies and changes. *International Journal of Psychoanalysis, 84*: 387–403.

Bhaskar, R. (1978). *A Realist Theory of Science*. Brighton: Harvester.

De La Puente, M. (1993). Sobre a palavra-conceito "conhecimento" para uso clínico. *Revista Brasileira de Psicanálise, 26*: 341–344.

Fédida, P. (1992). *Nome, Figura e Memória*. São Paulo: Editora Escuta.

Green, A. (1991). Preliminaries to a discussion of the function of theory in psychoanalytic training. Unpublished manuscript. Fifth International Psychoanalytical Association Conference of Training Analysts, Buenos Aires.

Herrmann, F. (1996). Análise didática em tempos de penúria teórica. *Jornal de Psicanálise, 54*: 33–42.

Israel, P. (1994). Some specific features of the psycho-analytic training. *Psychoanalysis in Europe, 42*: 29–37.

Kernberg, O. (1986). Institutional problems of psychoanalytic education. *Journal of the American Psychoanalytic Association, 34*: 799–834.

Kernberg, O. (1998). A concerned critique of psychoanalytic education. Unpublished manuscript.

Lakatos, I. (1978). The problem of appraising scientific theories: three approaches. In: *Mathematics, Sciences and Epistemology. Philosophical Papers, 2*. Cambridge: Cambridge University Press.

Langer, S. (1980). *Sentimento e Forma*. São Paulo: Editora Perspective.

Masur, C. (1997). The training analyst system: asset or liability? *Journal of the American Psychoanalytic Association, 46*: 539–549.

Meyer, L. (2003). Subservient analysis. *International Journal of Psychoanalysis, 84*(5): 1241–1262.

Mezan, R. (1991). O Bildungsroman do psicanalista. *Anuário Brasileiro de Psicanálise*. Río de Janeiro: Relume Dumará.

Michels, R., & Auchincloss, E. (1999). Keynote paper presented to the Nice Training Conference. Unpublished paper.

Mill, J. S. (1991). *Sobre a Liberdade*. Petrópolis: Vozes (originally published in 1859).

Rustin, M. (1991). *The Good Society and the Inner World*. London: Verso.

Widlöcher, D. (1997). Psychoanalysis: Challenges in university and research. *International Journal of Psychoanalysis, 84*: 387–403.

CHAPTER TEN

Training analysis as institutional enactment

Luiz Meyer

Over the past fifteen years, the training analysis issue, defined recently by Wallerstein (2010) as "psychoanalysis' perennial problem", whose history Balint (1948) classified as melancholic and around which an adverse literature continues to grow, has been of special interest to me. What first drew me to this was a bizarre happening of an anti-analytic nature: a colleague who had been in analysis for some years and finding it deeply beneficial, found himself obliged—actually, pressured—to change his analyst from the moment he decided to pursue his psychoanalytic training. He could do this only if he had an analyst who was recognized by the Institution. The violence of this situation led me to investigating this facet of training, and, related to this issue, I wrote various articles questioning its nature, its functioning, and the very need for it to exist (Meyer, 2002, 2003, 2007, 2008). The present work as a continuity to this critical posture aims to show how training analysis is structured and functions in the mode of enactment. The chapter comprises four sections.

In the first section (based on my former work), I describe, on the one hand, how training analysis is habitually perceived in the current literature and, on the other, my own way of conceiving its structure, *modus operandi*, and reasons for permanence.

In the second section, aiming to make clearer the distortion present in training analysis, I contrast it with the very basic and common aspects of analysis *tout court*.

In the third section, I summarise the best known descriptions of enactment. As a result of having this background to the concept, the reader can more readily appreciate the theme approached in the fourth section: enactment and training analysis.

Following these four steps, I provide information on the subject matter of this chapter so that, at its end, my own concepts and the conclusions I have reached arise logically from the articulation between the sections.

Training analysis: its polemic image, structure, and form of functioning

From the very start—that is, historically—training analysis presents itself as a category apart, superior, and the aristocratic aura with which it is enveloped promotes and sustains the creation of an oligarchic and authoritarian group. It gives rise not only to two types of analysis, but also to two types of analyst: those good enough for the simple paying patient and the really good ones who take care of the future members (Bernfeld, 1962). Therefore, its discourse, as the conveyor of "analytic truth", follows a model of educational messianism, bringing about the fusion of the idealization of the analyst with the School he follows and preaches, not uncommonly in a persecutory tone (not always veiled), to obtain the desired adhesion. Auchincloss and Michels (2003) shed light on the process, stating that "*the control* of educational structures remains the most important measure of intellectual and/or professional success for the majority of psychoanalysts" (p. 387, my italics). For these authors, excessive authoritarianism in psychoanalytic education is due mainly to "the complete condensation of all important professional functions into the single position of the training analyst, the attainment of which signifies eminence in all possible parameters of expertise" (p. 396). Thus, the position of training analyst as they put it, "entitles the person to claim authority and control over all intellectual, scientific, clinical, supervisory, pedagogic and administrative matters" (p. 396). They add further that our present system

> creates an overwhelming gap between the training analyst and the candidate[1] of a different and more serious kind as our candidates are educated to believe that the training analyst is not only all powerful but all knowing. (p. 397)

And, perhaps even more tellingly, they go on,

> In a world where . . . a single professional role is so venerated, ambitious students *are socialized* to imagine that they can close the gap between their relative ignorance and the omniscience of the training analyst not by inquiring into the nature of mental life but by striving to become training analysts themselves. As scientific curiosity collapses into professional ambition, the 'authority' of the training analyst position is further exalted. (Auchincloss & Michels, 2003, p. 397, my italics)

It is clear from this extract that this prescribed route—the socialization of candidates towards acquiring in the future the omniscience attributed to the training analysts—is independent of, and transcends, the personal characteristics constituting the candidate–training analyst dyad. The structure that organizes training analysis precedes and dominates individual particularities, as it functions ideologically. The extinction of scientific curiosity is not an epiphenomenon of the relation but, rather, a central element, necessary for maintaining the system that has its own reproduction as its aim.

Thus, the narrowing down of all pathways into that of power and prestige is favored in the direction of what Kernberg (2001) calls "the monolithic career path", which, according to Auchincloss and Michels (2003), "creates the experience of an overwhelming gap in professional status" between training and non-training members, between candidates and training analysts. Concomitantly, the power acquired by the training analyst facilitates his propensity to gratify his own emotional and narcissistic needs and the wish to be admired, for such availing himself of the candidate, to whom in this context he tends to turn into the severe and punitive judge or the absorbing seducer, presented as the ideal model, bearer of the right theory, and, in the event of victorious acceptance, tempting the candidate in return with a profitable future relation (McLaughlin, 1987; see also Greenacre, 1966).

When the focus is on the candidates' position, it is commonly observed that they seek analysis for training purposes, whereas patients *tout court* do so to be helped (McLaughlin, 1987). The candidate, in effect, plays the part of captive audience and font of survival (and identity) of the training analyst (Nacht, 1954). In contrast to the patient in analysis *tout court*, who can, and is seen to, express his discomfort and hostility towards the analyst abandoning or interrupting analysis at the peak of negative transference, the candidate linked with an institute hardly ever does so (Freud, A., 1938; Nacht, 1954). For the candidate, escape is practically impossible, as he is bound to analysis by needs that do not necessarily express themselves through the transferential channel. The dependence he experiences is not intrinsic to the dynamics of the analytic process as is, for example, that revealed in narcissistic wounding while confronting the constancy of the analytic attitude. On the contrary, it is linked with the candidate's need to reach his didactic aim (the candidate should not, or cannot, forget that he is "in training").

It is a type of analysis whose organization leads to personal identification of the candidate with his analyst (the expert), evading the conflicts inherent to the very creation of the analytic field. This identification, linked with the difficulty of working through the transference in training analysis, is one of the *leitmotifs* of the works consulted (Freud, A., 1938; Kernberg, 2000; McLaughlin, 1987). The research underscores that the identification of the candidate with the training analyst happens "in reality", bringing about a fusion between the infantile determinants of the transference and those inherent in the formal undertaking of the training analysis. One of the aspects of this reality is the need that each member of the dyad—"candidate in training" and training analyst—has of the other in ensuring their statutory position in the institution (Araico, 1992). An extra-analytic, mutual dependence is thus created, generating a continual negotiation towards keeping intact the "didactic" dynamics of the work under way (Whiting, 1996).

The admissions system (of the institutes in charge of training) also works so as to choose personalities that fit into the ongoing reproductive system.

By its very nature, training analysis allows for no path other than "success", the evaluation of which, incidentally, is carried out by domains external to it. The atmosphere enveloping the training analyst–candidate pair is one of coercion. There will be success for the training analyst if the candidate's analysis is successful. This situation, in its turn, puts the candidate in the position of interposed pawn, be it in the conflicts and competition or in the alliances that the training analyst experiences and establishes with his colleagues. If, for the candidate, it is required that analysis be with a training analyst, the latter, in his turn, receives from the institution the job of carrying it through and answering for it (which is not necessarily expressed in the regulations). This pressures the training analyst into measuring his production against that of his colleagues, a pressure that is passed on to the candidate, forcing him to act as showcase (Gomberoff, 2002) for the advances analysis is promoting in him. Actually, paraphrasing the renowned phrase of Freud's on mourning, it may be said that the shadow of the institution falls on training analysis (Araico, 1992), transforming it into the standard analysis (Herrmann, 1993) and the training analyst into the model analyst. Training analysis becomes, thus, a concrete representation of the split between explicit training objectives and actual models of administrative structures (Kernberg, 1992). In his passionate diatribe exposing training analysis to execration, presented in Chicago on November 10 1952, six months before his death, Bernfeld shows how, in the hands of the institution, training analysis had turned into a mere instrument for fulfilling legal contrivances, an activity regulated by decree, fostering and controlling the continual discovery of the already known. Its practice—reaching beyond all described above—ends up emptying the analytic relation of its essence, substituting it by formal, adapting, stratifying rules.

I shall now characterize those elements that make up the training analysis structure; that is, which characterize the dynamics of its functioning and can be detected, so to speak, through transparency, between the lines of criticisms directed at it in the series of works dealing with the subject.

We can see that training analysis brings to the foreground the institutional function and the mythical aspect of the analyst, relegating the analytic process *per se* to a secondary or instrumental position (Araico, 1992). Upon the training analyst's identity (turned functional in this case) being sustained by an organization, he finds himself obliged to speak for it. Thus, his word gains an authoritarian, extra-analytic connotation, which will tend to obscure and co-opt the work of analysis of transference.

If, in analysis *tout court*, the analyst works carefully towards the emergence and maintenance of conditions that favor the development of the analytic process, in training analysis this care is turned to the need to give to the analysis its didactic character. Put another way: the discovery of the analytic method, of its potential and transgressive action, tends, in training analysis, to be overshadowed by the repetition of the demands of the institute. Within this framework, training analysis gains the status of an autonomous reality, extrinsic to the pair, preceding and steering it. It is this *structural circumstance* that, in a certain way, invalidates the "good" criteria, meritocratic or democratic, for the selection or nominating of the training analyst. No matter what their good personal qualities, the "good" selected analysts will work within, and forcibly so, a culture ruled by the principles of the training analysis.

Analysis *tout court* is also immersed in a cultural universe with which it interacts and which gives it meaning. However, in the case of training analysis, there is yet another background, represented by the training analysis *project*, which tends to superimpose itself and reign supreme over all other influences.

It is unlikely that, of their own volition, the candidate–training analyst pair will separate, since, while remaining united, they hold a grand hope infused by mutual idealization which allows them the sense that together they can overcome Thanatos, since they possess or generate between them sufficient neutralizing Eros (Gomberoff, 2002). Here, separation (in the sense of awareness of ambivalent and/or negative feelings) would correspond to acknowledgement of limitations and the disruption of idealization. One of the obstacles present in training analysis previously described is the "realistic" character of transference, which forces identification of the candidate with the analyst, who is, most of the time, idealized. It might be objected that in an analysis *tout court* of a person interested in becoming an analyst, a similar identification can occur, since the analyst is also representative of an aspect of the patient's ego ideal. It so happens that the analyst *tout court* is not a specialist in the training of aspiring candidates and his practice is not linked with an institutional commitment. Analysis of this type is freer to concentrate on the transferential aspects related to this ego ideal and to questioning it. Such questioning is, however, hard to realize in training analysis, for, were it to arise, it would be directed at the very project that provides the *raison d'être* of the pair, threatening it.

Identification "in reality" refers to the verification that, in training, the training analyst is, in fact (institutionally), presented as an ideal object and the training analysis as a means of attaining analytic identity (Gálvez, 2002). Identification on the candidate's part happens with the person and the ideology of the training analyst, as well as the infrastructure supporting him. This is one of the ways in which the mythical aspect of the person of the analyst comes to the fore (as already mentioned), functioning as such as an obstacle to the introjection of the *analytic function*. It is this same perception of the structural aspect of training analysis that allows us to understand how innocuous is the proposal to examine in detail the intent or phantasy of the candidate in becoming an analyst. The problem does not lie in the subject's phantasy, but in the response this phantasy receives when the analysis is didactic. Inserted in an institutional, that is, regulatory, context, the ending point of the process is already defined from the starting point. Within this, the candidate under analysis simply revalidates the power with which the training analyst is invested, as well as the gamut of theories the latter professes. As such, a collusion is created by means of which the candidate inserts himself in the power scheme, guaranteeing for himself in the future the place which today belongs to the training analyst; the analyses repeat themselves like facsimiles (Herrmann, 1993).

The study of training analysis is fostered by a continual query: why is there this insistence on using a model repeatedly diagnosed as anti-analytic (Herrmann, 1993). Why is it that analysts claim they are searching for the new, the unknown (Herrmann, 1986) and yet organize a training that stifles creative and original research and thought? Why do they consider that the basis of the transmission is given through the development of insight and the education of affective sensibility and, nevertheless, codify it with norms and standards? I suggest two hypotheses, or interpretations, in the hope that they shed some light on these paradoxes and also unveil the nature of the forces that sustain the permanence of training analysis.

The hypotheses are: (1) training analysis is a fetish; (2) training analysis is an ideological construct.

Training analysis can be diagnosed effectively as the *non plus ultra* of syncretism (Auchincloss & Michels, 2003; Gálvez, 2002; Gomberoff, 2002; Sachs, 1992; Spruiell, 1983; Tagliacozzo, 1984). It is put forth as the harmonization of incongruence, engaged in integrating analytic practice with conceptions that negate its essence. The submission that pervades the formal rules inherent to the organization of training analysis is in opposition to the implicit project of psychoanalysis.

Training analysis creates and maintains (backed by institutional relations) a kind of idealized transference that is precisely what the practice of analysis *tout court* sets out to resolve. It seeks uncritically to conceal under the garb of necessity the ongoing dichotomy implicit to it, availing itself to that end, in its mode of operating, of presuppositions and actions that are conflicting, divergent, and irreconcilable.

The situation in which truth is seen at a glance but its being traumatic is disavowed without, however, being denied, resolving itself in an attitude which keeps both conflicting statements alive side by side but dissociated, is very well known in psychoanalysis. Thus, it takes only a small effort of association for us to conceive of training analysis as a fetish.[2] This, then, is the first hypothesis. Its symptomatic nature is revealed not only through its vested interest in emphasising what is incompatible, but also the pertinacity with which it does so (which, in part, explains its longevity), in its ambiguous belief in the analytic method, in its distorted way of practicing it, in its capacity for co-opting criticisms, in its rationalizing its presence as indispensable.

Castration anxiety, a condition of the construction of the fetish according to the classic Freudian discovery, develops on a substratum linked to a threat of castration, real or phantasized: it is this threat which gives efficacy to the vision, turned traumatic, of the female genitalia, leading to disavowal and the building of the symptom. In the analyst's case, this threat is represented by the unacceptable perception of the limits of analysis, of that to which he submitted himself and which he practices, of that of his colleagues, of his personal difficulties, of his symptoms, and of his idiosyncrasies. Training analysis, while a fetish, emerges as a product of the disavowal on the part of the analysts of the limits of the action of the analysis. The history of training analysis is, then, the history of the "legitimation" of a pathological dissociation. This assertion places the institution of training analysis more clearly in the field of perversion. This way of being is characterized not only by the kind of practice or even the violence that permeates it. What characterizes it fundamentally is representing the front as the back, the deviation as the norm, generating false equivalences that corrode the capacity for judgment and the discrimination of values.

Nonetheless, the creation of an analysis composed of split parts, one of them apparently linked to acceptance of the common analytical method (bowing to its limitations), and the other disavowing it precisely for being limited, setting out, thus, on an authoritarian and invasive appropriation of its functioning, is not yet sufficient to give to training analysis the character of super-analysis with which it has been presenting itself. A collective participation giving substance to the power of the fetish needs to be organized, one fostering and maintaining the shared belief in the power of the mechanism of disavowal. Its end is the continual reinforcement of the dissociation and syncretism. There is yet the further need of a container to receive the wounded narcissism of the analyst (Giovanetti, 1991), sanctioning the defensive form—the fetish—that he constructed.

Institutional bureaucracy (Baranger et al., 1978), with its retinue of standards and procedures, enters thus upon the scene. That which originally possessed the dynamics of a symptom gains the dimension and form of an ideology, having to be comprehended in accordance with the rules of power administration. This, then, is the second hypothesis. Ideology is the recourse to ideas for legitimating and justifying settled forms of domination (Chaui, 1980); in the case under study, training analysis and its bureaucratic intellectual domination. It presents itself as a coherent logic of representations and of concepts intending to substitute the real with a discourse about reality, obscuring its origin and disguising its sense. The ideological character permeating it is what allows training analysis to be presented as something essential and universal and which confers on it a prescriptive impress of repetitive speech shut into itself.

In ending this section, I wish to underscore that all the innumerable initiatives that, through time, have been suggested as means to extinguish the vices I have been describing have failed in their aim, essentially because they maintained the category of *training analysis*, of didactic analysis, as a *separate entity* with its extraterritorial significance in relation to analysis *tout court*. Rather than simply indicating analysis to the one who intends to become an analyst, there is the persistence in imposing on him a "differentiated" analysis, administered by the institution.

The civil analyst and his tout court *analysand*

To bring further to light the above depicted training analysis organization and functioning characteristics, I shall now, underlining the contrasts, describe those of analysis *tout court*.

The latter organizes a setting which functions as a container within which the patient's conflicts can be expressed and understood. As Steiner (2006, p. 315) writes, "Not only is it a space within which the patient should feel safe to bring his thought, feeling and actions to have them understood, but also it is part of our contractual relationship to provide the conditions in which an analysis can be conducted". Hanna Segal (1962, cited by Steiner, 2006, p. 316) says that

> . . . the analyst shall do nothing to blur the development of the transference . . . his function is to understand sympathetically and to communicate to the patient such relevant knowledge as he has acquired, at the moment when the analysand is most ready to understand it . . . through the relation.

As such, the analytic method, conjointly with the analytic *attitude* (my italics), represents a single opportunity for engaging with the other person, for exploring how his mind works (Steiner, 2006). In this setting, the projected identifications which build the transference and distort the figure of the analyst, turning him into the *de facto* representative of the internal world of the patient, can be recognized and interpreted, restoring to the analysand that which he split off of his personality. "All analytic models assume the presence of a constant tension between the expected behavior of the analyst and the expectations of the patient based on transferential phantasies" (Jiménez de La Jara & Fonagy, 2011, p. 15, translated for this edition). In analysis *tout court*, the analyst can, for example, be experienced transferentially as a figure of authority, but the setting is organized so that this construction and its likely origins can be traced and interpreted.

The feelings, beliefs, and desires of the analyst, solicited during the analysis, should remain in the background. The asymmetry and a discordant fit are necessary positions to be able to apprehend, in the interchange of the pair, that which is transference. The tension alluded to previously, as Borensztejn recalls (2009, p. 182, evoking the work of the Baranger couple, 1961), expresses itself through the "unconscious bipersonal phantasy, which is a phantasy that is built in the interplay of projective identifications of both members of the analytic dyad". This phantasy should reflect the field's ambiguity. As such, it favors the mobility of the transferential–countertransferential relations, reinforcing the asymmetry that is continually threatened. In analysis *tout court*, analyst and patient are continuously co-opted by the phantasy through the very fact that they are its co-creators. Nevertheless, if they "enter" it, they do so *to get out*, in a movement of recognition of the field involving them and of the composition, function, and constituting of this phantasy. Another way of describing this dynamic (Friedman, 2008) is to point out the extent to which the analyst and analysand need to abandon the behavior that governs the rationality of contractual relations. This happens when the analysand lets himself be taken by free association and the analyst by evenly floating attention. To do so, it is necessary to acquire a discipline. "In normal life attention and intention are fused: Intention directs attention and attention assigns priority to the intention" (Friedman, 2008, p. 438). In psychoanalytic practice, these two functions are split: (a) conscious attention is immobilized by free association; (b) unconscious intentions are freed and focused on the analyst; (c) attention is refocused on those intentions, revealed unwittingly, which escaped the control of attention. Therefore, in order that the process be efficient, it is necessary to interfere determinedly with the attention (free association), with the emergence of those intentions which attention had concealed (transference), and refocus attention on the "new" intentions made visible (interpretation and insight) (Friedman, 2008). The analyst must take on an ambiguous attitude (which allows him to become the targeted object of the transference and, at the same time, to detach himself from the object), that is, he must be abstinent. In analysis *tout court* all is real and, at the same time, transferential, as, for example, transference love. The analyst does not adhere to this love, but also does not dispel it (Friedman, 2006). The desires (intentions of the pair) need to be sustained in transference and both—patient and analyst—must experience them. This ambiguity impels the analysis and the pair moves towards keeping it, denouncing it, avoiding it, etc. What is asked—and expected—of someone who wishes to become an analyst is that he undergo this experience of the emergence of the unconscious in the transferential relationship.

In analysis *tout court*, the analyst must search constantly to leave the "center" (that is, he must constantly be cognizant of the transference) and free himself from the settling in of his own theories and beliefs. In sum, the analyst needs to keep continual contact with his internal objects, perceiving himself as separate from them and, therefore, in dialogue with them. This dialogue is a protection against narcissism and the condition for self-analysis. The analyst needs to perceive himself depressively, that is, that he is not who he thinks he is. Coherence in analysis *tout court* ensues from the recognition of this dialectic.

Evidently, what interests the pair is not the nature of the content that, previously hidden, is now revealed, but the reason for its being concealed (it is what Friedman (2008) calls "crystallization of knowledge in *status nascendi*"). Understanding this reason is what Freud called "working through". The ambiguous attitude creates an undefined atmosphere in the analytic *tout court* relationship, which becomes a stimulus for analytic work. Each time the "identification" is worked through, according, for example, to the Bionian model of preconception that transmutes into conception, a knowledge is revealed which serves as an incentive to continuing with the process. The autonomy achieved by the patient across work of this kind corresponds to the capacity reached in living with his conflicts and of recognizing the defensive moves that are the symptomatic solutions he creates when faced with such conflicts.

What is expected is that, at the end of the process (Soler, 2004), the analysand introjects the analytic function and, making use of it, proceeds with his self-analysis, and that the analyst, free of the transference, perceives that his identity, separate from that of the patient's, carries the function that the analysand knew how to introject.

Describing enactment

The descriptions of the procedures in training analysis and in analysis *tout court* prepared the field for presenting enactment. This chosen sequence should facilitate visualizing its presence and function in each of these forms of analysis.

Enactment, etymologically, carries the idea of theatrical representation, acting a part, putting on stage. In analytic enactment, both participants, analyst and patient, are bringing to the stage characters and stories that, although enacted, are, as it were, concealed. The enactment is something that happens *between* patient and analyst with the ongoing participation and contribution of both. It is an intersubjective behavior: "Nothing happens in one member of the pair that does not reflect on the other" (Cassorla, 2013a, p. 18, translated for this edition).

Jimenez de La Jara and Fonagy (2011) synthesize elegantly its characteristics:

1. The patient expresses the desire that the analyst join him in the suspension of disbelief characteristic of the game.
2. An action or representation arises whose end is to persuade or force the other into reciprocated action (McLaughlin & Johan, 1992, cited by Jimenez de La Jara & Fonagy, 2011). Here, the mutual coercion character shows clearly.
3. It is co-construed and shared.
4. Its functioning entails moments of entanglement between the personal experiences of the patient and the analyst. The asymmetry is lost; the analyst then moves on to thinking about the happening and what his contribution is towards this loss.

Cassorla (2013a, p. 84) defines enactment as

> an intersubjective phenomenon in which from the mutual emotional induction the analytic field is overtaken by discharges and/or behaviors involving both members of the analytic dyad, without their being able to be sufficiently aware of what is happening and which takes to situations in which verbal symbolization is impaired. (Translated for this edition)

The dynamics of enactment point to the projection by the patient on the analyst of unthought-of or not thought out elements (because, to him, they are unthinkable) that then complementarily hook on to aspects of the analyst also not thought out or worked through. In this description, what immediately draws attention is the establishment of a complementarity that, in functioning as collusion, sacrifices the fundamental element of the field: asymmetry. Cassorla (20013a) highlights emphatically that both elements of the analytic dyad feel themselves as extensions of one another. He calls this mirroring, in which a mutual and silent submission happens, "chronic enactment".

The same author, along the lines of Bion and Ogden, conceives the analyst as having the function of leading the patient to transform his non-dreams (that which above I called the elements unthought-of because unthinkable) into dreams. When "entanglement", collusion, and, consequently, loss of asymmetry occur, "patient and analyst discharge and/or repeat conducts compulsively without perceiving what is happening" (Cassorla, 2013a, p. 189, translated for this edition). For him, it is a defensive maneuver which aims to immobilize "traumas embedded in the non-repressed unconscious, including transgenerational facts. The analytic field is overtaken by archaic configurations built by both members of the pair, without their being aware" (Cassorla, 2013a, p. 194, translated for this edition). This chronic enactment is described as "non-dreams-for two".

It may be said that when the chronic enactment becomes saturated and some aspect of the solicited complementarity is no longer satisfied, a conflict arises, most of the time exacting and disruptive, which exposes the ongoing dynamics, the agreement, its nature and function: this is acute enactment. In analyses *tout court* this irruption on unveiling the collusion offers a chance to recompose the analytic frame and its capacity for verbalization/symbolization.

As the analytic situation, due to its technique and nature, entails privation, words take the place of action, functioning as acts or incitements to action (McLaughlin, 1991). Levenson (2006, p. 322) writes that enactment is the "behavioral component of what is being talked about". The author emphasizes that both parts experience the happenings taking place in the relationship of the dyad as being due to the behavior of the other, even if the attempt at influencing and thinking is mutual. Enactment, then, occupies the place of psychoanalytical thinking (Goldberg, 2002) by means of an agreement wherein the distortion that is being practiced is not questioned. Chused (1997, cited by Maroda, 1998) underlines that what we are dealing with here is an interaction conjointly created and fed into by unconscious psychic forces of both the patient and the analyst. A silent conspiracy develops through which each participant is taken to the splitting or disavowal of a personal area that is complementarily problematic: they agree then implicitly on removing it from the perceptive and dialogic field. Although nothing is formally disrespected, the founding elements of the analytic situation are being disregarded. The psychoanalytic process seems productive (Cassorla, 2013a) but awareness of certain transferential configurations pertinent to the relation is blocked due to an intense unconscious collusion between analyst and patient. Even if the analyst engages himself in the enactment unwittingly and even if the enactment is seen as initiated by the unconscious effort of the patient to persuade or force the analyst into a reciprocal complementary action, the enactment entails a playing out of the most fundamental internal configurations of the patient which have found an echo in the analyst (Hirsch, 1998).

Sandler (1976, cited by Hirsch, 1998) in his classic article on responsiveness, underscores the extent to which the analyst—dragged in by the very nature of the setting—can not only comply with the role the patient attributes to him, but also integrate it into his mode of responding and relating with him.

As Steiner (1996, p. 1080) writes,

> In recent years we have become much more aware that the analyst's own needs interact with the patient's needs in complex ways. *It is when their defensive needs coincide that a stuck situation is particularly likely to go unrecognized and to become chronic.* (My italics)

Another way of putting it is pointing to the emergence or construction of narcissistic bastions by the dyad along the analysis. Analysts have identified and studied these impasses, seeking ways of unblocking them, centering their focus on the interpersonal patient–analyst link. But this stance demands acknowledgement that the aspects that needed to be split off came to the fore within the analysis, on its being developed.

None of this is surprising in so much as we know that, in an analysis, intrapsychic conflicts linked to the organization of the objectal traumas of both patient and analyst are revised and updated. It is understandable also that both seek to avoid awareness of these conflicts within the transferential–countertransferential movement, owing to the traumatic nature and suffering they cause.

Thus, the breach in the line of conduct present in enactment must be understood in light of that which the analyst had set out to follow. The enactment emerges then as a neoformation of/in the analytic field which distorts the comprehension of the patient and orients the interpretive activity of the analyst (effected now not through understanding the transference and countertransference, but following the involvement with the patient), immobilizing, by its stereotyping, the development of the analytic process.

Enactment and training analysis: a model of chronic infiltration

In this part of the chapter, I show that, in constituting itself as a separate form of analysis, training analysis has not only distanced itself from the current analytic practice, such as described in our addressing analysis *tout court,* but also, in subjecting itself to the sponsorship of the institution, has turned itself into a singular form of chronic enactment.

In analysis *tout court,* the discrimination of the separate identities of the dyad making up the analytic pair, that is, the continual interpretation of transference coupled with contact with countertransference, is experienced as a productive trauma, which engenders knowledge of both psychic content and functioning. This discrimination is inherent to the analytic activity: a work-in-progress, never terminated or terminable, worked through in each session, which goes on allowing the subject to discover the nature of his relations with the object.

In training analysis, on the contrary, this discrimination needs not to be conquered as it is offered at the very outset and as a functional principle by the institution. The training analyst is not the "other person" of the transference; he is always the *same person,* sustained by the institutional function. It suffices to recall here what I said in the first part about the identification with the training analyst taking place "in reality". In this context, the identities of the pair do not need to be constructed, since they are provided ready-made, from the outside in. Seen from the outside, at face value, what emerges when we contemplate the pair is an analyst working with his analysand (and *vice versa*). Structurally, however, we are confronted with a candidate-aiming-to-become-an-analyst interacting with a training-analyst-destined-to-train-him. The pair needs to operate within this range to maintain their objectives, which must coincide with the fixing of pre-established roles. The complementarity necessary to the fulfillment of the task is typical of enactment, just as is the subservience to this complementarity.

Training analyst and candidate repeat compulsively a form of communication aimed at maintaining the nature of the bond that sustains their common, extra-analytic objective. On offering themselves to carry out the role they were actually recruited for, they follow a path that does not allow deviation, "fitting into", as such, a chronic enactment that will take them to the sought-for destination.

I wrote above that chronic enactment reveals itself—and, to an extent, is resolved—through the emergence of acute enactment. The latter, as an abrupt confrontation between patient and analyst ensuing from the loss of chronic enactment efficacy, turns into an opportunity for understanding the why of its presence and the nature of its defensive function. It is for this that many authors consider enactment a productive occurrence towards recomposing the analytic process: it would allow silent impasses and paralyses to be identified and enable resuming the work at a more evolved level.

However, the training analysis is organized to impede the emergence of these acute, revealing episodes that would bring to light the nature of the agreement which allows its functioning. In the case of the pair, their agreed submission to the imposing, *fixed* character of the triangle formed by the candidate–training analyst–institution cannot surface: it cannot become acute. Thus, it cannot be contrasted with the oedipal triangle usually sized up in psychoanalysis *tout court*, which is fluid and mobile. The training analyst is there to meet the candidate's desire to become an analyst, and, with this, ratify his own desire to remain a training analyst. The acute enactment (or that which corresponds to it) will then be dislocated, in a substitutive form, out of the field of enactment of the pair. We shall discuss this a little later in the chapter.

In training analysis, the anxiety triggered by the possibility of the emergence of acute enactment, induced by the revelation and disclosure of the truncated mode of analysis being practiced, pressures the threatened pair even further to recover their functional identities. There is a subtext underlying the communication between candidate and training analyst which, in this genre of enactment, can in no way surface, since this would put to question not a blind spot in the relationship, but the whole conceptualization of the work, putting its continuity at risk. This has been described already in the first part of this chapter, when we spoke of training analysis as a fetish and as an ideological construct.

For this subtext to stay split off and the enactment to continue, the vigilance that each member of the dyad maintains over the other, obstructing any detouring from the path, is central: it is mandatory that the ongoing verbalization remains attuned to the prefixed roles they are playing. In this closed interplay (chronic enactment), the analyst endorsed by the institution (the training analyst) is reappraised in his role of authority by the candidate who, in doing so, has his role as candidate appraised by the training analyst. It is as though we were before a melancholic version of the grand finale of Carrocelo

Napolitano (Napolitan Carousel): "Tu dai una cosa a me; io do una cosa a te" ("You give me something; I'll give you something").

We have already seen that the enactment present in analysis *tout court* seeks to protect the dyad from awareness or acknowledgement of an element that it considers disturbing and which emerges *during the analytic work in progress*, being thus its product. It is, therefore, *post factum*, the outcome of the analytic process. In its turn, the enactment characterizing training analysis begins simultaneously with it, or, better, is known beforehand, *ante factum*, established by the series of prescriptions, goals, and limitations specific to this sort of analysis that precede the encounter. Yet, as the entire process was naturalized (a concealing typical of enactment), not only is this distortion not perceived but, under the form of codified rules, is adopted as model. In analysis *tout court*, the analyst seeks to keep a critical distancing from his ideological standing; training analysis, in its turn, is ruled by an ideology which defines the relation as one of candidate–training analyst, which must be continually reappraised. It is sustained by a non-analytic "common ground": the "mission", wherein the personal theory of the analyst is not, in truth, a relevant factor, since, whatever it may be, it will be at the service of this "common ground". This mission manifestly puts in check the very notion of analysis whose central mark is not to predetermine its end.

Thus, training analysis is delegitimized by its lack of analytic coherence, being, however, paradoxically designated as representative of the analytic ideal. This is one of the singularities of the enactment present in didactic analysis.

Steiner (2000) underscores that the analyst must pay attention not simply to the words of the patient, but to their context and the "non-verbal cues that accompany them". Aron (2003), in his turn, recalls Sullivan's maxim that we are what we do more than what we say. Paraphrasing Friedman (2008), it could thus be put that what is disquieting here is not only what is happening, but what is kept from happening.

The context of training analysis imposes on the pair a listening that determines not only what must be heard, but also what needs to be excluded. This attitude is not, however, a defensive outcome of the operating transferential–countertransferential dynamics as happens in "common" enactment: it has its origin in the *ante-factum* prescriptions accepted by both. The interplay of projective identifications loses its expressive dimension to function as a mere role-fixating element. What is striven for finally is to impede the analysis *tout court* from erupting within training analysis, as this emergence would work in the mode of an acute enactment, putting in check the category candidate–training analyst and calling for its substitution by that of analysand–analyst.

This acute enactment, or, better, its latency, is then split off and projected into the institution, which, being guarantor of the training analysis, offers itself as container to shelter and "absorb it". In this context, we are no longer being confronted with enactments ensuing from the transferential–countertransferential experiences of the pair. The taking in of these projections by the institution is an active movement whose end is not only to maintain the tie between it and training analysis, but also to reinforce the model character of the latter. While this taking in promotes the introjection by the pair of the "training facet" of the analysis, it deters the likely ensuing and emerging analytic facet, thus facilitating the splitting off and parceling into the institutional relations of those conflicting analytic aspects whose emergence in the analysis could lead to questioning its "didactic" orientation. The ambivalent feelings experienced by the pair in relation to the didactic standing of the analysis are dissociated, that is, projected on other analysts, other institutions, other theories, boosting the idealization of training analysis and validating the *modus operandi* sustained by the institution (Gálvez, 2002). Thus are then formed the group rivalries of a narcissistic bent, the charismatic schools, the practitioners of the true psychoanalysis, the gossips, the oblique political maneuvers. What is construed is not only a chronic enactment, but also a standardized enactment.

We stand before a hypostatized analysis: while attributing to its analytic nature a central role, in truth this is only peripheral to its didactic character. An interaction is conjointly created which sets out to create an analysis in which analysis *tout court* cannot erupt. The "disentangling" of which Cassorla speaks (2013a) cannot take place: what pervades is a "non-dream-for- two".

Skeptical about analysis, analysts through the institution decided to create a respectable analysis. Mistrustful of the unconscious—and of its emergence—they proposed identification with an ideal subject and practice. Training analysis is, as such, a singular illustration of the battle of psychoanalysis against itself.

Post scriptum

Cassorla (2013a, p. 191) writes that even in the full activity of enactment, it must be assumed that "in a parallel area the analytic process is developing apparently productively" (translated for this edition). In this parallel area, the "explicit alpha function" continues active. In another article of the same year, Cassorla (2013b, p. 343) states that during "the obstructive collusion an implicit development of the symbolic network is happening in areas parallel to the obstruction". The "parallel area" concept is not developed in the texts, its probably being the outcome of *a posteriori* observations. If, however, we apply it to training analysis, we have it then that outside or in the periphery of the process, in moments of distraction (or relaxation), in spurts and subterraneously, candidate and training analyst allow themselves the exercise of analysis *tout court*.

All goes on as though the unconscious, in a tropism inherent to it, sought to be psychoanalytically listened to by the training analyst, even if against his will; in point of fact, in opposition to, or challenging, him. To know that the ontological density (Herrmann, 1991) of the psychoanalytic method confers on it this degree of resistance, compactness, and consistency should not serve as an excuse to ignore the extent to which we try to disfigure it.

Notes

1. Besides that already mentioned by them, between training and non-training analysts.
2. Gálvez, in a commentary on the first draft of this chapter, suggests that the expression "exclusive statements" would be more precise than "conflicting statements". He does so taking into consideration the transferential impasses inherent to training analysis that are usually evaded.

References

Araico, J. R. (1992). Lá escisión en el campo de la transferencia–contratransferencia en el análisis didática [Splitting in the transference–countertransference field in training analysis]. *Revista de Psicoanálisis (Arg.), 49*: 373–386.

Aron, L. (2003). The paradoxical place of enactment in psychoanalysis. *Psychoanalytic Dialogues, 13*: 623–631.

Auchincloss, E., & Michels, R. (2003). A reassessment of psychoanalytic education: controversies and changes. *International Journal of Psychoanalysis, 84*: 387–403.

Balint, M. (1948). On the psycho-analytic training system. *International Journal of Psychoanalysis, 29*: 163–176.

Baranger, M., Baranger, W., & Mom, J. (1978). Psicopatologia del processo didático [Psychopathology of the training process]. *Revista de Psicoanálisis (Arg.), 35*: 181–190.

Baranger, W., & Baranger, M. (1961). La situación analítica como campo dinâmico [The psychoanalytic situation as a dynamics field]. In: *Problemas del campo psicanalítico*. Buenos Aires: Kargieman.

Bernfeld, S. (1962). On psychoanalytic training. *Psychoanalytic Quarterly, 31*: 453–482.

Borensztejn, C. L. (2009). El enactment como concepto clinico convergente de teorias divergentes [Enactment as a clinical concept converging divergent theories]. *Revista de Psicoanálisis (Arg.), 66*: 177–192.

Cassorla, R. M. S. (2013a). Afinal, o que é esse tal enactment? [After all, what is enactment?]. *Jornal de Psicanálise, 46*: 183–198.

Cassorla, R. M. S. (2013b). When the analyst becomes stupid: an attempt to understand enactment using Bion's theory of thinking. *Psychoanalytic Quarterly, 82*: 326–360.

Chaui, M. S. (1980). Ideologías autoritarias e filosofia [Authoritarian ideologies and phylosophy]. Palestra pronunciada no 32. Reunião da Sociedade Brasileira para o Progresso da Ciência, Rio de Janeiro. Manuscrito.

Chused, J. F. (1997). Discussion of "observing-participation, mutual enactment, and new classical models" by Irwin Hirsch. *Contemporary Psychoanalysis, 33*: 263–277.

Freud, A. (1938). The problem of training analysis. In: *The Writings of Anna Freud (Volume IV): Indications for Child Analysis and Other Papers, 1945–1956*. New York: International Universities Press.

Friedman, L. (2006). What is psychoanalysis? *Psychoanalytic Quarterly, 75*: 689–713.

Friedman, L. (2008). Is there life after enactment? The idea of a patient's proper work. *Journal of the American Psychoanalytic Association, 56*: 431–453.

Gálvez, M. J. (2002). Notas sobre aspectos atuais da transmissão da psicanálise [Notes on current aspects of the transmission of psychoanalysis]. *Revista Brasileira de Psicanálise, 36*: 679–702.

Giovanetti, M. F. (1991). O divã e a medusa [Medusa and the couch]. *Ide, 21*: 64–69.

Goldberg, A. (2002). Enactment as understanding and as misunderstanding. *Journal of the American Psychoanalytic Association, 50*: 869–883.

Gomberoff, M. (2002). Crisis y analisis didactico [Training analysis and crisis]. Apresentado no XIX Pré-Congresso Didactico—I Pré-congresso de Institutos, Fepal, Montevideo.

Greenacre, P. (1966). Problems of training analysis. *Psychoanalytic Quarterly, 35*: 540–567.

Herrmann, F. (1986). Sobre a formação, sobre um velho desabafo [About training, about an old anger]. *Ide, 13*: 12–13.

Herrmann, F. (1991). *Andaimes do Real: livro primeiro, o método da psicanálise* [Scaffoldings of the Real: Volume 1, The Psychoanalytic Method]. São Paulo: Editora Brasiliense.

Herrmann, F. (1993). Análise didática: uma história feita de críticas [Training analysis: a story composed of criticisms]. *Jornal de Psicanálise, 26*: 29–69.

Hirsch, I. (1998). The concept of enactment and theoretical convergence. *Psychoanalytic Quarterly, 67*: 78–101.

Jiménez de La Jara, J. P., & Fonagy, P. (2011). Un ejercicio en psicoanálisis comparativo: el concepto de enactment en algunos autores orientaciones desde la perspectiva de su fenomenologia [An exercise in comparative psychoanalysis: the concept of enactment in some authors, orientations from the perspective of its phenomenology]. *Revista chilena de psicoanálisis, 28*: 8–17.

Kernberg, O. F. (1992). Autoritarisme, culture et personnalité dans la formation psychanalytique. *Revue internationale d'histoire de la psychanalyse, 5*: 341–354.

Kernberg, O. F. (2000). A concerned critique of psychoanalytic education. *International Journal of Psychoanalysis, 81*: 97–120.

Kernberg, O. F. (2001). Some thoughts regarding innovation in psychoanalytic education. Paper presented to the IPA Executive Council Meeting in Puerto Vallarta, 7 January.

Levenson, E. A. (2006). Response to John Steiner. *International Journal of Psychoanalysis, 87*: 321–324.

Maroda, K. J. (1998). Enactment: when the patient's and analyst's pasts converge. *Psychoanalytic Psychology, 15*: 517–535.

McLaughlin, J. T. (1987). The play of transference: some reflections on enactment in the psychoanalytic situation. *Journal of the American Psychoanalytic Association, 35*: 557–582.

McLaughlin, J. T. (1991). Clinical and theoretical aspects of enactment. *Journal of the American Psychoanalytic Association, 39*: 595–614.

McLaughlin, J. T., & Johan, M. (1992). Enactments in psychoanalysis. *Journal of the American Psychoanalytic Association, 40*: 827–841.

Meyer, L. (2002). Análise subaltern [Subservient analysis]. *Revista Brasileira de Psicanálise, 36*: 145–159.

Meyer, L. (2003). Subservient analysis. *International Journal of Psychoanalysis, 84*: 1241–1262.

Meyer, L. (2007). A análise didática deve ser mantida? [Should we keep training analysis?]. *Revista Brasileira de Psicanálise, 41*: 33–40.

Meyer, L. (2008). Pensando a análise didática enquanto fetiche e Formação ideológica [Thinking of training analysis as a fetish and an ideological construct]. *Jornal de Psicanálise, 41*: 121–129.

Nacht, S. (1954). The difficulties of didatic psychoanalysis in relation to the therapeutic analysis. *International Journal of Psychoanalysis, 35*: 250–253.

Sachs, D. M. (1992). What makes a training analysis "good enough"? Freud's science and the syncretistic dilemma. *International Review of Psychoanalysis, 19*: 147–158.

Sandler, J. (1976). Countertransference and role-responsiveness. *International Review of Psychoanalysis, 3*: 43–48.

Segal, H. (1962). The curative factors in psycho-analysis—contributions to discussion. *International Journal of Psychoanalysis, 43*: 221–233.

Soler, C. (2004). Qué se espera del análisis y del psicoanalista [What is expected of analysis and of the analyst?]. *Revista Psicoanálisis, Asociación Psicoanalítica de Buenos Aires, 26*: 779–794.

Spruiell, V. (1983). Kuhn's "paradigm" and psychoanalysis. *Psychoanalytic Quarterly, 52*: 353–363.

Steiner, J. (1996). The aim of psychoanalysis in theory and in practice. *International Journal of Psychoanalysis, 77*: 1073–1083.

Steiner, J. (2000). Containment, enactment and communication. *International Journal of Psychoanalysis, 81*: 245–255.

Steiner, J. (2006). Interpretative enactments and the analytic setting. *International Journal of Psychoanalysis, 87*: 315–328.

Tagliacozzo, R. (1984). Analisi didatico. *Rivista di Psicoanalisi, 30*: 611–621.

Wallerstein, R. S. (2010). The training analysis: psychoanalysis' perennial problem. *Psychoanalytic Review, 97*: 903–936.

Whiting, C. (1996). Psicopatología de una denominación: análisis didáctico [Psychopathology of a name: training analysis]. *Revista Latino-america de Psicoanálisis, 1*: 15–19.

CHAPTER ELEVEN

Still crazy after all these years

Robert Pyles

Introduction

Yes, it really *was* previously a school for embalmers. I am referring to the massive mansion at 15 Commonwealth Avenue in Boston, the home of the Boston Psychoanalytic Society and Institute (BPSI) where I began my psychoanalytic training in 1967.

It contained a magnificent men's room, by far the largest I had ever seen, which was reputed to have been the embalming room. Massive in size, it had eight stalls and twelve urinals. Intimidating to say the least, but at least the sheer size made it less likely to wind up at a urinal next to a training analyst!

I report this partly in jest, but the anxiety for a beginning candidate was certainly real enough. Much later, I also came to appreciate that this, in an uncanny way, seemed a fitting metaphor that symbolized the essential organizational and educational dilemma for the whole profession.

What follows is a chapter in two parts. The first was written in 1984, at a time when my new institute, the Psychoanalytic Institute of New England East (PINE) had been in existence as a "provisional institute" for the mandatory five years required in order to be considered for permanent status by the American Psychoanalytic Association. This final approval had just been obtained, which meant that the institute was now approved to begin appointing new training analysts.

PINE had formed five years earlier, the product of a "split" at BPSI. After some years of conflict, the causes of which were quite opaque to us candidates, seven senior analysts broke away to form PINE. Some recent graduates, most of whom had been leaders in the candidate group, were invited to join the new group.

As soon as PINE had become official, however, to my intense disappointment, and that of many of the younger faculty (recent graduates, most of us), the senior training group formed their own Training Analyst Committee and began processing potential new TAs in the exact manner of every other analytic institute, including the one we had just broken away from, quite the opposite of what we had been led to expect.

I also came to understand that whatever the various stated reasons for the conflict at BPSI had been, the root cause was the same as it usually is everywhere else—who's in, and who's out. There was an "in-group", consisting of senior TAs, but the membership was largely excluded from faculty and TA appointments. The body of members at BPSI eventually became large enough that they began to push for appointments.

In retrospect, the "split" was unusual, in that the more conservative TAs were the ones that broke away to form PINE. The siren song for my group of recent graduates was that PINE was going to be an institute without walls, without hierarchy, an "ideal" of academic freedom. We could not possibly have been more wrong.

Because I felt strongly that we were about to duplicate all the mistakes that had plagued most institutes in the USA, often resulting in "splits", I wrote the following paper, as noted, in 1984. I should also mention that I wrote this paper *before* I was a training analyst. At the time, I was aware that I was writing it at considerable personal risk.

When I presented the paper, it created such a firestorm among the senior TAs that I realized two things: (a) the system was not going to change, and (b) there was no point in trying to publish it, so I just put it away. Until now.

I must beg the reader's indulgence, because there are a number or points in Part I that will seem dated. And that is because they *are* dated. I have chosen to present this part unchanged, exactly as I wrote it in in 1984. My reason for doing so is that I want to underline the point that the disadvantages of the training analyst system that have so plagued us, especially in recent years, were perfectly obvious thirty years ago.

In fact, looking at some of the articles in the references section, the problems were clear even thirty years before that. So, it could reasonably be said that for at least sixty years we have struggled with this albatross around our collective necks, with only the occasional article drawing attention to it.

So we must ask, how could that be true? What is going on?

How could a group of dedicated psychoanalysts not only fail to deal with the issue, but fail to even ask the relevant questions?

My answer is that I feel we have been blinded by a group belief system, the powerful roots of which can be found in the very nature of the training system itself. It has been self-perpetuating and self-sustaining from one analytic generation to another, from training analyst to candidate to training analyst, so on and so on, *ad infinitum*. How can something be successfully analyzed that is an integral part and parcel of the very core of the system itself?

The most damning and compelling evidence can be found in the almost total prohibition of even a *serious discussion* of the training analyst system. I do not think it is overstating the case to say that there has been an unconscious and prolonged conspiracy of silence, a quasi-religious taboo, on any such discussion.

Consider, for example, the American Psychoanalytic Association, where an attempt to bring the TA system to the floor of BoPS for discussion led to a million dollar (plus) lawsuit, to prevent such a discussion.

So why does this issue come up now? What is so pressing about it?

The answer is that we can no longer afford it, or its disastrous effect on our profession.

Psychoanalysis is under siege from a number of outside threats. Government and political intrusion, shorter-term therapies, and competition with other analytic groups have led to dramatically declining numbers of patients and candidates. In APsaA, almost one half (thirteen of twenty-nine) of our institutes are poised to go the way of PINE. Our archaic educational and organizational practices are making it difficult to survive, crippling our ability to protect our patients and our profession. We *must* do better.

When I presented this paper, I predicted that if we continued down this road, PINE would most likely fail. And, largely, it has, but more about that later. Here is the 1984 paper.

Part I (1984)

History of the training analysis

As we all know, the history of the analyst being analyzed begins with Freud's self-analysis, a remarkable achievement, incomplete as it might have been. Freud felt strongly about continuing self-analysis, and came to feel that an analysis "with someone with expert knowledge" was necessary for *doing* analysis. This was not, however, as was later assumed, a justification for a training analyst system. Neither Freud himself nor his analysands operated within a formal training system.

Balint's review of training is one of the first serious considerations of this topic. He puts particular emphasis on the second period of "proper analysis" initiated by Ferenczi, apparently out of reaction to his own analysis with Freud. Ferenczi's further writing led to a period of "super therapy", still ongoing, in which a lengthy training period has placed the training analyst in an enormously powerful position and, as he put it, "an atmosphere . . . strongly reminiscent of primitive initiation ceremonies", introjection of the over-idealized analyst, and a displacement of negative feelings onto the society and theoretical issues, leading to "power politics and hostility".

The formalization of the requirement for training analysis was made at the Budapest Congress in 1918 by Nunberg, and in 1925 was adopted as a requirement by the International Psychoanalytical Association.

History of the training analyst system

Prior to 1920, there was no formalized training institution. Plans to form an institute in Budapest, funded by Von Freund, had fallen through due to political considerations. In 1920, Max Eitingon, with his own funds, began the Berlin Institute. In reviewing the "Ten Year Report of the Berlin Institute, 1923–1933", several things stand out. The idea of not only a training analysis, but a designated training analyst seems to have been in place from the beginning. Hans Sachs was imported from Vienna to be the first training analyst and was joined later by Sandor Rado. The training program is described in some detail and it is remarkable in the fact that the tripartite system, the administrative structure, and the curriculum seem to be exactly the same as we now use, to the point of being a little unnerving. The training system was shorter, three years including analysis, and included courses from the humanities. The group apparently also spent a considerable amount of time on what they call "propaganda", namely lecturing at universities and various citizen groups to educate the public as to the nature of analysis.

It is made quite clear in this report that the Berlin system has become the model for other institutes established in Europe at that time, and later in the other regions. Another somber note is the slightly eerie feeling in reading this material, written in 1933, knowing that within three years, the nephew of Herman Goering would be installed as the head of the Berlin Institute, and that all of the writers, Horney, Sachs, and others would be scattered to other countries.

Certainly, while the issues facing our profession are of nowhere near such a catastrophic nature, nevertheless some parallel with the sense of being overtaken by environmental forces pertains.

It seems that the training analyst system did not arise out of any unique educational or analytic necessity to do it in that particular way, but was, in fact, a natural consequence of the German educational system and methods of child-rearing, which were particularly regimented and hierarchical, or, to use Sigfried Bernfeld's term, "Prussian". This view in turn seems to rest on the nineteenth century German philosophical view of man as an animal full of primitive instincts, who must be "trained" into civilized behavior.

In *The Birth of an Institute,* Ives Hendrick (1958) described the founding of the Boston Psychoanalytic Society and Institute, BPSI, which was approved as a training institute in 1932. In an unpublished paper, Sanford Gifford makes a convincing case for these early difficulties being a result of Hendrick's insistence on a rigid central control that resulted from his "idealized picture of the Berlin Institute". Gifford feels that what Hendrick was able to achieve was a rigidity of structure considerably greater than that in Berlin. On the other hand, Hendrick writes of the establishment of the "faculty principle", that is, central control, as being a great achievement. Other writers, however, have considered this to be the paradigm of the "teacher centered," as opposed to the "student centered" form of education.

A number of splits were reviewed in researching this paper, but, in summary, it seems clear that the splits and dissensions are nearly always over the training analyst issue. This cycle of a small power group, increasingly numerous excluded members, and eventual open conflict is endlessly repeated, and yet no alternative structure seems to have been attempted. No article examining pros and cons of the TA system seems to have been written. Instead, the Berlin system seems to be mindlessly reproduced, preserved, and reified by the training analyst system.

Dynamic problems of the training analyst system

In considering Freud's self-analysis, Wilhelm Fliess might be seen, at least transferentially, to be in the position of being the first training analyst. Freud's over-idealization of Fliess, his inability to question the scientific productions of Fliess, and his desperate attempt to blame himself in the Irma dream, rather than recognizing any fault in his mentor, is hard to miss. Eventually, when Freud was able to admit to himself the flaws in Fliess' thinking, the result was a rupture of the relationship—a split. This pattern is seen as a paradigm for Freud's earlier relationship with Breuer, and for his later difficulties with Jung, Adler, and others. Freud attempted to deal with this problem of repeated splits and schisms by reducing the number of his trusted colleagues to a small secret society, "The Committee", but even this proved a failure for reasons that Freud could never quite grasp. Neither has any other analytic organization since that time been able to understand this problem.

Bernard Fine reports that Eitingon, who was analyzed by Freud, was so fanatically devoted to Freud that he never attempted to write any articles on his own, on the grounds that everything worthwhile had already been said by Freud. It is highly likely that this compliant, idealizing transference was operating when he undertook, with missionary zeal, to spread the word of the master to Berlin and set up the Berlin Institute, as mentioned, at his own expense. In addition to the sociological factors mentioned earlier, one suspects that the training analyst system's springing into existence, apparently *de novo*, may well have been the reincarnation of his idealized analyst, from the very beginning. Eitingon's other achievement, and one of which he was reportedly even more proud, was establishing and becoming head of the International Training Commission of the International Psycho-Analytic Association. Fine (1979) reports that his conduct of this central controlling body was so unyielding as to be a major factor in the revolt and eventual independence of the American Association in 1938. Thus, here we have a prime example of compliance and idealization leading to rigidification and control of others, which in turn produces conflict and eventual splitting.[1]

The opposite side of the coin seems to be represented by Ferenczi, who reproached Freud repeatedly for "having failed to give him a complete analysis" in that Freud, in Ferenczi's view, failed to deal with the negative transference. Ferenczi attacked Freud's more casual manner of approaching training analyses, called for "proper analysis", and eventually for what Balint refers to as "super therapy". This emphasis on extended training then set the stage for what Balint referred to as excessive compliance among candidates in Institutes, and the problem that Fine referred to as "education versus indoctrination".

Thus, we see compliance in the case of Eitingon and rebellion on the part of Ferenczi, both leading in the direction of establishing coercive training systems and requirements for analytic generations to come.

Hendrick's history of BPSI also provides a fascinating example. Franz Alexander was the first training analyst at BPSI in 1931–1932, before leaving for Chicago, when Hans Sachs succeeded him in 1933. Sachs was Alexander's analyst and Alexander was Hendrick's. Hendrick describes with enthusiastic joy the arrival of Alexander in Boston. This is contrasted with the viciousness with which he takes occasion in this historical survey to attack the character of Sachs, and to point out what a troublemaker he was, not only in Boston but also in Berlin. The trouble that Sachs promulgated seems to have been that he was firmly opposed to the "faculty principle", committed to a much less structured training system, and, not being an MD, agreed with Freud that psychoanalysis should not ally itself primarily with medicine. Hendrick seemed to regard Sachs as his particular boogieman and took every opportunity to demolish him with special zeal, even post mortem. Interestingly, also in Hendrick's 1955 presidential address to the American Psychoanalytic Association, he apparently felt that the lay analysis issue was settled once and for all and remarked, "Happily, I find this no suitable occasion for re-arguing the tattered dialectics of the lay analysis problem."

A host of articles on the "central problem of the training analysis" point out the essential incompatibility between the therapeutic and training function. Greenacre, Tartakoff, and several more recent authors point out the essential impossibility of analyzing issues when the transference is contaminated by real aspects of the analyst–patient relationship, which, in effect, serve to re-enact infantile conflicts. The result is often collusion between analyst and patient to avoid the negative transference, resulting in a narcissistic idealization of the analyst, identification with him, and a desire to become like him and protect his beliefs against all comers. The negative affects are then displaced on to colleagues, theoretical issues, etc. Thus, the training analysis at its worst and even unavoidably, to some extent, at its best, becomes an instrument of inducing compliance to a degree at which a corporate president could only marvel.

Many authors were reviewed on the problems of the termination phase of a training analysis, about which there is the old truism that, rather than saying "good-bye", the candidate says "hello". In effect, there is no real termination, and it is ironic to consider the emphasis that the American Psychoanalytic Association has recently been placing on the termination phase in the certification process. The Committee on Certification quite correctly, in my opinion, holds that if there is no proper termination phase, there can reasonably be considered to have been no analysis, as the termination phase provides the opportunity for ultimate renunciation of infantile wishes toward the parent. And yet in the training analysis, the termination phase is hopelessly compromised.

On the basis of the foregoing, I feel that it could be reasonably concluded that the training analyst system produces a situation which is essentially anti-analytic, seriously compromises the quality of the analysis, and creates large areas of unanalyzed material, particularly those relating to training, analytic, and organizational matters, which probably goes a long way toward explaining the endless political conflicts in most of our analytic groups.

Another aspect that should not be overlooked is the regressive effect of the training analyst system on both the training analyst and the non-training analyst alike, resulting in exacerbation and exaggeration of narcissistic and genital conflicts. For those who fail to become like their analyst, the result is depression, lowered self-esteem, hopelessness, rage, and eventual disengagement from the organization. For those who do succeed in becoming training analysts, and, therefore, like their own analyst, the effect is also withdrawal, isolation, and increasing constriction on the number of meetings to which they can or will go. There is often a dramatic conservative shift in philosophy as the burden of becoming a "keeper of the flame" is felt, and ever greater numbers of internally oriented rituals are evolved.

I cannot avoid the analogy to the Oriental rulers described by Freud, whose movements become so increasingly constricted that Freud regards their plight as an expression of the ambivalence of the people—to be adored on one hand but hated and punished on the other.

Case histories

I mention a personal note here referring to the days of training at BPSI when the candidate group felt themselves to be so victimized at the hands of what seemed to be a baroque hierarchy that three candidate colleagues and I bestirred ourselves to resurrect the then defunct Candidates' Council, in what I think was a positive attempt to deal with some of the negative factors about our training. Several questions impressed themselves upon me at that time which I have never forgotten. One was to be puzzled by how such exciting intellectual ideas as Freud wrote about could be made into something so phenomenally dull and lifeless. Another was a comment made by a recent graduate of that time, who remarked, "If I never see that G__ d____ place again, it'll be too soon." I can now understand, in retrospect, that what we were feeling was the result of a system that engenders enormous rage, and also crushes the life out of any creativity, except that which is permissible in a very narrow range.

When the controversy began to boil in what eventually became the split of the two Institutes, I participated in many of the meetings, and was appalled and depressed at the vindictiveness and viciousness with which the faculty members treated each other. Here were my ego ideals behaving in such a way as to make me question the very work of analysis. I was also chagrined at the failure of leadership, the passivity among influential analysts who could have had enormous influence in dealing with the controversy, but instead chose to retire, similar to Freud's turning over the International Psycho-Analytic Association to Jung in 1910.

I was deeply disturbed about this for quite some time until I began to realize that there must be (1) unrecognized group factors operating, and (2) only some artifact of the training analysis could possibly explain such intensity of emotion.

In joining PINE, it appeared that there was an opportunity to start over, so that these mistakes of the past possibly could be avoided, given what we all should have learned from that experience. Though initially in PINE there were battles and defections within the top rank, that is, among the training analysts, what evolved was a two-tier system, with the established training analysts on one side, and the very junior faculty on the other, with essentially no middle group. This happy circumstance had the effect of creating a "honeymoon" period in which all were united in trying to reduce the negative hierarchical effect of the previous system. The very successful co-teaching technique was developed, with a junior faculty member teaching with a senior analyst. There was a general assumption, even stated specifically, that all of the junior faculty would, in a natural manner, and in good time, become training analysts.

PINE existed for some time in this happy oblivion; then came accreditation by the national Association, which then led to consideration of appointing new training analysts. These first several appointments began to shake the solidarity of the group somewhat, and one could sense the competitive juices beginning to surge, as small nastinesses began to increase. When the TA Committee guidelines came out, particularly in the "from the top" manner in which they did, with no consultation to the faculty, it was a re-affirmation of (1) the re-institution of the hierarchical system, (2) the shattering of the widespread belief that all eligible faculty members with sufficient clinical experience would one day be named TAs, based on service, and (3) made it clear that training decisions were considered to be the exclusive province of training analysts.

Confusion ensued as members recognized the name of this game—how to please the elders. It becomes a "true self–false self" issue, how to become the kind of person that would be approved of enough to gain the prize. Service and teaching to the organization over the many years appeared to not be valued, only one's performance on this "test".

The group regression was very noticeable, resulting in decreased morale, decreased attendance at meetings (since they did not seem to be valued), and more guardedness. The competitive jousting at meetings began to take an increasingly ugly tone. The candidates remarked that scientific meetings seemed to be primarily for the purpose of sword-play among the faculty and also of competitiveness among their own ranks, as the effects filter down, as would be expected from the well recognized principle of social psychology, the Staunton–Schwartz phenomenon (covert and unrecognized conflict among the senior staff results in the "acting out" of the conflicts by the younger members). Talk of resigning, returning to BPSI, forming another group, began to occur.

At this point we seem to be in the position of considering cancelling our colloquia on the grounds that no one can safely and openly present any sensitive material. (Note: I was the first to present, got roundly attacked by a senior TA, then was defended by my supervisor, another senior TA. No one else would volunteer to present after that.)

It is reminiscent of the anthropological study done by Colin Turnbull of the regressive behavior of the African Ik tribe (1972), which turned upon its own people when faced with an apparently insoluble social problem.

We are beginning to see an increasing the sense of disparity between the training analyst and non-training analyst, in the fact that newly appointed training analysts are instantly never again seen at regular faculty functions, such as the Curriculum Committee meetings. Teaching also is becoming split between the clinical courses, taught by training analysts, and, therefore, apparently more valued, and the rest of the courses taught by non-training analysts.

I suppose that it should be no surprise, in retrospect, that we wound up re-creating what we came from (possibly even worse), as has every other analytic institute, with undoubtedly the same unfortunate results, but what I find particularly galling, for us as analysts, is that we seem to have done it so unthinkingly.

Again, in retrospect, we did quite well as long as we, in effect, had no training analyst system. The minute one was announced, we hit the same rock that everyone else has hit. I suspect that when each of us joined PINE, we each had a deeply held personal vision about what our own ideal institute would be like. We were able to continue this until the re-institution of the training analyst system smoked out everyone's true philosophy.

It may be that these philosophies that we hold are incompatible. But, for me, the tragedy that our organization faces is that we have been unable to air them, discuss them, and examine the issues. This was precisely what happened at BPSI, and it would appear that we have not learned much.

Specific effects of the training analyst system

First and foremost, the TA system compromises every phase of the tripartite system. The effect on the training analysis has already been discussed. Within the faculty, every act or interaction becomes weighed, based on how personally exposing it is. A climate of hostility, suspiciousness, and competitiveness is created that transforms any kind of open presentation or discussion into a sterile and guarded exercise. Referrals of cases for institute analysis are reduced, due to the concern that previous psychotherapy will be criticized. Undertaking any kind of action on behalf of the organization is avoided, both on the basis that it is not valued, and also because such noticeable behaviors make one into a target for the group's displaced rage.

Regressive behavior on the part of both training analyst and non-training analyst becomes increasingly obvious, with greatly increased narcissistic behavior and unpleasantness on all sides. There is an increasing involvement with internal matters, developing rituals, procedures, which absorb the energies of the group so totally that no external issues can be addressed. All energies are turned inward, and even survival issues, such as ways to generate patients, policy matters of educating insurance companies and the public about psychoanalysis, liaison with other medical disciplines, the increasing irrelevancy of psychoanalysis economically and medically, are all ignored.

Probably the worst effect, but perhaps the most intangible, is that people simply do not enjoy each other any more. Meetings become unbearable burdens, because of both the interpersonal friction and the endless irrelevancies that are addressed.

Positive effects

Two primary arguments have been advanced to justify the training analyst system. The first, of course, is quality control, and the second is that there simply is no other alternative. As to the first point, as can be seen from the foregoing, I feel that the system insures mediocrity and sterility, not quality. In *Monograph #4* of the IPA, the Argentinian group reports a system that, in effect, does away with the training analyst system, though the term is still used. The effects of this, as reported, has been no decrease in quality, a demythologizing of the training analyst's position, a shift of training analyses toward a more therapeutic effect, and a more lively and creative scientific exchange—all of these being, I think, what one would reasonably expect.

As to the argument of no other alternative, it is simply the case that none has been tried, examined, or written about. Neither has the effects of the current system been studied. There is virtually a total absence of articles considering the training analyst system from the point of view of really evaluating it, and, with two possible exceptions (Kernberg and Wallerstein), none suggesting alternatives.

Two further arguments should be addressed: one is that it is a naïvely equalitarian approach to believe that the skill of each analyst is equal, and, therefore, there must be a way of insuring that the best analysts are the ones who analyze the candidates, thereby guaranteeing the best analyses and education.

Obviously the need to preserve quality is not at issue—everyone is interested in that. The question is, how should this quality best be achieved? As I tried to illustrate, I believe the training analyst system is destructive to quality. I believe that if candidates were allowed, with some education, to select their own analysts, they would try to select those people who were considered the best analysts. The only danger in this would be in the occasional charismatic, destructive analyst, who should certainly be dealt with by other, more direct means. I believe that in this way, the only thing that would be sacrificed would be control, not quality.

The other argument is that "everyone wants to be a training analyst" because of Oedipal issues. One of our unfortunate habits as a group is our tendency to diagnose each other, rather than deal with the issues. I am afraid that I am inclined to regard this as a kind of analytic name-calling, particularly unfortunate because, for one thing, there are enough diagnoses to go around, and second, it diverts us from the issue.

Our particular selection system

1. All of the above negative effects apply, but in much more dramatic fashion. The damage, I believe, is proportional to the length of the process.
2. The particular method we have is literally eight to ten times more extensive than most selection systems, resulting in even more polarization and exaggeration of the effects described above. The number of interviews with assessors is running 18–30 and more, as compared to two or three at BPSI. To this must be added committee, travel, case write-up time, etc. It must be borne in mind that all of this is designed to evaluate colleagues who have worked, thought, talked, taught, and presented together for many years.
3. The system is enormously time and energy draining, diverting us from vital tasks facing us. Just out of interest, figuring conservatively, converting the person hours into fees, it would appear to cost an average of $55,000 to evaluate each applicant. The five applicants evaluated so far amount to a total cost of $275,000.
4. There is an intolerable sense of humiliation involved in suddenly being judged by one's peers with whom one has worked for twenty years.
5. The out-of-town interviews are understood as an attempt to objectify the process. However, one wonders why we need to be protected from each other, either from one of our own members "blackballing" an applicant, or the need for the evaluating members to have "a blank cartridge", so that the applicant cannot be sure who did it to him.
6. There is a fantasy of objectivity in what is inevitably a primarily subjective selection process.
7. I believe that it is also a fantasy that clinical work can be assessed fairly in this way. As one former non-training analyst remarked, what is delivered in such a test situation is "BS" (excrement of a bull). Inevitably, the presenter will be guarded and select the least problematic cases and material. Working and thinking together over a period of time would appear to be a much more sound basis for evaluation.
8. The destructiveness to group morale and purpose is incalculable.

Conclusions

In the plenary address of the May (1984) meetings of the American Psychoanalytic (also appears in IPA *Monograph #4*), Kernberg states that psychoanalysis is suffering from a "serious illness." He presents four educational models, feeling that current educational systems most closely resemble that of a combination trade school and religious seminary. He comments at great length on the transference contaminants produced by the system, which I have enumerated earlier, bringing about seriously compromised analyses, as well as an arid educational climate. He suggests we should move toward an art school/university model. I very much agree with his diagnosis but feel that his prescription is too simple. The power of the unconscious issues involved is such that no cosmetic solution can have significant effect.

I would propose that the training analyst system, and the hierarchical educational structure that has derived from it, be considered from the point of view of a neurotic symptom, a compromise formation, a solution in action of unanalysed, ambivalent, transferential issues. Like any neurotic defense, it brings about the very thing it seeks to prevent. It insures, by its essentially abusive nature, its own destruction, engendering hostility, and guaranteeing attack from succeeding generations. The constant re-creation of the precise same system no matter how many times it does not work, the inability to consider alternatives, or to even examine the system itself, can be seen as a classic repetition compulsion.

It certainly could be argued that calling this organization phenomenon a "neurosis", could well be "diagnosing up". It may be that it more closely resembles an organizational "character disorder", on the grounds that there is no conscious discomfort on the part of those infected with it.

To look at our life history of PINE is revealing. Having been spawned out of what I believe we would all agree was a bad educational system, after a period of health, we have now succeeded in re-creating, and perhaps even in an even more extreme form, the very system that time and again has proven to be disastrous—the return of the repressed. The structure that we have evolved, without much in the way of conscious realization, is the most constricted possible structure—a self-selecting, self-perpetuating Education Committee of training analysts, presiding over the non-training analyst faculty, with a proposed appendage society, the very same prescription which led to such educational sterility at BPSI.

The only two mistakes that we have not yet made, though both are under some consideration, is the creation of a society composed of yet a third level of citizenship, and to re-institute the practice of the reporting training analyst.

Mark Twain remarked that the "primary difference between education and a massacre, is that a massacre is more sudden". I believe that what he had in mind was not true education, but the inexorable intellectual hemorrhage created by control structures, which are really designed to reassure the teachers, rather than to meet the needs of the student.

In describing the "ideal institute", Freud seems to have visualized the ideal analyst as being a kind of "Renaissance" individual. Cecil Rhodes seems to have had a similar idea in mind in defining his Scholar:

> literary and scholastic attainments; truthfulness, courage, devotion to duty, sympathy for and protection of the weak, kindliness, unselfishness, and fellowship; exhibition of moral force of character and of instincts to lead, and to take an interest in one's contemporaries; physical vigor as shown by fondness for a success in sports. (Johnson, 1916, p. 11)

This also embodies the Greek ideal of the well-rounded individual. We could do worse than to follow this model.

It seems difficult to justify the training analyst system on educational grounds. Training analysts, non-training analysts, and candidates alike seem victimized and imprisoned by the system. Regardless of the certainly honorable intentions of all involved, the system is, in its very essence, a political and coercive structure, and as such is profoundly antithetical to the spirit and ideals of both education and analysis. No method of selection can change that essential fact.

Perhaps it is more accurate to suggest that what is really at issue here are two essentially different and deeply held views of man. During the Continental Congress debates to determine our form of government, Alexander Hamilton represented one side, when he argued that government was "too important to be left in the hands of the people", and informed Thomas Jefferson, that "Your people, sir, are a great beast." Jefferson, on the other hand, felt that small power groups of even honorable men would inevitably become self-serving, and that the better hope over the long term lay in investing an educated populace with the decision-making capability.

Recommendations

1. I believe that it would be a courageous and creative act to do away with the training analyst system in fact, and ideally in name, and consider alternative possibilities. I believe that it is very difficult for any other than a young institute to do this. Bureaucracies become self-perpetuating and vested interests become binding very soon in the history of an organization. I believe at this point we have what is possibly our last opportunity to consider this alternative. It may already be too late.

   I feel, however, that we are not only in a unique position in terms of our organizational history, but also from the point of view of our position with the American Psychoanalytic Association. We are positively regarded, and I think accurately, as a serious, committed, talented, analytic organization. A proposal by us, well presented, would have a very good chance of being approved, at least, on a provisional basis. We have an opportunity not only to free ourselves, but to free analysis from this albatross, which has been with us since 1920. I really do not believe that it is overstating the case to feel that it may be the system or us that has to go.
2. If the training analyst system is retained, then I would have the following recommendations, the purpose of which would be to reduce the idealized position and actual power of the training analyst appointment, in order to minimize the damage to the training analyses and education.
   (a) Most importantly, the By-laws should be revised to make the Education Committee a sub-committee of the faculty. The educational process should be governed by all the faculty, with training analysts being simply regarded as serving a specialized function.
   (b) The important EC sub-committees, such as Progressions, Admissions, Curriculum, Committee of Training Analysts, and the EC itself should be balanced with equal number of non-training analyst faculty.

(c) The number of candidate analysands by any one training analyst should be limited to three (3), a rule followed by many institutes, including BPSI.

(d) The training analyst selection process should be reduced to as simple and time/energy saving procedure as possible. BPSI's method of one short write-up and two to three interviews seems reasonable, based as it is on the assumption that the applicant is already well known, and the interviews can be expected to clear up only a few remaining questions.

(e) No separate society should be considered at this time. If a society is needed for political reasons with the American, we can create a society that is synonymous with the faculty.

(f) One model, of course, would be the "Argentinian option", which would involve much less formalized faculty division into senior faculty and associate faculty, with the training analyst designation applying as one moved from one tier to the other, this being based on service to the organization, teaching contributions, etc.

(g) It should be recalled that on the last occasion at which the guidelines were discussed, the meeting ended with the very serious proposal, which probably would have passed at that time, to end the training analyst system at PINE. I believe that it was (another colleague) and I who felt this might be premature at that point, and perhaps as unilateral as were the guidelines, given the fact that as a group, we had not thought the problem through sufficiently.

The current guidelines remained in place in a *de facto* manner, which, in retrospect, might have been a serious mistake. It seems to me that the very least that we should try to accomplish now would be to recommend a termination of those guidelines and put an immediate freeze on any applications in process, on the grounds that we need to assess what we are doing before we proceed too far down that organizational road from which there appears to be no return.

The sentiment is often expressed by those applying to become training analysts that they will "get in" and then change the system from inside. I believe this is a rationalization. I think that once one becomes a training analyst, such a price has been paid to get there the tendency is to preserve and re-enact it.

I believe that it is quite possible that we could continue as an organization for the foreseeable future in a crippled and truncated fashion. I even think that it is possible we could continue for long enough that most of us would have come to the end of our professional life. However, I also think that it is a fact that our system even now is beginning to degenerate into the unrelenting mediocrity which I think is inherent in the system from which we sprang. We have increasingly little to offer candidates over BPSI. All we ever had to offer was the excitement and creativeness of our faculty, which I think is now being extinguished. I think we have a responsibility to future generations of analysts, if there are going to be any, to "bite the bullet" and address this very difficult issue, which no organization before us has yet been able to do. If we do not, I think it is likely that PINE will gradually fade away, in the foreseeable future.

Discussions with colleagues about their training analyses reveals a surprising number who feel that rigid and doctrinaire attitudes on the part of the training analyst resulted in conscious compliance and withholding, which contaminated their analyses to a significant degree. Certainly, this suggests that this question should be looked into more systematically, as difficult and touchy as it may be. The quality of training analyses and its consequent educational value might have an undeservedly high reputation, especially given the fact that there is no actual data available on the matter.

That the first analysis is for the institute, and the second is for one's self, has become something of a truism. The way Grete Bibring put it,

> By virtue of his position the training analyst loses the role of neutral and understanding parent and turns into the dreaded judge. For this reason a second analysis, after graduation and membership have been attained, is often easier and more fruitful. (1954, p. 169)

The "problem of the training analysis" is not that the therapeutic function of analysis is incompatible with the educational function of analytic training. The therapeutic function *is*, however, incompatible with the training analyst system, which is inherently hierarchical. The "problem of the training analysis" (and the consequent organizational problems) are considered, therefore, to be not inevitable, but iatrogenic (self-created).

Freud wrote in 1926, describing his ideal institute,

> what is known as medical education appears to me to be an arduous and circuitous way of approaching the profession of analysis . . . a scheme of training for analysts has still to be created. It must include elements from the mental sciences, from psychology, the history of civilization and sociology, as well as from anatomy, biology, and the study of evolution . . . I am merely setting up an ideal . . . but an ideal which can and must be realized. (1926e, p. 252)

Freud was very clear about what his "ideal institute" would be. We have paid little heed to his vision, and less to discovering and discussing what each other's and our own personal visions are.

My ideal institute would be a community of dedicated scholarship, in which we would truly concentrate on the educational, scientific, and reality issues facing analysis, and would communicate to each other our true thoughts and feelings as directly as possible, secure in the knowledge that these ideas would be received, not necessarily with agreement, but with respect, consideration, and even kindness; an institute where petty rivalries and backbiting competitiveness would be minimized in the service of the greater good; an institute where our considerable energies and talents would not be dissipated in procedures, ritual, and conflict, but, to paraphrase Freud, would be utilized in productive collegial interchange and creative mutual work.

I do not feel that this is an "ideal" in the sense that it is unrealistic or unreachable. PINE began in that spirit. I believe that our first step in recovering that goal is to return to that point before we had evolved the framework which prevents us from operating with the common decency we all possess, and begin again.

Part II (2016)

Training analyst system: organizational consequences

Since this is a case study, I will pick up the action in 1984, right after it became clear to me that nothing was going to change at PINE. I was so disappointed in what PINE had become, I decided to pursue my career elsewhere. I had seen an advertisement from the Medical University of South Carolina describing two analytic positions, one clinical, and one academic. I applied for the academic one. A very knowledgeable Medical Director wrote back and said, in essence, if you are an academic, why are you not a training analyst?

Thus, it became clear to me that I had to get that credential in order to relocate. So, I applied and I became "certified", which is a test required by the Board on Professional Standards of the American Psychoanalytic Association, in order to become a training analyst. This is no easy matter, as it requires extensive case write-ups, and, sometimes, case presentations.

Once that was done, I began the process, which required a great many interviews, with three different senior psychoanalysts, two from PINE, and one from an out of town institute.

When I was seeing one of the interviewers from PINE, a close friend of mine, in addition to hearing my case, said to me, "Bob, don't you think writing that TA paper was neurotic?" I said, "Neurotic? It was f——- suicidal." And then I explained to him the play that I used to dread when I played high school football, a play called "student body right". I explained to him that is where everyone who possibly can gets in front of the ball carrier and comes around your side. Your job is to throw yourself in front of them, so that somebody behind you can make the tackle. I said that is what I was trying to do with PINE, because I thought we were making a terrible mistake.

I was duly appointed a training analyst, and I think to everyone's credit they did not hold the writing of the paper against me. However, during the process, I made sure to drive my son's Toyota to Education Committee meetings, rather than drive my own Porsche 911.

By the time I had become a TA, the lawsuit against the American Psychoanalytic and the IPA had occurred, because of the practice of excluding non-physicians from training in APsaA. I thought APsaA was completely on the wrong side of the case, and wrote the then-president, Dick Simons, a letter telling him so, and suggesting that we change law firms to try to achieve a settlement.

Apparently, he had been thinking along the same lines himself and, interestingly, came up with the same law firm I had suggested.

He asked me if he could, in appreciation, appoint me to a committee in the Association. I told him I would like a committee that was on the "cutting edge of change". He appointed me to the Committee on Non-medical Clinical Training, which had been formed to process non-physicians for training in the Association.

To make a long story short, I became increasingly involved in the American Psychoanalytic, mainly because I felt it would be easier to create change in the national organization than in my local group.

I shall return to this part of the story later, but I want to turn now to a follow-up on the fate of PINE. It took many years longer than I had thought it would, but PINE did indeed gradually deteriorate, and eventually was able to draw no candidates to train. PINE had come to be seen in the Boston community as by far the most rigid and restrictive of the three local institutes. Of those three institutes, the independent psychology institute seemed do reasonably well in drawing candidates, BPSI did moderately well, but PINE did very poorly.[2]

Eventually, bowing to the inevitable, the PINE faculty decided, in essence, to close PINE. This was precipitated by the great majority of the training analysts deciding to transfer from PINE back to BPSI. It should be noted that this group of training analysts was the same group that had continued the extremely conservative practices at PINE. In my view, this group was, in many ways, largely responsible for PINE's demise. However, I would doubt very much if any of them would feel that that was the case, or that their policies had anything to do with PINE's difficulties.

At this point, a group of younger faculty has decided to continue PINE and try to revive it, and I have considerable hope that PINE might be able to return to its original philosophy. If so, I think it would have a good chance of not only surviving, but flourishing.

To return to the adventures at APsaA, again to make a long story short, I became increasingly involved in the organization, and became president of the organization twice, once from 1998–2000 and more recently from 2012–2014.

Like PINE, the Association had developed along very narrow, inward-looking lines. The twin goals were candidate education and sponsoring scientific programs for members. I felt that there was no question that we were in the midst of a worsening crisis for psychoanalysis, with steadily declining numbers of candidates, and analytic patients, and yet we seemed helpless to do anything about it.

I ran during my first term with the goal of trying to help the organization begin to engage the external forces that were threatening us, which were increasing regulation and interference by the government and insurance companies, and a community uninformed about psychoanalytic treatment.

During my first term, we were indeed able to become increasingly effective in political advocacy, use of the media, and direct outreach to the public. We were fortunate in that my brother, James Pyles, was a founding partner in a health law firm in Washington, DC, and he became our legislative representative on Capitol Hill.

At the same time, we hired a professional public relations person to help educate the public and legislators about the nature of psychoanalysis. Both of these efforts seemed to work extremely well.

I eventually ran for a second term because of continuing conflict within the Association, around this very issue that we are discussing. The organization had continued to have difficulty attracting students. It was also reported by the Committee on Institutes that thirteen of our twenty-nine institutes, nearly half, were very close to going the way of PINE.

I felt that the twin lightning rods of the training analyst system and certification were, to some degree, responsible for it. Certainly, no one would argue that doing away with the training analyst system would solve all of our problems. But at least I thought it might prevent us from participating in a system that seemed to bring out the worst in everyone.

Accordingly, two colleagues and I, Rick Perlman and Warren Procci (who was president just before me), wrote a proposal that came to be known as the "PPP Proposal". What we were calling for was a thorough discussion and evaluation of the training analyst system, to be done within the Board on Professional Standards (BoPS).

Little did we know that this was to ignite yet another firestorm, similar to the one that occurred in my local institute (PINE) when I tried to get the TA system discussed. The leadership of the Board on Professional Standards managed for three years to prevent *any* discussion of the PPP Proposal, except for a token fifteen minutes. Using every parliamentary trick in the book, the leadership was able to prevent it from coming to the floor. It seemed startlingly clear once more that even the mere *discussion* of the TA system was incredibly threatening to the BoPS leadership.

A few words about the very unusual organizational structure of APsaA are necessary here, and I beg the reader's indulgence. As opposed to every other psychoanalytic society in the world, APsaA is divided into two separate and distinct sections, the training part, which is the Board on Professional Standards (BoPS), and the membership part, which is the Executive Council. It also happens that the Executive Council is the Board of Directors for the entire Association. Training institutes send representatives to BoPS, and societies send representatives to the Executive Council. Hence, membership and education is often kept separate at the local level as well.

However, to return to the action, at this point the Executive Council, in frustration, passed a resolution, in essence directing BOPS to develop "objective and verifiable" guidelines for the selection of training analysts.

The response from the leadership of BoPS was swift and decisive. Without discussion or warning, seven leading members of BOPS filed a lawsuit against the Association.

This lawsuit was a very serious and expensive one, and cost our Association a very large amount of money. To the surprise of many of us, the judge decided that our bylaws gave BOPS exclusive jurisdiction over education. The judge stated that even though our Executive Council (the Board of Directors) supposedly oversaw the whole Association, it could not interfere with, or oversee, educational policies. The judge further commented that if we wanted that to change, we would have to change our bylaws.

The framers of the bylaws, in 1946, had apparently done their job well.

Accordingly, since I had become president at that point, I appointed a task force to develop a bylaw which would clearly establish the jurisdiction of our Executive Council over all matters in our Association and, finally, after sixty plus years, unite our Association under one roof, essentially like every other group in the IPA.

Predictably, the Bylaw Proposal itself quickly became a flash point, as both sides realized that if it passed, we would finally be able to have Association-wide discussions about educational matters, including the TA system and certification.

A word explaining the peculiar politics of APsaA is in order here. In 1938, the insistence of APsaA on training physicians only led to a near split between APsaA and the IPA. The compromise reached at that time granted APsaA semi-independent status over training, as long as APsaA adhered to the minimum standards of the IPA.

The reason for this odd arrangement goes, again, back to 1938, when the Association developed policies for training only physicians and set up a "certification" test similar to the medical specialty board examinations. The goal was to ensure that educational practices would be free-standing and permanently insulated from possible adulteration by the membership side, including the Executive Council (the Board of Directors). We have been plagued with the legacy of these ancient shibboleths ever since.

As a part of the embracing of the "medical model" for training, the Board on Professional Standards (BoPS), as said, developed an examination ("certification", as it is called), based on the medical specialty examinations in the USA. This would not have been a problem, except that BoPS decided to make this test a mandatory requirement for becoming a training analyst. No comparable test exists in any other society in the world.

This has rightly been called "the politics of exclusion". The original purpose was to exclude non-physicians from training, and this policy continued until 1988, when settlement of the famous lawsuit brought by a group of non-physicians began to allow for the training of other mental health professionals. APsaA was exceedingly fortunate to have as its president, Dick Simons, who, in the face of considerable opposition, was able to achieve this historic agreement.

Ironically, this settlement, which was so vociferously resisted by many, has been the salvation of our Association, allowing the inclusion and training of so many talented mental health professionals. We were, quite literally, saved from our own hubris. But the spirit of the original exclusionary policies has continued with the BoPS leadership until the present day, making it almost impossible to include other quality independent analytic groups in our Association.

It might seem as if I am being a bit harsh in my comments about the leadership of BoPS. However, it is an undeniable fact that those officers have been in the forefront of APsaA exclusionary policies for the past sixty years. There are two reasons for that. The first is that candidate education, and who may be allowed to be trained, has, from the beginning, been considered to be the exclusive province of BoPS. Therefore, BoPS, until very recently, has had a complete stranglehold on training.

That part of the problem is organizational, and may soon be remedied. The second part of the problem is at once deeper and more profound. It could be stated as a question: "How can reasonable people be co-opted to go to such extreme lengths to protect such a coercive system?"

The answer, all too often, is, become a training analyst. It seems to change people, to maximize latent narcissistic issues, not always, but often. I have even known several colleagues who now wanted to be called by the more formal versions of their names. Part of becoming a TA seems to be that one has become a "Keeper of the Flame". To become an officer of BoPS seems to have the most toxic effect, because now one has become, in effect, a high priest entrusted with protecting the "Holy of Holies". And, as Freud noted in *Group Psychology and the Analysis of the Ego* (1921c), the self-observing ego seems to be lost as the price of admission to group leadership.

The other major group dynamic to consider is what happens to any group that is allowed to operate for sixty years, entirely on its own, with no equilibrating or correcting feedback. As the Founding Fathers of the USA's Constitution understood, better than we have, such a group is almost certain to gather increasing power to themselves, until they are convinced that they are privy to a higher truth than their constituents. It was for that very reason that they designed a government in three parts, each to act as a "check and balance" on the others.

The training analyst system and "Certification" have become the two major points of contention in the ongoing political struggle within APsaA. As it has become increasingly likely that the Bylaw Proposal may pass, allowing both our Board of Directors and our members to have a full and open discussion of both the TA system and Certification, the leadership of BoPS has come up with a desperate measure to preserve both.

That measure is "externalization". What that means is that independent and free-standing organizational entities would be set up to oversee Certification, possibly TA appointments, and the accreditation of institutes as well.

The "independent" status is something of a fig-leaf, as the Boards of those entities would be staffed by the same people as the leadership of BoPS has been. What would be different is that these functions would be finally and permanently freed from the threat of oversight by the Board of Directors and the membership of APsaA.

What the threatened danger of the splitting off of the more conservative institutes has led to, however, is an effort by the Executive Committee to craft a compromise. Our Executive Committee consists, essentially, of the nationally elected officers, plus the officers of BoPS. The compromise is the "Six-Point Plan", and we are told that it has to be approved in its entirety, with no changes, in order to keep the peace.

The problem is that the "Six Points" were written so vaguely by the Executive Committee that it is difficult to know what is really in it.

However, what has begun to emerge is that the Plan would result in major changes in the essential nature of our Association.

Just to take two major points that, in my opinion, are extremely problematic. Our Association has always had the twin missions of education and membership. This plan would put education into independent bodies, outside the oversight of our members and our Board of directors, and transform the Association into a "membership only" body.

Since the education of candidates has always been a source of great pride and "moral gravitas", this would split our Association right down the middle, and cut the heart out one of our two major functions.

Second, the Association would commit to the use of the Eitingon Model exclusively, no other models of education being permitted. This would enshrine the training analyst system permanently.

Between these two provisions, this "Plan", if passed, would put permanently in place the major provisions considered vital by the BoPS leadership. Efforts to change these very policies were what started the conflict in the first place.

If these provisions are approved, the future of our Association, in my opinion, will be very problematic.

Late breaking news

Quite literally, as this chapter was going to press, the following events took place.

Latest development. A little background. As described above, one of the most remarkable developments in this struggle occurred when our Board of Directors attempted to direct BoPS to consider the use of objective measures for the selection of training analysts. The reaction of some of the BoPS leadership was to file a lawsuit against our Association. This lawsuit eventually cost our organization over a million dollars in legal fees (fortunately, covered by insurance). To the surprise of many, the Court decided twice in favor of the BoPS leaders. The Judge ruled that our Board on Professional Standards, and not our Board of Directors, was solely in charge of education (and, therefore, the TA system). In her decision, she said if we wanted it to be different, we would have to change our bylaws. So, as president, I immediately formed a Task Force to rewrite the bylaw. This was put on hold by the new adminstration. However, a bylaw can be independently introduced by fifty members, and that is what happened.

In APsaA, it is almost impossible to get a substantive bylaw changed or passed, because it requires a two thirds majority.

Hardly anyone thought the new bylaw proposal would pass, because it would require 66%. However, members were angry about the lawsuit, and the vote just occurred. The new bylaw passed by 69.3%. So now our Board of Directors is in charge of everything, including education. The response from the BoPS leadership? They are continuing to try to move the regulatory functions into two independent external bodies (which could be done, since neither would be within the purview of our organization), to protect it from oversight!

This is quite literally a revolution in our Association, and changes the whole nature of our organization. For the first time since 1946, we have a fully functioning Board of Directors. For the first time, the entire membership can be involved in discussions of education. And, finally, for the first time in seventy years, we can have an authentic discussion of the training analyst system. This is a truly historic development.

This is where we now stand, and it is important to note the desperation and the extreme measures that some will go to not only preserve the TA system, but to prevent even a discussion of it.

The point I am trying to make here is that these internal conflicts preoccupy us to the point where we cannot devote our energies to doing what we should be doing, which is to bring psychoanalysis as much as possible into the public realm, and to acquaint potential candidates with the usefulness of psychoanalytic thinking in a whole variety of areas.

It is clear to everyone that psychoanalysis is in terrible trouble. Our institutes are dying. There are ever fewer candidates and analytic patients. We are getting out-recruited by other analytic groups. We are under increasing pressure from government and insurance regulation. Private practice is under siege, and is directly in the crosshairs of politicians as a major cost-driver of health care. It took twenty years to bring in even our first independent analytic group, the William Alanson White.

Our response to this? We fight with each other. We even sue each other. We have continual splits. We ignore the external threats to our profession. But the one thing we cannot seem to do is talk with each other. And this has been the pathetic legacy throughout our analytic history.

I am reminded of a story that a former president, Marvin Margolis, used to tell. When the Romans surrounded Jerusalem in 70 ad, there were three or four different groups of Jews in Jerusalem, each of whom felt they had the best way to deal with the Romans. They began fighting and killing each other. The Romans simply waited until they were done, marched into the city unopposed, killed all the men and sold all the women and children into slavery.

The striking similarity to religious conflicts, of course, has to be noted. Here, I harken back to my first two paragraphs regarding beginning my training at BPSI and the essentially tribal nature of these battles. The two groups involved each feel that the fate of psychoanalysis is at stake, and if their point of view does not prevail, psychoanalysis will die.

For this reason, I must point out that, although there have been many powerful and scholarly presentations on this critical fault-line in our associations over many years, no change has occurred. Not even the threat of annihilation of our profession has had significant impact.

I am forced to conclude, therefore, that the only approach that is likely to save us is to combine these worsening external threats, and potent scholarly arguments, with another ingredient-courage, translated into determined political will, or even political muscle, if necessary. As many have noted, from Cincinnatus to Martin Luther King, Jr, very few ever give up power voluntarily.

I am sure it is clear that I think the training analyst system is a terrible one. It is anti-analytic, anti-educational, and very close to being unethical, in my opinion. If we were starting analysis from scratch, without the authoritarian legacy of our past, I feel sure that if someone suggested this system, we would think they needed medication.

But one thing I am very sure of. We cannot keep behaving in this manner if we want psychoanalysis to survive. We have to begin acting like responsible adults. Maybe even like *real* psychoanalysts!

Epilogue

Educational and organizational aspects of the training analyst issue

Basically, the thesis is this: there is very significant evidence to suggest that the training analyst system, far from enhancing quality, by its very nature produces serious and inevitable deterioration in the quality of science, education, and analysis.

To aid in our consideration, I have listed below some of the specific effects.

1. Negative
   (a) Effects on the training analysis
      - Contaminated transference producing unanalyzable elements because of intruding reality factors (Greenacre, 1966).
      - The "setting" of analysis seriously compromised (Limentani, 1974).
      - Termination phase inevitably compromised.
      - True neutrality even more difficult to achieve.
      - Frequent compliance of the analysand, with issues kept out of the analysis.
      - Idealization of analyst, and displacing of negative affects onto colleagues: splitting and organizational conflicts.

   (b) Effects on the training analyst
      - Isolation from faculty and other TAs.
         - Keeper of the flame—conservative shift.
         - No longer able to present clinical material.
         - No longer have access to supportive meetings with openness and interchange.
         - Unable to attend many faculty functions, parties, and other meetings.
         - Denied feedback, cut off from candidates, faculty, and even other TAs.
      - Skewed and limiting selection of patients.
      - Isolation of the work is made even more difficult.
      - Isolation from economic and scientific realities.
         - Appointment amounts to tenure and sinecure.
         - Often the only way to have a full analytic practice.
         - Able to disregard such things as the lack of analytic patients.
      - Identification with his own idealized TA—one has become a "knower"—the center of our system. In our system, a TA is the only worthwhile thing to be. Our system is centered

in the idea that there are those who know and those who do not—enormous energy in distinguishing the better people from the lesser people—results from inappropriate use of intrapsychic theory; Greben (1952–1953)—"The TA starts with the fantasy of his superiority over his analytic brothers".

- Net result: tendency to increase narcissism, grandiosity, and regression, emphasizing the worst aspects of personality. Almost inevitably, a noticeable change in those appointed, unrealized by themselves, and generally not told because of the power of the new position.

(c) Effects on non-TA faculty

- Similarly, increased regression because of failure to become like one's TA-parent.
- Repression, lowered self-esteem, internally directed rage, passive compliant depression, tendency to blame self, like an abused child identifying with the aggressor, or taking the passive victimized position.
- Tendency to avoid exposure, vulnerability, such as meetings, presentations, referrals – passive withdrawal.

(d) Effects on educational and organizational aspects

- Destructive of group cohesiveness as central beliefs of group are eroded; group begins to become not a *real* group, but a collection of individuals.
- Inadvertent but inherent in the system is the centralization of power, with no checks, balances, or feedback. This leads to inevitable politicization and polarization, in that the system, by its very nature, is inherently political.
- Regressive behavior on all sides, leading to decreased trust, an increased competitiveness, and suspiciousness. Conformance rewarded and difference penalized.
- Decreased involvement in meetings, teaching—passive compliance, low profile, activity avoided because (i) perceived as not valued, (ii) reluctance to risk exposure, and (iii) depression saps energy.
- Decreased referrals because of concern about exposure of one's psychotherapy.

- Increased barrenness of scientific presentations and discussions (especially clinical), cessation of colloquia and other clinically oriented meetings.
- Decreased trust and enjoyment of each other.
- Elaboration of energy absorbing internal rituals, turning away from productive and creative attempts to address educational issues and external challenges (i.e., lack of patients, etc.); increased misperception of control as representing quality.
- Group becomes energy consuming, not really a group giving anything back, but a "black hole".
- Result: antithetical to spirit of education, science, and analysis itself.
- While currently system still has not effected candidate education, this is likely to erode, as negativity affects every phase of the tripartite system as it had before PINE began.

2. Positive
   (a) Tradition: this is not to be taken lightly. Group traditions and rituals are important cohesive mechanisms, so long as they express a value system that is positive and generally compatible with the members. The question is—does our tradition really reflect our values, or are we subordinating our values to a tradition which no longer quite fits? Are we riding the horse, or is the horse riding us?
   (b) The argument is that quality control is best served by having the best analysts analyzing those who are to be analysts. This is best articulated in Ferenczi's comment that it is intolerable for a patient to be better analyzed than the therapist. However, the problems here are many and complicated, as were the motivations for Ferenczi's comment.
   - It is highly dubious that the best analysts can be selected by any known method, or, at least, so the record would suggest.
   - The very concept of "best" introduces a power structure antithetical to the spirit of analytic inquiry.
   - The quality of training analyses may very well not be as high as that of therapeutic analyses – for the reasons mentioned above.
   - It has been repeatedly demonstrated that quality under such a system decreases, rather than increases.

Notes

1. While freeing themselves from the IPA, the American carried within itself the seeds of its own destruction, and proceeded to institute a system more rigid than that against which they rebelled. PINE, in splitting away from BPSI, also seems to have followed this pattern, as will be commented on later.
2. Thomas Szasz (1958):

> It is important to note here that-as is the case with so many revolutions with which one is familiar-even though the revolution starts out with the officially avowed aim of "making things more democratic", once it becomes successful, the old drama is re-enacted exactly as before, only with different "actors". The formerly rebellious group now becomes the possessor of power and wields it usually even more forcibly than did its predecessor. The roles of those who have power and those who do not remains unaltered; only the identity of the specific individuals who comprise the two groups changes.

> No attention is paid to the social organization of the group.

Bibliography for the 1984 paper

Alexander, F., & Selesnick, S. (1966). *The History of Psychiatry, 1891–1964.* New York: Harper & Row.

Arlow, J. (1982). Psychoanalytic education: a psychoanalytic perspective. *Annual of Psychoanalysis, 10*: 5–20.

Atkins, N. (1970). The Oedipus myth and the successions of generations, *Journal of the American Psychoanalytic Association, 18*(4): 860–875.

Balint, M. (1948). On the psychoanalytic training system. *International Journal of Psychoanalysis, 29*: 163–173.

Balint, M. (1954). Analytic training and training analysis. *International Journal of Psychoanalysis, 35*: 157–162.

Benedek, T. (1954). Countertransference in the training analyst. *Bulletin of the Menninger Clinic, 28*: 12–16.

Benedek, T. (1955). A contribution to the problem of termination of training analysis. *Journal of the American Psychoanalytic Association, 3*: 615–629.

Bion, W. R. (1961). *Experiences in Groups and Other Papers.* London: Tavistock.

Blum, H. (1981). The forbidden quest and the analytic ideal: the superego and insight. *Psychoanalytic Quarterly, 50*: 535–556.

Bruzzone, M., Casaula, E., Jiménez, J. P., & Jordan, J. F. (1985). Regression and persecution in analytic training: reflections on experience. *International Review of Psycho-Analysis, 12*(4): 411–418.

Cabernite, L. (1982). The selection and functions of the training analyst in analytic training institutes in Latin America. *International Review of Psycho-Analysis, 9*: 398–417.

Calef, V. (1954). Training and therapeutic analysis. *Journal of the American Psychoanalytic Association, 2*: 175–178.

Calef, V. (1982). An introspective on training and non-training analysis. *Annual of Psychoanalysis, 10*: 93–114.

Calef, V., & Weinshel, E. (1973) Reporting, non-reporting, and assessment in the training analysis. *Journal of the American Psychoanalytic Association, 21*: 714–726.

Curtis, H. (1982). Educational prerequisites for analytic training. *Annual of Psychoanalysis, 10*: 21–28.

D'Amore, A. (1981). Psychoanalysis in America: 1930–1939. *Psychoanalytic Quarterly, 50*(4): 570–586.

Dorn, R. (1982). Training analyst's selections: the need of criteria. *International Journal of Psychoanalytic Psychotherapy, 9*: 961–704.

Eckstein, R. (1955). Termination of the training analysis within the framework of present-day institutes. *Journal of the American Psychoanalytic Association, 3*: 600–614.

Eckstein, R. (1960). A historical survey on the teaching of psychoanalytic technique. *Journal of the American Psychoanalytic Association, 8*: 500–516.

Eckstein, R. (1969). Thoughts concerning appointment and election procedures for training analysts and other faculty members. *Journal of Nervous and Mental Disease, 149*(2): 208–212.

Eisold, K. (2004). Psychoanalytic training: the 'faculty system'. *Psychoanalytic Inquiry, 24*: 51–70.

Eissler, K. (1965). *Medical Orthodoxy and the Future of Psychoanalysis*. New York: International Universities Press.

Ferenczi, S. (1911). On the organization of the psychoanalytic movement. In: *Contributions to the Problems and Methods of Psychoanalysis* (pp. 229–307). New York: Brunner/Mazel, 1980.

Freud, A. (1950)[1938]. The problems of training analysis. In: *Writings of Anna Freud, Volume IV*: (pp. 407–442). New York: International Universities Press, 1968.

Freud, A. (1971). The ideal psychoanalytic institute: a utopia. *Bulletin of the Menninger Clinic, 35*(4): 225–239.

Freud, S. (1887). *The Origins of Psychoanalysis*, A. Bonaparte, A. Freud, & E. Kris (Eds.). New York: Basic Books, 1954.
Freud, S. (1910). The future prospects of psychoanalysis. *S. E., 11*: 141–151. London: Hogarth.
Freud, S. (1912). Recommendations to physicians practising psychoanalysis. *S. E., 12*: 111–120. London: Hogarth.
Freud, S. (1914). History of the psychoanalytic movement. *S. E., 14*: 7–67. London: Hogarth.
Freud, S. (1937). Analysis terminable and interminable. *S. E., 23*: 211–253. London: Hogarth.
Gaskill, H. (1979). Bridges to the future. *Journal of the American Psychoanalytic Association, 27*(1): 3–26.
Gifford, S. (1978). Psychoanalysis in Boston: Innocence and experience. Introduction to panel discussion, April 1973. *Psychoanalysis, Psychotherapy, and the New England Scene* 1894–1944. G. Gifford, Jr., New York: Scientific History Publications.
Gifford, S. (1983). The first 50 years, 1933–1983. *Psychoanalytic Newsletter*, 5–7.
Gifford, S. (1985). Depression or sea change (Fenichel's *Rundbriefe* and the political analyst of the 1930s). *International Journal of Psychoanalysis, 66*(3): 265–272.
Gitelson, M. (1954). Therapeutic problems and the analysis of the "again normal" candidate. *International Journal of Psychoanalysis, 35*: 179–183.
Goodman, S. (1977). Psychoanalytic education and research. COPER Report. *American Journal of Psychoanalysis, 33*: 877–879.
Greben, S. (1982–1983). Some sources of conflict within psychoanalytic societies, *International Journal of Psychoanalytic Psychotherapy, 9*: 657–678.
Greenacre, P. (1966). Problems of training analysis. *Psychoanalytic Quarterly, 35*(4): 540- 567.
Greenson, R. (1969). The origin and fate of new ideas in psychoanalysis. *International Journal of Psychoanalysis, 50*(4): 503–515.
Grinker, R. (1977). Twenty years of psychoanalysis: retrospect and prospect. *Journal of the American Academy of Psychoanalysis, 5*(1): 79–94.
Grotjohn, M. (1954). About the relations between training and psychoanalytic therapy. *International Journal of Psychoanalysis, 35*: 254–262.
Hall, L. (1984). Some reflections on our professional standards. *Journal of the American Psychoanalytic Association, 32*(2): 421–426.
Herrigel, E. (1971). *Zen in the Art of Archery*. New York: Vintage Books.
Hiemann, P. (1954). Problems of the training analysis. *International Journal of Psychoanalysis, 35*: 163–168.

Holzman, P. (1976). The future of psychoanalysis and its institutes. *Psychoanalytic Quarterly*, *45*(2): 250–273.

Joseph, E. (1978). Ego ideal of the psychoanalyst. *International Journal of Psychoanalysis*, *59*: 377–385.

Joseph, E., & Widlöcher, D. (1983). *The Identity of the Psychoanalyst. Monograph 2. International Journal of Psychoanalysis* (articles by M. Gitelson and D. King).

Kairys, D. (1964). The training analysis: a critical review of the literature and a controversial proposal. *Psychoanalytic Quarterly*, *33*: 485–511.

Keiser, S. (1984). Private communication.

Kernberg, O. (1996). Thirty methods to destroy the creativity of psychoanalytic candidates. *International Journal of Psychoanalysis*, *77*: 1031–1040.

Kernberg, O. (2004). Discussion: problems of power in psychoanalytic institutes. *Psychoanalytic Inquiry*, *24*: 106–121.

Kirsner, D. (2000). *Unfree Associations: Inside Psychoanalytic Institutes*. London: Process Press.

Klauber, J. (1982). Psychoanalytic societies and their discontents. *International Journal of Psychoanalytic Psychotherapy*, *9*: 675–689.

Kolansky, H. (1971). Some reflections on a psychoanalytic core curriculum. *Bulletin of the Philadelphia Association for Psychoanalysis*, *1*(2): 59–69.

Kovacs, V. (1936). Training and control analysis. *International Journal of Psychoanalysis*, *18*: 346–354.

Lampl-DeGroot, J. (1954). Problems of psychoanalytic training. *International Journal of Psychoanalysis*, *35*: 184–187.

Lewin, B., & Ross, H. (1960). *Psychoanalytic Education in the United States*. New York: W. W. Norton.

Lorand, S. (1976). The founding of the psychoanalytic institute of the State University of New York Downstate Medical Center. An autobiographical history. *Psychoanalytic Review*, *62*(4): 675–735.

Lothane, Z. (2007). Ethical flaws in training analysis. *Psychoanalytic Psychology*, *24*: 688–696.

McLaughlin, J. (1967). Addendum to a controversial proposal: observations on the training analysis. *Psychoanalytic Quarterly*, *21*(4): 697–726.

McLaughlin, J. (1973). The non-reporting training analyst, the analysis, and the institute. *Journal of the American Psychoanalytic Association*, *21*: 697–712.

Myerson, A., & Epstein, G. (1976). The psychoanalytic treatment center as a transference object. *Psychoanalytic Quarterly*, *45*: 274–287.

Nelson, M. (1976). Paths of power: psychoanalysis and sorcery. *Psychoanalytic Review*, *63*: 333–360.

Oberndorf, C. P. (1953). *History of Psychoanalysis in America*. New York: Grune & Stratton.

Orgel, S. (1982). The selection and functions of the training analyst in North American institutes. *International Review of Psychoanalysis, 9*: 417–434.

Palacios, A. (1984). Changes in the training analyst: characteristics, requirements, prerequisites. *International Psychoanalytical Association Monograph 4*, pp. 47–51.

Pyles, R. (1991). Sigmund Freud: the secrets of nature and the nature of secrets. *International Review of Psychoanalysis, 18*: 143–163.

Pyles, R. (2003). Psychoanalysis in the age of managed care. *Journal of the American Psychoanalytic Association, 51*(Suppl.): 22–41.

Rangell, L. (1972). Aggression, Oedipus, and historical perspectives. *International Journal of Psychoanalysis, 53*(3): 3–11.

Rangell, L. (1976). Lessons from Watergate: a derivative for psychoanalysis. *Psychoanalytic Quarterly, 45*: 37–61.

Rangell, L. (1982). Transference to theory: the relationship of psychoanalytic education to the analyst's relationship to psychoanalysis. *Annual of Psychoanalysis, 10*: 29–56.

Reeder, J. (2004). *Hate and Love in Psychoanalytic Institutes*. New York: Other Press.

Rudnytsky, P. (2015). Freud, Ferenczi, Fromm: the authoritarian character as magic helper. *Fromm Forum, 19*: 5–10.

Sachs, H. (1925). Metapsychological points of view in technique and theory. *International Journal of Psychoanalysis, 6*: 5–12.

Sachs, H. (1947). Observations of a training analyst. *Psychoanalytic Quarterly, 16*: 157–169.

Semader, E. (1983). Some aspects of the training analysis. *International Review of Psychoanalysis, 10*: 145–157.

Settlage, C., & Brockbank, R. (1985). Toward a philosophy of psychoanalytic education. In: *New Ideas in Psychoanalysis: The Process of Change in a Humanistic Science*. Hillsdale, NJ: Analytic Press.

Spruiell, V. (1983). Kuhn's 'paradigm' and psychoanalysis. *Psychoanalytic Quarterly, 52*: 353–363.

Stainbrook, E. (1974). Psychoanalysis: the analysis of behavior and some aspects of the sociology of science. *Journal of the American Academy of Psychoanalysis, 2*(2): 101–112.

Sterrin, H. (1975). The problem of the training analysis. *Annual of Psychoanalysis, 3*: 259–267.

Terman, B. (1972). Dependency and autonomy in a student situation. *International Journal of Psychoanalysis, 53*(1): 47–48.

Wahgh, M. (1962). *Fruition of an Idea: Fifty Years of Psychoanalysis in New York*. New York: International Universities Press.

Wallerstein, R. (1981). The psychoanalyst's life: expectations, vicissitudes, and reflections. *International Review of Psychoanalysis, 8*: 285–298.

Wallerstein, R. (1984). *Changes in Analysts and Their Training*. IPA *Monograph 4*. London: IPA Press.

Weigert, E. (1955). Special problems in connection with termination of training analysis. *Journal of the American Psychoanalytic Association, 3*: 630–640.

Weinshel, E. (1982). The functions of the training analysis and the selection of the training analyst. *International Review of Psychoanalysis, 9*: 434–444.

Zimmerman, D. (1983). Relationships among training analysts. *Annual of Psychoanalysis, 11*: 99–122.

References

Bernfeld, S. (1962). On psychoanalytic training. *Psychoanalytic Quarterly, 31*: 453–482.

Bibring, G. (1954). The training analysis and its place in psychoanalytic training. *International Journal of Psychoanalysis, 35*: 169–173.

Cooper, A. (1984). Psychoanalysis at 100: beginnings of maturity. *Journal of the American Psychoanalytic Association, 32*(2): 245–268.

Fine, B. (1979). *A History of Psychoanalysis*. New York: Columbia University Press.

Freud, S. (1921c). *Group Psychology and the Analysis of the Ego*. *S. E., 18*: 65–144. London: Hogarth Press.

Freud, S. (1926e). The question of lay analysis. *S. E., 20*: 179–258. London: Hogarth.

Gifford, S. Unpublished paper of Dr. Ives Hendrick, Berlin Institute and Boston Psychoanalytic Society and Institute.

Hendrick, I. (1955). Presidential Address: professional standards of the American Psychoanalytic Association. *Journal of the American Psychoanalytic Association, 3*: 561–589.

Hendrick, I. (1958). *The Birth of an Institute*. Freeport, ME: Bond Wheelwright.

Johnson, J. (1916). *Qualities of a Scholar*. Rhodes Trust, the Rhodes Scholarships. Oxford: Oxford University Press.

Kernberg, O. (1984). Organizational problems of psychoanalytic education (plenary presentation), American Psychoanalytic Association (taped). In: *Monograph 4* (pp. 56–61). International Psychoanalytical Association.

Limentani, A. (1974). The training analyst and the difficulties in the training psychoanalytic situation. *International Journal of Psychoanalysis, 5*(1): 71–83.

Szasz, T. S. (1958). Psycho-analytic training—a socio-psychological analysis of its history and present status. *International Journal of Psychoanalysis, 39*: 598–613.

Turnbull, C. (1972). *The Mountain People*. New York: Simon & Schuster.

CHAPTER TWELVE

Can organized psychoanalysis create an optimal education?

Robert S. Wallerstein

Over my professional lifetime in psychoanalysis (1949–2014, sixty-five years), I have mostly become known via two central perspectives: (1) my involvement, from the very start, in formal and systematic process and outcome research in psychoanalysis and psychoanalytic therapy (see 1986), and (2) my later focusing theoretical and clinical psychoanalytic attention on the issue of our burgeoning metapsychological pluralism, and what warrants the search for common ground within it that would give us to claim a shared psychoanalytic identity to which we all subscribed (see 1988, 1990). What has been, I think, less seen as central over my career, perhaps because of its more variegated and piecemeal expression over time, is my ongoing concern with the nature of psychoanalysis as a discipline, its status (or not) as a basic science of the mind (in its normal and aberrant functioning), and in the properly constructed research by which science incrementally tests and expands its knowledge base, and then in the educational structure within which psychoanalytic aspirants can be best trained.

It was in this context that I responded positively to Dr. Zagermann's invitation to express my updated views in this volume devoted to "the reforms of psychoanalytic training". On reviewing my own prior contributions to this large landscape of psychoanalytic education from its earliest days, its vicissitudes over this time span, now almost a century and a quarter, with my perspectives on its accomplishments but also on its inadequacies, with its many calls for reforms, including with that the nature of psychoanalysis itself as a discipline, science or not, and, if science, the kind of research that could best advance it, I found that over a span of forty-four years (1968 to 2012), I had published a total of twenty-five separate accounts, and that they had pursued a somewhat zigzag course as my focus shifted over time, or as the *Zeitgeist* seemed to change in terms of the sociocultural and political surround within which psychoanalysis is intellectually embedded. In this chapter, I attempt to present a unified and coherent present day picture of what I think psychoanalysis as a discipline, and as a professional practice, and the education for it, should and (if not currently) can, one hopes, become over time, in order to best address the question with which this chapter is titled.

Since psychoanalysis, perhaps more than any other discipline, is the product of the thought and the work of a single genius, Sigmund Freud, with aid, of course, from a surrounding small circle of gifted adherents, I begin with his disquisitions on this particular subject, which, though few in number, have been strongly influential long past Freud's own lifetime. From the very start, Freud, based probably on his own prior neurological and neurophysiological training, conceived of psychoanalysis as a science, framed within the natural science structure of the end of the nineteenth century, evolutionarily derived and biologically based. But, for whatever reasons, which are not at all clear to me, Freud never embraced the related conviction that science, any science, grows and amplifies its knowledge base by properly tailored systematic research, and, to my knowledge, he only once mentioned, and actually favorably, a piece of formal psychoanalytic research, when, in a 1919 footnote in a revision of his 1900 dream book, he remarked positively on the 1917 publication, in Vienna, of Otto Pötzl's (psychoanalytically based) experimental studies of subliminal perception (Freud, 1900a, footnote added in 1919, pp. 181–182). And when the American psychologist Saul Rosenzweig, in Saint Louis, wrote to Freud in 1934, describing his laboratory support for some of Freud's central psychoanalytic concepts, Freud responded tersely and dismissively, stating that such confirmatory evidence was not needed, since psychoanalysis rested on such a wealth of positive clinical experiences. Freud ended acerbically with: "Still, it can do no harm" (Shakow & Rapaport, 1964, p. 129). (Parenthetically, this attitude of Freud's played a large hampering role in delaying the start of significant formal and systematic psychoanalytic research, and also, of course, in its slow acceptance as a vital and necessary activity within organized psychoanalysis.)

But I think certainly that Freud's steadfast commitment to psychoanalysis as science played a role in his lifelong sense that the natural home for psychoanalysis should be the university, called by Walter Lippman (1966), "that ancient and universal company of scholars", a home to which Freud aspired lifelong, but was always denied, except for the University of Vienna allowing him, over 1915–1917, to present his series of *Introductory Lectures* (Freud, 1916–1917). An early direct statement by Freud of his own hopes for psychoanalytic education was in his 1919 paper, "On the teaching of psycho-analysis in universities", which was published first in Hungarian, to mark the March 19, 1919 installation by the Bolshevik government which briefly controlled Hungary, of Sandor Ferenczi as Professor of Psycho-Analysis in the medical school at the University of Budapest (Freud, 1919j).

In that short paper, Freud stated that

> This [medical] training has been quite rightly criticized during the last few decades for the one-sided way in which it directs the student into the fields of anatomy, physics and chemistry, while failing, on the other hand, to make plain to him the significance of mental factors in the different vital functions as well as in illnesses and their treatment. (p. 171)

And he added further on, "Psycho-analysis, in fact, more than any other system is fitted for teaching psychology to the medical student" (p. 172) (clearly not just in the teaching of mental illness within the department of psychiatry). He ended with "To sum up, it may be asserted that a University stands only to gain by the inclusion in its curriculum of the teaching of psycho-analysis" (p. 173).

This led Freud to state that "The inclusion of psycho-analysis in the University curriculum would no doubt be regarded with satisfaction by every psycho-analyst" (p. 171). Unhappily, Freud's vision on this issue was one-sided. He did not picture, at the time, the enduring benefits in the reverse direction, to psychoanalysis, for its education, and for the accompanying systematic psychoanalytic research for which he never felt the need. Of these potential goods, Freud said dismissively, "At the same time it is clear that the psycho-analyst can dispense entirely with the University without any loss to himself" (p. 171).

Freud's fullest statement of his own model structure for psychoanalytic education was set forth only in the latter part of his professional lifetime, in "The question of lay analysis" (Freud, 1926e), and then in the context of his spirited defense of the psychoanalytic *bona fides* and impressive credentials of a favorite non-medical adherent, Theodor Reik. In that monograph, he ventured his ideal prescription for training in the new discipline of psychoanalysis as follows:

> If – which may sound fantastic today – one had to found a *college of psycho-analysis*, much would have to be taught in it which is also taught by the medical faculty: alongside of depth-psychology, which would always remain the principal subject, there would be an introduction to biology, as much as possible of the science of sexual life, and familiarity with the symptomatology of psychiatry. On the other hand, analytic instruction would include branches of knowledge which are remote from medicine, and which the doctor does not come across in his practice: the history of civilization, mythology, the psychology of religion and the science of literature. Unless he is well at home in these subjects, an analyst can make nothing of a large part of his material. By way of compensation, the great mass of what is taught in medical schools is of no use to him for his purposes. (Freud, 1926e, p. 246, my italics)

A few pages further on, Freud stated this university-like conception even more tersely:

> A scheme of training for analysts has *still to be created*. It must include elements from the mental sciences, from psychology, the history of civilization and socioloty, as well as from anatomy, biology, and the study of evolution. (p. 252, my italics)

Embedded in these statements is Freud's implicit acknowledgement of the insufficiency of the already established part-time and private practice psychoanalytic institute structure created just a half decade earlier by Max Eitingon and his colleagues, first in Berlin in 1920, and, by the time of Freud's writing, already spreading across the central European heartland—Freud's acknowledgement evident in the 1926 quotation: "a scheme of training for analysts has still to be created".

Clearly, Freud's stated ideal could be realized only within the academic university structure. As presented by Freud, it seems distinctly a call for the creation of a full-time (postgraduate) psychoanalytic training institute—full-time would be necessary if Freud's programmatic message was to be fulfilled—to which psychiatric physicians and other properly qualified individuals would come for education in this new discipline and identity of clinical psychoanalysis. But nothing in it specifies Freud's vision of the particular relationship of the analytic training enterprise to the existing medical school structure, or to the cognate disciplines of human mental functioning within the broader university context. But, altogether, without explicit reference to the university, Freud's 1926 statements are clearly his plea for what he considered the optimal educational placement of this new discipline to be.

However, because of the scandalous nature of Freud's doctrine of childhood sexuality and the oedipal vicissitudes in early twentieth century Victorian Vienna (and in Victorian Europe more broadly), and also the almost official anti-Semitism of the Austro-Hungarian empire, this new "Jewish science" could not win a place in the medical world or the wider academic university world at the time, and the psychoanalytic training structure had to evolve as a private and part-time activity of dedicated individuals with the time and money provided then by their full-time professional practices. This was, of course, the independent psychoanalytic institute with its tripartite structure, the personal (training) analysis of the aspirant, the didactic sequence of theoretical and technical seminars, and the conduct of (control) analyses under the monitoring of senior supervising analysts, started first by Eitingon and his colleagues in Berlin in 1920, as already stated, and then spreading rapidly over Central Europe—Vienna, Zurich, Budapest, and Frankfurt—followed over the years since by Western and Scandinavian Europe, then, in the 1930s and 1940s, by North America, followed from just before the Second World War and ever since by Latin America, Australia, Asia (first in India and Japan and today China and South Korea as well), Israel, Turkey, South Africa, Russia, and the former Soviet Union East European nations. Over the close to a century from its beginnings, this training has become more formalized, and significantly lengthened and deepened.

Yet, from close to the beginnings, serious questions were raised about the difficult problematics of this training program, both its structure and its venue. Very early, these centered around the nature and the purpose of the training analysis, the difficulty posed by its variously constituted and seemingly irreconcilable components, the therapeutic (directed at the personal neurotic and character problems of the candidate analysands), and the educational (directed at conveying the working of psychoanalytic techniques), dubbed by Lewin and Ross (1960) the "syncretistic dilemma". In my own full-length article on the problems of the training analysis (Wallerstein, 2010), I reviewed in detail the early, very telling critiques by a group of very prominent and esteemed early psychoanalytic contributors, Anna Freud (1938), Michael Balint (1948, 1954), Siegfried Bernfeld (1953, but not published until 1962), and Otto Fenichel (1942, but not published until 1980).[1]

Anna Freud's critique centered around many aspects of the educational needs of the training analysis and its setting within the institute training structure, all of which would be looked upon as serious violation of the conditions of the "ordinary" therapeutic analysis; Balint's even more sweeping critique focused on the authoritarian and infantilizing pressures within the training analysis structure, leading to submissive, or oppositely in some cases, rebellious, students; Bernfeld went to the extreme of calling for the destruction of the entire psychoanalytic training apparatus as totally unanalytic in its way of operating and for a return to the original, totally voluntary training method, with the many extraordinary psychoanalytic products of those informal (and chaotic) beginnings; and Fenichel, in responding oppositely to the perceived problems of the training analysis, advocating a longer and deeper totally "therapeutic" analysis, expressing opposition to what most felt at the time to be Sigmund Freud's own feeling that all that was necessary for the candidate was a short "didactic" analysis that served to acquaint the analysand with the workings of the unconscious.

Actually, when Balint wrote his 1948 paper decrying all the many problems he saw in the training analysis system, secretiveness, dogmatic and inhibited thinking, authoritarian techniques on the part of the teachers, matched by the respectful and submissive behaviors of the students, he expressed his surprise that, "in over twenty-five years [from the start in 1920] one of the most important problems of psychoanalysis, the training, has not been discussed adequately in print, indeed hardly at all" (p. 164)—despite being, by then, very much remarked in corridor conversations at analytic meetings. Following these original four statements, a widening critical literature began, mostly in basic agreement among not only prominent training analysts, but also a growing chorus of analytic members, and also candidates declaiming from their perspective. Thus, over the years, pressures arose to somehow alter the training analysis system in an effort to mitigate these adverse effects.

The one significant alteration over all the decades since came as a consequence of what I label (Wallerstein, 2010) "The great debate: Fleming vs. Kairys", over the span of the 1960s to the 1980s. Joan Fleming, the often-hailed "dean" in America among psychoanalytic educators at the time, propounded, in 1973, a full defense of the existing Eitingon model of psychoanalytic education, that not only could the training analysis simultaneously serve both goals, therapy and education, but that it was necessary to do so in order to be most helpful in furthering the candidate's capacities for his/her psychoanalytic career. Fleming's position was attractively optimistic and persuasive. In regard to the complexities created by being a real object as a major determining voice in the progression of the candidate's professional career as well as a fantasy object in the candidate's psychic space, Fleming declared that,

> Reality events, in my experience, have enabled the patient to experience the world of affect more completely when I have not warded off the reality perception but instead, encourage associations activated by the reality. (p. 284)

And if the analyst is neutral or uninvolved in these educational issues of the analysand, the analyst is clearly shirking his/her educational responsibilities. Fleming had many supporters of her stand, among them, very strongly, Calef and Weinshel (1973).

Fleming's posture was a full-throated response to an earlier clarion call by David Kairys (1964) who, after a careful review of the, by then, sizeable literature on the problems of the training analysis, recommended, as a remedy, the elimination of any reporting by the training analyst of any part of the analytic work to any of the institute's educational bodies. Kairys called this a controversial proposal, "to divorce the training analysis completely from the rest of the student's training" (p. 506, all in italics). He based this recommendation on the conviction that the essential hopelessness of the attempt to really carry out the "dual function of the training analyst who tries at the same time to treat the candidate's neurosis and to be one of his educators" (p. 487) because, necessarily, "the training analyst does exactly what we all insist must never be done" (p. 488) in an ordinary therapeutic analysis, and, thus, renders any effort to maintain this combined task detrimental to both. Therefore, the training analyst should be converted from his, up to then, customary operation as a reporting training analyst (RTA) to that of a non-reporting training analyst (NRTA), only informing the institute of the starting date, the weekly frequency, and, at the end, the termination date, whether by mutual agreement or not, plus the total number of hours. Because the analysis would still be in the normal "hot-house atmosphere" under the institute's auspices, significant problems could still remain, but Kairys was optimistic that one large problem would be eliminated: the analytic transference would no longer be contaminated.

Over the decades of the 1960s to the 1980s, as more institutes became troubled by the increasing awareness of the problems of the training analysis, the tide of psychoanalytic opinion gradually shifted in Kairys's direction, so that, by now, the non-reporting stance has become much more the norm. Occasional voices have been raised around the new problematics that this has occasioned. Patrick Casement (2005), for example, struck a cautionary note about the possible detrimental impact of the massive shift from the reporting to the non-reporting stance. He stated his conviction that the training analyst knows the candidate's problems and capacities better than anyone else (in agreement with Fleming) and that removing the training analyst completely from the decision-making process leaves the educational fate of the candidate wholly in the hands of less knowledgeable others (teachers, supervisors) who might well be pushed into judgments based on "wild analysis in committee" (p. 1148). But there is by now a preponderant body of psychoanalytic opinion that feels oppositely, that the training analyst is less well equipped than teachers and supervisors to render *objective* judgments about the candidate's educational issues and progress.

This newer, now dominant, NRTA position has been strengthened by the growing worldwide psychoanalytic awareness of the post Second World War development in the francophone psychoanalytic world (originally in France, but adopted as well in French Switzerland, French Belgium, and French Canada) of a training system markedly different in salient aspects from the original Eitingon model. One central difference is the requirement that one can only apply for candidacy after at least two years of personal therapeutic analysis, with any qualified analyst of whatever psychoanalytic institute (there were two IPA member institutes in Paris when the French system arose) and even by candidates conducting supervised analysis. Without asking even the name of the treating analyst, the process of admission to candidacy would be based on interviews designed to determine whether the aspirant was enough in an ongoing, seemingly solid analytic experience to be capable of working successfully in a training sequence of seminars and supervisions (the latters also with marked differences from the Eitingon model). Here, there is even more truly a total separation of the personal analysis from the professional training and career.

Since there has been, by now, the almost worldwide establishment of the NRTA position in the overall psychoanalytic world, there has been minimal effort towards the refinement or further alteration of the training analysis itself, even though there is still a very widespread current feeling that the many problems noted early, and increasingly, of an oligarchic self-perpetuating power elite centered in the training analysis structure, with all the issues of secrecy, authoritarianism, and infantilization, leading to indoctrinated submissiveness or rebellious fighting of the candidates, though somewhat mitigated, are far from truly resolved.

One recent suggestion by Robert Michels (cited by Masur, 1998) and Welsh (2008) has been to increase further the separation of the personal analysis from the training setting by urging institutes in large metropolitan areas, where two IPA member institutes may be in the same geographic area, to trust the work of their sister institutes sufficiently (which has not always been the case) to accept candidates for training who are in analysis with analysts of the other institute and to allow them to stay with those analysts for the progression of their personal analytic experience. I know of at least one city where this is allowed (San Francisco), and this is, of course, permitted within the francophone training system.

However, all these changes—to whatever extent—to the venue and the conduct of the training analysis have addressed only part of the many problems in the psychoanalytic educational structure that have been noted for so long, and increasingly over the, by now, almost a century of formal psychoanalytic training (since 1920, starting in Berlin). It was Bernfeld's sweeping critique in 1953 (published in 1962) which was the most fundamentally challenging of the entire structure and the most radical in calling for the total destruction of institutionalized training, as being, in its essence, totally incompatible with basic psychoanalytic conceptualizing. Bernfeld advocated a full return to the earlier days of psychoanalysis, when education was essentially self-motivated and willing students and adherents essentially sought mentorship and taught themselves.

He called on Freud's legacy in full support.

> From the first to the very end, Freud kept his didactic cases absolutely free from interference by rules, administrative directives, or political considerations. His teaching was completely student-centered (to use my pedagogical terminology) or more simply he acted as a psychoanalyst should. He continued this long after the establishment of institutes, to the dismay and embarrassment of the authorities, as he sometimes, and a little ironically, referred to them. (p. 462)

Bernfeld illustrated his argument by how Freud brushed aside his need for a personal analysis by declaring, "Nonsense. Go right ahead. You certainly will have difficulties. When you get into trouble, we will see what we can do about it"—and only a week later, Freud sent him his first case.

Bernfeld stated his own conviction most directly.

> My thesis is this: the training program that is conducted in our professional schools distorts some of the most valuable features of psychoanalysis and hinders its development as a science and as a tool by means of which to change behavior. (p. 458)

He went on to describe the twin major faults of infantilization and authoritarianism as inevitable concomitants of the working of the "teacher-centered" (rather than "student-centered") educational system, with its centralization of unrestricted power in the hands of the training analyst cadre. Bernfeld saw this structure as a defensive response to the solid opposition of the German medical establishment, operating within "the spirit of the Prussian army" (p. 479), to the new science of psychoanalysis. But, to Bernfeld's surprise, "the psychoanalysts themselves desired respectability. They wished to set themselves up as part of the medical profession, and in order to achieve this aim they felt they had to have clinics, professional schools, and professional societies" (p. 466). Also, with Freud's long illness and eventual death in 1939, the analysts "became very eager to establish a solid claim against heterodoxy, as they now felt themselves responsible for the future of psychoanalysis" (p. 467)—all of which strengthened the tenets of rigid educational control.

With his counterthrust, Bernfeld set himself squarely against this institutionalized totality. He wished to abolish the entire training apparatus and return to the days of totally informal training, when you mentored people who interested you, brought them to meetings, introduced them to colleagues, and helped them gradually to absorb the fervor of the analytic pioneers. He averred that "Of course some people learn psychoanalysis in any setting. That does not prove that we have to invent the most unfavorable situation in which to teach psychoanalysis" (p. 480). He could also point to the many extraordinary psychoanalytic products of those informal (and chaotic) beginnings (with returning the required "training analysis" to a voluntary expression of desire or need)—not all of them necessarily well-balanced individuals. This is, of course, the most extreme of the changes to our educational system that have been espoused, and, as far as I know, no serious psychoanalytic thinker has since proposed that we take up Bernfeld's radical suggestions for totally dismantling it. As already stated, this was, in 1953, Bernfeld's last presentation to the San Francisco Psychoanalytic Society, of which he had been one of the founding members, and after that, true to his principles, he resigned from the Society and Institute and then died shortly thereafter. It took nine years before the paper could be published (in 1962).

It was not until the salvo by Otto Kernberg in 1986 (three to four decades after the initial broadsides of Balint and Bernfeld) that the nature—and the flaws—of our entire educational structure became a matter of systematic (and increasingly widespread) published attention within organized psychoanalysis, and Kernberg followed his initial 1986 article with a further, increasingly documented, ten more over the following quarter century.

In Kernberg's first, 1986, article, after describing the various unhappy attributes he saw in psychoanalytic training in its present form(s) (a paranoiagenic atmosphere, a selfperpetuating training analyst power elite, indoctrination, a closed environment with regressive group processes, fostered idealizations and/or an aroused defensive de-idealization, arbitrary enforcements, and, ultimately, what he felt to be diminished creative thinking and scientific productivity, with a severely narrowed intellectual frame, dubbed by him "cross-sterilization" (p. 806)), Kernberg characterized all this as the inevitable outcome of the improperly evolved relationship between what he called the primary declared educational tasks of our psychoanalytic discipline and the administrative structure created to realize them.

Kernberg here famously differentiated four possible administrative models for psychoanalytic institutes (and comparable educational institutions): (1) a technical or trade school, to acquire a skill; (2) a university college, to acquire new knowledge and advance science; (3) an art academy, to foster individual creativity; (4) a monastery or religious seminary, to enhance faith and the search for immutable truths. He stated that the optimal structure of a psychoanalytic institute would be some admixture of the second and third, the university college and the art academy, but that what had unhappily developed was an admixture of the first and the fourth, a trade school that, at best, makes a competent clinician, and a monastery endowing that clinician with full faith in the tenets of Freud and his adherents. Unfortunately, he stated that the monastery also squelches the critical questioning that might lead to individual creativity and to the accretion of the new knowledge needed to continuously advance our science and to enhance its clinical application.

In a follow-up article six years later, Kernberg (1992) detailed a variety of corrective measures designed to move our institutes in the direction of greater transparency, more open communication, and wider participation in administration and governance, all with the intent to demolish the centralized power of an arbitrary and secretive training analyst elite. Training analysts in the transformed program Kernberg envisioned would now openly communicate their own clinical work in the educational context, while fully segregating their candidate training cases from the educational administrative structure. These measures, taken together, would, in the words of his earlier paper, tend to

> strengthen the university college and art academy models at the expense of reducing the technical school and, especially, the monastery

> or religious retreat models [which] should go a long way in reducing the pervasive idealization and persecution processes that plague psychoanalytic institutes. (Kernberg, 1986, p. 833)

Kernberg (1996) then added to this overview with his widely remarked paper, "Thirty methods to destroy the creativity of psychoanalytic candidates", a sardonic commentary detailing the extreme consequences (in many cases not so very exaggerated) of the many faults he had previously identified as intrinsic to the current operations of our analytic training system. Kernberg's whole cascading series of articles in pursuit of his proclaimed goals have drawn marked attention and considerable concurring praise, but I think it fair to say that there has been little real shift in identifiable institute operations over the almost three decades since his initial exposition. Rather, the more central psychoanalytic concern with our educational structure over all these years has been with the increased looking at the issue of its venue, and of its possible placement within the medical school and/or the wider university world in pursuit of Freud's original idealized home. Although not central to his proposals, Kernberg did support these concerns about university placement as well, and, for me, they have been basic and fundamental from the beginning, as I have pursued my own zigzagging course in this quest.

The first expression of this university possibility came in the wake of the Second World War when the tide of pre-war psychoanalytic Hitler refugees came to America, joining with the American adherents who had earlier gone to Europe to be trained, now together a majority of the world's active psychoanalytic practitioners, and together creating the first American institutes on the Boston–New York–Philadelphia–Baltimore–Washington axis, plus in Chicago. I, of course, was not party to the organizational events of those days, and I do not know the extent to which the decisions that were made, and the history that they then determined, were self-consciously thought out and planned, in terms of the full array of consequences that then ensued. Perhaps, as is more likely, they were more the result of only partial and partisan perspectives imposed upon events, leading, through contention and compromise, to outcomes in part foreseen, and, for the rest, perhaps only dimly thought out, and, to that little extent, entitled to be called planned. But certainly in retrospect, it was as if a major strategy was deliberately evolved and pursued for psychoanalysis to follow a path in America different from the proud but lonely isolation that had marked it in Europe. The strategy was, in effect, for the newly institutionalized psychoanalytic world in America to capture organized psychiatry and its formal training centers in medical schools, hospitals, and clinics, to then become its prevailing psychological theory under the banner of dynamic psychiatry, or psychodynamics, and, thus, to be planted firmly in the midst of medicine, the medical school, and, via that route, in the university.

It was this effort to transform the departments of psychiatry in the various medical schools and hospitals of our nation into bulwarks of psychodynamic thinking and practice that was so stunningly successful during the heyday of the psychoanalytic tide within American psychiatry all through the early post Second World War years, and for a full two decades into the 1960s. Then, as one after another of the Adolf Meyer-trained generation of psychobiological leaders[2] retired from positions of leadership, they were regularly replaced by psychoanalysts, or by psychoanalytically sympathetic psychiatrists, determined, with the help of psychoanalytic clinicians recruited to teaching and supervising roles, to make the teaching and learning of psychoanalytic principles, and psychoanalytic psychotherapy, the central activity of the departments of psychiatry in the nation's hospitals and medical schools.

A logical extension of this campaign was the conception, in some centers, of the university-based psychoanalytic institute as an administrative division, autonomously governed, within the medical school's department of psychiatry, with some, if not all, of its psychoanalytic teachers part of the full-time academic faculty of the department of psychiatry. The new psychoanalytic institutes at Columbia, Cleveland, Denver, Downstate (since moved to New York University), and Pittsburgh were all in that wave of university-based institutes in those first post Second World War decades. They have been followed more recently by Emory (originally sponsored by Columbia) in Atlanta, though two of the original group—Pittsburgh and Cleveland—have, for different reasons, since left their university homes and reverted to the more usual independent institute status. (See Wallerstein 2011, p. 627, for the declared reasons for these separations.)

These institutes, the first in university placement, have posed an alternative educational model for psychoanalysis. They have had the putative advantages of a university base, at least some full-time faculty (but with commitments, of course, to the overall mission of the parent department of psychiatry), access to department of psychiatry resources for research support, and opportunities for cross-disciplinary contact and mutual enrichment, certainly within the medical school and, to a variable extent, within the wider university community, including the social and behavioral sciences and even the humanities, and, in recent years, neuroscience. However, the clinical psychoanalytic training itself is still a part-time activity, much of the faculty are still private practice based volunteers, giving their extra time, and, apart from the proportion of the student body working within the department of psychiatry, the candidates are also involved in full-time private clinical work to support their living and training costs.

Therefore, over these same post Second World War years, other schemes have been advanced in the literature, or to whatever extent possible, given the circumstances of their creation, brought into being to further, or to better, embed psychoanalysis within the university. The first total university model was that of David Shakow (1962), strongly supported by David Rapaport. It was proposed particularly for the training of behavioral and social scientists for careers in psychoanalytic scholarship and research. Shakow's proposal was simple and radical; unhappily, when proposed, it was even less realizable than the idea of psychoanalysis embedding itself enduringly in medical school departments of psychiatry. Shakow began by stating that our training institutes, organized as part-time activities, whether independent or based in medical school departments of psychiatry, were not able to train proper cadres of scholars and researchers in psychoanalysis.[3] He pleaded, therefore,

> not only for the greater recognition by institutes of the importance of research in psychoanalysis, but for emphasis on educational programs that are oriented toward the development of persons who can contribute effectively to research . . . Suppose medical schools over the country no longer had basic science faculties, merely faculties consisting of medical practitioners who devoted a part of their time to teaching. How long could medical schools prevent themselves from becoming vocational schools . . . rather than professional schools, to say nothing of centers of research and scholarship? (pp. 151–152)[4]

Shakow's solution was to move psychoanalysis, and psychoanalytic education, into the university more generally, which he considered a better and more logical home for our discipline than the medical school department of psychiatry. He considered the latter an improvement over the independent institute, but still far from what was optimal or even sufficiently necessary. His proposal was that, "The psychoanalytic institute should be an independent institute in the university setting associated with both the graduate school and the medical school" (p. 155), since

> the optimal arrangement would be an autonomous institute intimately related to the graduate school and the medical school . . . The psychoanalytic institute could then be an important center of intercourse between those who are primarily clinically oriented and those who are primarily theoretically oriented. (p. 156)

He went on to adduce an array of clearly beneficial consequences for this arrangement.

Shakow, given his political savvy regarding the academic world, was strangely optimistic about the practical possibilities for such a development. "Because of the reluctance of universities to set up independent institutes [in any realm of knowledge] on their campuses", he said,

> . . . and because the suggestion here is that the institute have considerable autonomy and especially close relations with the two quite separate parts of the university, it is most important that the administration of the university as a whole, and that of the medical school and the graduate school in particular, be strongly committed to such a program. (p. 157)

He did not address the need for such commitment to be able to endure despite the shifting priorities and obligations of departmental administrations over time, or the issue of such a major financial involvement by the university in these days of increasing budgetary pressures.

Another proposed model was Anna Freud's prescription (1971) for what she called, "The ideal psychoanalytic institute", and then dubbed, in her subtitle, "a utopia". She began with a disclaimer, describing her own childhood preference for stories that "might be true" (p. 225), as against those with unrealistic or supernatural elements. In this light, she said, "The Ideal Psychoanalytic Institute . . . claims my interest only in so far as it is capable to becoming true. Accordingly, there will be nothing in my description of it which excludes this possibility" (p. 226). The most distinctive aspect of her proposal was her vision of the ideal institute as a full-time training center, an independent institute—not necessarily in the university but very much full-time—on the model of her own Hampstead Clinic (renamed the Anna Freud Centre after her death), which has indeed approximated her ideal in the specific realm of clinical training for child analysis. She contrasted the kind of training possible in such a setting with that currently available in our institutes, whether independent or university based. Of our current training situation, she said,

> As it was done fifty years ago, candidates still spend their working days in nonanalytic surroundings and nonanalytic pursuits. They still arrive for their clinical and theoretical seminars and lectures in the evenings or on weekends, i.e. tired out and unreceptive, at times when, by right, they should be at leisure and pursue their personal lives and interests with their families. They are still lectured to by senior members of the profession, who devote some off-time to teaching, often against their real inclination, and only too often without having developed any teaching skills. Candidates still have little or no time left for reading, apart from the most urgent course requirements, or for pursuing spontaneous theoretical interests. To the best of my belief, there is no other serious and ambitious discipline where part-time training schemes of this type are adopted, or where they are expected to be effective. (p. 230)

Anna Freud contrasted this with the ideal institute with "full-time students, able to pursue their psychoanalytic studies intensively, leisurely, and with enormously increased profit" (p. 230), and she ended with the acerbic statement, "the present part-time system seems as out of date to me as if church services were still conducted in catacombs since this is where the early Christians were obliged to meet" (p. 230).

The balance of her article detailed the advantages that would accrue to our science in such a full-time educational institution. These include the sharing of clinical material in group settings with faculty and fellow students, and participation in workshops that pursue topics of scholarly and scientific interest:

> By formulating, dissecting, summarizing, and evaluating their data, and by placing them in analytically meaningful categories, they will learn to turn the undigested mass of items as they are elicited in every

> analysis into materials which can be profitably assimilated, understood, and used by every analyst. (pp. 232–233)

Shakow, of course, would have added to Anna Freud's formula a formal psychoanalytic research component offering courses in philosophy of science issues relevant to psychoanalytic theory and scholarship, as well as courses in empirical research strategies appropriate to the subjective data of our consulting rooms.

The one major obstacle to implementing this plan (as with Shakow's proposal), the lack of an identifiable funding base, Anna Freud left for her concluding paragraph:

> I trust that I have kept my promise and that there is nothing in this blueprint of the Ideal Institute which will prevent the Utopia of today [she did not refer to her own Hampstead Clinic as representing an organized effort at present day fulfillment of that Utopia] from becoming a reality of tomorrow. The only serious obstacle which will have to be met is the financial one. Here I am confident in the idea that money is usually found for worthwhile purposes and that the training of true analysts, equally versed in human understanding, clinical insight, therapeutic skill, and searching exploration, ranks high among these. (1971, p. 239)

Actually, there was a time, certainly in the 1950s through the 1970s, when those of us active at the Menninger Foundation (which had its own intramural Topeka Institute for Psychoanalysis) viewed that major center of residential and outpatient treatment for the full spectrum of the treatable mentally ill, both adult and child, as potentially the kind of psychoanalytic training and research center that Shakow and Anna Freud envisioned (see Wallerstein, 1983). It lacked at the time only the vital university linkage to both the natural sciences (via the medical school) and the social and behavioral sciences (via the graduate school facilities), and there were thoughts then of overcoming that lack through an affiliation with the nearby University of Kansas and its school of medicine.

However, such a connection was never accomplished, and, as time went on, it seemed ever more difficult to attain. Ultimately, the increasing pressures for cost containment exerted by private and governmental reimbursement sources, and the concomitant lure of lower-cost treatment using psychoactive drugs and/or shorter and simpler psychotherapy paradigms, weakened the Menninger Foundation's finances to the point where it had to close its doors in Topeka. To survive, it found an affiliation with a willing medical school department of psychiatry in another state, and it relocated there, but having to sacrifice its intramural psychoanalytic institute.

Such is my account of the trajectory until now of the institutionalized analytic training experience starting with its initial formulation in 1920, with all of its problematics as they emerged close to the very beginnings, and have been increasingly dissected since the first descriptive papers after the first quarter century, the authoritarian self-perpetuating training analyst elite, with its paranoiagenic and infantilizing aspects, its independent, part-time night school setting for a complex theoretical and clinical learning, its isolation from a proper embedding within the appropriate medical school and wider university academic world, and with the still paucity and still uncertain acceptance of the systematic formal research by which all sciences steadily test and enlarge their established knowledge base.

Various reform efforts have been advanced over the years, but only one, the change of the training analyst's stance from the reporting posture of having a major role in the career-deciding educational decisions about his/her candidate (RTA) to the current non-reporting position (NRTA), has been more or less widely accepted within our training institutes, and there has been the additional proposal to allow the personal analysis to be totally excluded from even the awareness of the training institute's educational structure, adopted only within the training system of the francophone institutes, and perhaps a few other world places where the geographic propinquity of at least two institutes in some of the largest metropolitan centers in the world makes this a feasible possibility. Nevertheless, though heralded as a major step in removing the candidate's personal analytic experience from involvement in his/her life progression, the overall difference in the total training experience has been less than hoped for. The training analysis is still conducted mostly within the "hothouse climate" of the institute educational structure with its analytic siblings and parent generation, its colleagueships and competitions, and its constant personal interchanges. For the rest, the psychoanalytic training system remains essentially as it was created nearly a century ago with all of its successes in developing—despite its problems—generations of competent psychoanalyst clinicians, but with its many enduring problems still all too present, even in the differently organized French (and the Uruguayan, a third training structure, quite akin to the French) systems devised as overall alternatives to the Eitingon model.

This is what I have been party to, and involved in, over my own sixty-five years (1949–2014) in organized psychoanalysis worldwide. I came with my own commitments (like Freud) to psychoanalysis as a biologically based science of the mind, in both its normal and its aberrant functioning, but (unlike Freud) with the linked commitment to formal, systematic research as the way to test and enlarge that science's knowledge base, albeit by methods appropriate to its subjective data. I was trained uncritically within the rigidities and the constraints of the dominant classical Eitingon training model as the established and, seemingly, only feasible method to achieve the proper educational goals. It was a training within what Kernberg (1986) described as the mixture of the trade-school and monastery educational conceptions rather than the more desirable, and more truly psychoanalytic, university and art academy models. But with my commitment also to the university as the best organized venue for the teaching and the research growth of scientific knowledge, abetted by my own training and working (over seventeen years, from 1949 to 1966) at the Menninger Foundation, a full-time salaried clinical structure, I indeed welcomed the American post Second World War innovation of the medical school based department of psychiatry psychoanalytic institute as an important first step in the desired direction of ultimate full university embedding with all of its promised advantages for both training and research.

Unhappily, to the initial cluster of five departments of psychiatry based psychoanalytic institutes (Columbia, Downstate, Pittsburgh, Cleveland, and Denver), only one (Emory, originally sponsored by Columbia) has been subsequently added in the more than half a century since the first wave, and in two of them (Pittsburgh and Cleveland) the emplacement broke down within two to three decades, over struggles between the priorities of the institute and of the parent department of psychiatry. And the educational and research gain, to whatever extent significant, proved less than hoped for with these university based psychoanalytic institutes, which were like the independent majority, still only part-time, with mostly private practice based, unpaid, voluntary teachers and supervisors, and the cross-involvements with cognate disciplines of human mental functioning also less than hoped for, and, as well, the desired research essential developing far less intensely than both sides desired, but also that both sides inhibited out of structured impediments and ideological misgivings.

When I saw, over the span of years, the stagnation of foreseeable progression towards a true and full university placement over my own projected professional lifetime, I swung about a decade ago into giving up on the university quest in favor of welcoming the creation (recently arising in some American metropolitan areas), independent of the university, of the psychoanalytic center concept, an effort at development potentially as university-like and university-linked as given local conditions in each setting could make possible. This I described comprehensively (Wallerstein, 2007) as an eight-fold compartmental structure with a governing board holding legal and fiduciary responsibility (with non-psychoanalysts among its members, public citizens, attorneys, financial experts, etc.) and a full-time psychoanalyst director, responsible to the governing board for directing and implementing policy.

The full eight needed components would be:

1. The psychoanalytic training institute itself
2. A psychoanalytic psychotherapy training program for interested mental health professionals, some of whom might well go on to full psychoanalytic institute training.
3. Professional affairs, the psychoanalytic society scientific meetings, the library, and postgraduate educational programs as the psychoanalytic interests of the members develop.
4. Outreach and collaboration, including a low-fee clinic (for the supervised psychoanalytic candidates) and courses for mental health professionals, educators, lawyers, pediatricians, etc.
5. Interface with academia, sharing educational programs with psychoanalytically aware university academics interested in mutual learning and mutual involvement.
6. A research component, again sharing, to the extent possible, with university academics involved in psychoanalytically related research questions.
7. A fundraising foundation, appealing, partly through the governing board, to the potentially supportive, psychoanalytically interested philanthropic community.
8. An essential long-range planning arm.

Such a plan for an overall independent psychoanalytic center, linked to the extent possible in each venue to the psychoanalytically interested faculty of the university (and, within it, the medical school) as shared interests in teaching, scholarship, and research would make possible, was actually in the planning or construction phase in half a dozen major metropolitan areas in the USA (including San Francisco), each with as many of my idealized cluster of the eight component structure as locally seemed possible at the time that I was assembling my 2007 description of this effort. It was what, at the time, was the best I could think of in planning what I felt could be the best possible (or the most feasible) educational structure for psychoanalytic training that I could at least settle for when the road to full university deployment seemed to have no realistic opportunity for advancement. It is now much too early to tell both how far and how well these psychoanalytic centers have indeed established themselves within this ambitious framework and how successfully they have been able to secure a modicum of the inherent university advantages within such an independent framework.

That is where my thinking had come to rest until I received the invitation to present a paper at a symposium on "Psychoanalysis in the university" to be held in November 2007 at Emory University, co-sponsored by the university and the American (and IPA) Psychoanalytic Associations. Emory had, of course, one of the four currently existing psychoanalytic institutes within its medical school department of psychiatry. It also had gone furthest in integrating the psychoanalytic presence within the fabric of the university, with psychoanalytic scholar Sandor Gilman as Director of its program in Psychoanalytic Studies, for graduate students in the arts and sciences interested in psychoanalytic scholarship in relation to their own area of cognate degree study, under the Emory college dean, Robert Paul, a professor of anthropology, who himself had full clinical psychoanalytic training.

The conference was opened by a brief introductory paper by the university president, James Wagner, an engineer by training. Wagner (2009) used the history of engineering in relation to the university as the springboard for his talk entitled, "Psychoanalysis and its place in the evolutionary chain of academic disciplines". Wagner began with the roots of higher education and liberal learning. Early liberal learning was available only to the free man, essentially from the aristocracy, whose future was assured and therefore had no need to earn a livelihood. Four central academic disciplines evolved over time, each with its own degree, theology, medicine, law, and philosophy, the last of these for theoretical studies. Wagner's own discipline, engineering, had grown outside the academic structure, with originally two major components, military and civil, given initial major impetus by the needs of the Roman empire for military equipment, arms, carriages, roads, bridges, and aqueducts to hold and protect its far-flung domain. Only when West Point was established by the USA in 1802 did engineering begin to be taught here, military engineering to begin with. When Yale opened what became the Sheffield Scientific School, in 1847, students were not allowed to sit in chapel with regular academic students. At Dartmouth, science students attended classes only in wintertime when the regular students were off campus earning money as tutors. Eventually, this pattern of resistance to welcoming the sciences and engineering began to change in partnerships with corporate leaders, progressive educators, and the federal government establishing the land grant college system in the newly emerging western states.

Wagner held forth a similar developmental vision for psychoanalysis. Compared with the discussion of the long struggles of the advocates for applied sciences and engineering, Wagner sensed an unusual degree of self-awareness, if not fully open self-criticism, with psychoanalysis. His optimistic message was that in time, but over time, psychoanalysis could anticipate the same ultimate destiny, that it would indeed enter the academic canon, the canon populated by fields that formulate and pose the questions and not so much by the library titles that purport to contain all the known answers. It was this resetting of the time dimension for psychoanalysis and the vision of ultimate fulfillment of the proper (in my mind) university placement that gave me warrant to reset my own perspectives, and gave me the impetus to reframe all of my disparate thinking about the many issues of psychoanalytic education, and to fashion my current crystallized conception of an ideal psychoanalytic education, overcoming as best as possible all the serious and contentious problems that have bedevilled our educational structure for all of its existing years until now.

I begin, of course, with the issue of the required training analysis, still burdened by its many problems (noted by at least some from its very start), as essentially the expected fundament of the entire training enterprise. Of all those who have written of its problems, only Bernfeld (1962) has seen fit to call for its being completely abandoned as a requirement, actually the initial requirement. Bernfeld's call, as one of the first generation of psychoanalytic educators within an institutionalized educational system, was actually a most radical call, to not only abandon the requirement of the initiating training analysis, but, far more sweepingly, the abolition of the entire structure of organized psychoanalytic training. What he advocated so intensely in this final paper was the wholesale destruction of the whole formal apparatus for psychoanalytic education, by then (1953) deeply entrenched, and a return to the earliest days of a voluntary, self-motivated, and self-executed training model.

Bernfeld's entire polemic—abandon the training analysis and destroy the whole organized training structure—was indeed widely noted, but nowhere implemented. As far as I could determine, there has been only one psychoanalytic contributor, Samuel Lipton (1988) who has echoed one aspect of Bernfeld's wholesale assault, that of making the personal analysis a totally voluntary proposition. Lipton stated that although the training analysis could indeed have personal and educational values, it had been made a beginning requirement of training principally, he felt, because it served as a "screening method" (p. 13) for candidates and, thus, "While marginally the preliminary personal analysis was the only effective method of screening, there are now other methods which can take its place" (p. 17), such as intensive psychoanalytic case supervision. Lipton added that neither the personal nor the educational value of the training analysis explained

> why it must be mandatory. The elements of coercion, judgment and selection cannot be of any advantage in an analysis and can be serious obstacles. It is true that such obstacles become subject to analysis just as other obstacles are in other analyses, but the fact that obstacles can be overcome does not argue in favor of their introduction. (p.13)

In Lipton's scheme, the fact of personal analysis, when, where, and for how long, should be a totally personal decision, completely apart from the educational training program, which would have its own stepwise training criteria. Clearly, an endorsement of Bernfeld's call concerning the mandatory training analysis, but not of his wider abolition of the entire institutionalized training structure.

Which brings me up to date with my currently crystallized views after their somewhat zigzagging course, as my predilection for the university as the natural home for psychoanalysis, its scholarship, its training, and its research, has seemed ultimately properly possible, if not inevitable. Acknowledging that in today's sociocultural and budgetary world, this is not now directly feasible, I take heart from Wagner's (2009) encouragement about the long-term gravitational thrust of serious scholarly disciplines into inevitable university placement alongside their cognate disciplines. In this—ultimate—ideal placement, let me first bring up for serious consideration and, I am sure, debate, a return to a single, though central, aspect of Bernfeld's (1962) long ago call for the total demolition of the entire training structure that was inaugurated by Eitingon and his colleagues in 1920. I am not advocating a return to the earlier, totally voluntary, informal, and haphazard acquisition of psychoanalytic knowledge and competence that prevailed in the first days of psychoanalysis. I do believe, ever more firmly, in an organized and rigorous training structure for psychoanalysis in the same way as for any other formal academic and/or healing discipline.

This would include, in fact, taking the theoretical and clinical seminar sequence much more seriously than we currently usually do, with appropriate examinations and required papers, as every university discipline exacts. This would be far different from the devalued status that this didactic education now mostly enjoys; I do not remember ever witnessing or hearing about a psychoanalytic educational progression that was hampered, let alone halted, by a failure in the formal course sequence. The supervision experience would, of course, also continue, and be as central as it is today, even more so, with a more universally accepted agreement on how much (satisfactorily accomplished) clinical experience would be deemed essential in terms of number and kinds of cases, of what age groups and gender distribution, total supervision hours, and actual demonstration of achieved clinical competence, by written examination and/or oral presentation or written case description. And, of course, I would embed research needs and possibilities as an integral component of the educational program.

Personal analytic therapy started before or during training would, however, be as Bernfeld advocated, completely voluntary in terms of self-felt need or wish. Bernfeld expected, perhaps too optimistically, that every aspirant analyst would come to want such a personal therapeutic experience. Some might not. But many of us have encountered psychologically gifted individuals who, with intensive course instruction and good psychoanalytically guided supervision, but without personal analysis, have come to do substantial psychoanalytic therapy, not readily distinguishable from that done by their trained psychoanalyst colleagues. How rare such circumstances are, I cannot say. My proposal is a gamble, an experiment, but not an unreasoned one.

Such a recommendation as I am now making would have been unthinkable by me and by the overwhelming majority of my confreres, and our elders, during my own training days in the 1950s, when it was the accepted wisdom that the personal training analysis was the fundament of the training, inextricably linked to the other two components of the tripartite training structure, geared to produce together the properly competent, well-trained psychoanalyst. And, as I have stated, it is only Lipton (1988), a highly respected, somewhat maverick, psychoanalyst in Chicago, who has raised a voice in full explicit support of this same recommendation and he did so marshalling a detailed and comprehensive argument, with two major components, on its behalf.

The one component was that no one has really established the necessary linkage of the personal treatment to the professional education, or, put differently, that only those in personal training analysis could achieve the psychological resources to properly master the necessary training (even if the training were as rigorously carried out and monitored as I have just briefly indicated). The second component, to which Bernfeld had also called attention, was that there was a first psychoanalytic generation, a galaxy of gifted contributors to our discipline, who were not analyzed, and it is not evident, as disturbed even as some of them clearly seemed to be, that their psychoanalytic competence and productivity was less than that of subsequent generations of formally trained and graduated psychoanalysts. In fact, what some (Kohut, 1970) have seen as a progressive drying up of psychoanalytic creativity might be one consequence of our current training analyst centered and dominated educational system, certainly according to many of the contributors to our literature that I have reviewed.

There is, at present, no certainty as to which direction—the current one with the obligatory training analysis, or the trial of a voluntary personal therapy regime—would create a better qualified and more creative body of psychoanalytic scholars and practitioners and would also better protect the public that seeks psychoanalytic treatment. What I am suggesting, and I trust not rashly, on the way to the ultimate full-time university placement for our discipline, is a trial by at least some established psychoanalytic training entity of such a system as I propose: the voluntary psychoanalytic treatment, as desired or felt needed by the candidate, combined with the strengthened, more rigorous educational program of theoretical and clinical seminars, and together with intensive, properly long psychoanalytic supervisions of an adequately diverse set of control cases—all this under an intensive, years-long monitoring and research study of achieved outcomes in terms of the demonstrated theoretical and clinical competence of the graduates. And all of this while trusting again in the long-term ultimate embedding of the entire psychoanalytic training structure within the university, where such a program as I am proposing would, I think, best thrive.

If successful, such a system should overcome the deleterious consequences of the obligatory training analysis system within the presently operating educational structure as it now exists: for the individual candidate, in the sense of the possibility of a more open, and more honest, personal analysis for all those who have it (and without the need or desire that members not infrequently now have, for a second analysis "for me" after the one "for the institute"), and for the whole psychoanalytic training system, in the sense of a psychologically freer, less constrained and intimidated student body, opening the door to, one hopes, enhanced productivity and creativity, all the while better safeguarding the interests of those who become our psychoanalytic patients.

I feel it to be a trial and an end very much worth working towards.

Notes

1. Bernfeld's paper was his last talk at the San Francisco Psychoanalytic Society, following which he resigned from the Society in protest at what he called its unpsychoanalytic training methods (the Eitingon system structure), and, several months later, he died. It could only be published nine years later, in 1962, strongly propelled by Rudolf

Ekstein. Fenichel's paper was privately mimeographed and circulated in the Topeka Society in 1942, but he declined to publish it at the time out of fear of its possible hurtful impact on the consolidating psychoanalytic movement. When published in 1980, it had preambles by Merton Gill and Joan Fleming.

2. "Psychobiological" is used here in Adolf Meyer's designation of close attention to the remembered total life experience of the patient, with the effort to causally relate significant events, both traumatic and normative, to the concomitant unfolding of the patient's psychiatric symptomatology. This approach differed significantly from the successor psychoanalytic perspective, in the absence of the determining role of unconscious conflict, or of any conception of the transference. This sense of psychobiological is quite different from the current use of the word to refer today to the coequal consideration of biological and psychological factors in the psychiatric patient's illness picture.
3. For a good statement of the reasons for the difficulty in training for psychoanalytic research within the present institute structure of psychoanalytic training, see the *cri de coeur* of George Engel, an eminent psychoanalytic psychosomatic researcher (1968), and the response by Wallerstein (1968).
4. Implicit here is that psychoanalysis seems to be the only serious scholarly discipline that thinks of itself as a growing science, that has an educational system resting entirely on a volunteer, essentially unpaid, teaching staff, with the exception of the few faculty members in medical school based institutes with salaried full-time positions. Our system is reminiscent of the way American medical schools were functioning before the famed, devastatingly critical 1910 Flexner report, which led to the rapid transformation of the nation's medical teaching structure into the full-time academic system that prevails today.

References

Balint, M. (1948). On the psycho-analytic training system. *International Journal of Psychoanalysis*, *29*: 163–173.

Balint, M. (1954). Analytic training and training analysis. *International Journal of Psychoanalysis*, *35*: 157–162.

Bernfeld, S. (1962). On psychoanalytic training. *Psychoanalytic Quarterly*, *31*: 453–482.

Calef, V., & Weinshel, E. M. (1973). Reporting, nonreporting, and assessment in the training analysis. *Journal of the American Psychoanalytic Association, 21*: 714–726.

Casement, P. (2005). The emperor's clothes: some serious problems in psychoanalytic training. *International Journal of Psychoanalysis, 86*: 1143–1160.

Engel, G. L. (1968). Some obstacles to the development of research in psychoanalysis. *Journal of the American Psychoanalytic Association, 16*: 195–204.

Fenichel, O. (1980). Theoretical implications of the didactic analysis with preambles by Merton M. Gill and Joan Fleming. *Annual of Psychoanalysis, 8*: 21–35.

Fleming, J. (1973). The training analyst as an educator. *Annual of Psychoanalysis, 1*: 280–295.

Freud, A. (1938). The problem of training analysis. In: *The Writings of Anna Freud, Volume IV* (pp. 407–421), New York: International Universities Press, 1968.

Freud, A. (1971). The ideal psychoanalytic institute: a utopia. *Bulletin of the Menninger Clinic, 315*: 225–239.

Freud, S. (1900a). *The Interpretation of Dreams. S. E., 4–5*. London: Hogarth.

Freud, S. (1916–1917). *Introductory Lectures on Psycho-Analysis. S. E., 15–16*, p. 239 and 16, pp. 248, 496. London: Hogarth.

Freud, S. (1919j). On the teaching of psycho-analysis in universities. *S. E., 17*: 169–173. London: Hogarth.

Freud, S. (1926e). The question of lay analysis. *S. E., 20*: 177–258. London: Hogarth.

Kairys, D. (1964). The training analysis: a critical review of the literature and a controversial proposal. *Psychoanalytic Quarterly, 33*: 485–512.

Kernberg, O. F. (1986). Institutional problems of psychoanalytic education. *Journal of the American Psychoanalytic Association, 34*: 799–834.

Kernberg, O. F. (1992). Authoritarianism, culture, and personality in psychoanalytic education. *Journal of the International Association for the History of Psychoanalysis, 5*: 341–354.

Kernberg, O. F. (1996). Thirty ways to destroy the creativity of psychoanalytic candidates: an inquiry. *International Journal of Psychoanalysis, 77*: 1031–1040.

Kohut, H. (1970). Scientific activities of the American Psychoanalytic Association. *Journal of the American Psychoanalytic Association, 18*: 462–484.

Lewin, B. D., & Ross, H. (1960). *Psychoanalytic Education in the United States*. New York: W. W. Norton.

Lippman, W. (1966). The university. *New Republic*, 28 May.

Lipton, S. D. (1988). An argument in favor of making training analysis voluntary rather than mandatory. *Annual of Psychoanalysis, 16*: 11–17.

Masur, C. (1998). The training analyst system: asset or liability? *Journal of the American Psychoanalytic Association, 46*: 539–549.

Shakow, D. (1962). Psychoanalytic education of behavioral and social scientists for research. In: J. H. Masserman (Ed.), *Science and Psychoanalysis 5* (pp. 146–161). New York: Grune & Stratton.

Shakow, D., & Rapaport, D. (1964). *The Influence of Freud on American Psychology*. New York: International Universities Press (Psychological Issues, Monograph 13).

Wagner, J. W. (2009). Psychoanalysis and its place in the evolutionary chain of academic disciplines. *International Journal of Psychoanalysis, 90*: 1097–1101.

Wallerstein, R. S. (1968). Discussion of "Some obstacles to the development of research in psychoanalysis", by George Engel. *Journal of the American Psychoanalytic Association, 16*: 215–222.

Wallerstein, R. S. (1983). The Topeka Institute and the future of psychoanalysis. *Bulletin of the Menninger Clinic, 47*: 497–518.

Wallerstein, R. S. (1986). *Forty-Two Lives in Treatment: A Study of Psychoanalysis and Psychotherapy*. New York: Guilford Press.

Wallerstein, R. S. (1988). One psychoanalysis or many? *International Journal of Psychoanalysis, 69*: 5–21.

Wallerstein, R. S. (1990). Psychoanalysis: the common ground. *International Journal of Psychoanalysis, 71*: 3–20.

Wallerstein, R. S. (2007). The optimal structure for psychoanalytic education today: a feasible proposal? *Journal of the American Psychoanalytic Association, 55*: 953–984.

Wallerstein, R. S. (2010). The training analysis: psychoanalysis' perennial problem. *Psychoanalytic Review, 97*: 903–936.

Wallerstein, R. S. (2011). Psychoanalysis in the university: the natural home for education and research. *International Journal of Psychoanalysis, 92*: 623–639.

Welsh, S. S. (2008). A new model for psychoanalytic education. *The American Psychoanalyst, 42*(4): 18, 22.

CHAPTER THIRTEEN

Changes and transformations in psychoanalytic training*

Sara Zac de Filc

Current challenges to psychoanalysis

Numerous changes have occurred in every sphere of human life since Freud discovered the unconscious and created psychoanalysis. Particularly in the past three or four decades, new social movements have emerged, the old geopolitical balance has been altered, new technologies have developed, communications, capital, and labor have been globalized, and nationalisms and fundamentalisms have spread. Such transformations have affected human life at every level—social, economic, political, and cultural—engendering suffering and violence that constantly threaten individuals' mental stability and give rise to new and more serious pathologies than we had known so far.

At the same time, the advance of computer technologies has brought about deep transformations in social relations, the construction of identities, and the ways in which knowledge is produced and circulated. These transformations have generated many advantages in

* Translated by Judith Filc.

terms of knowledge and experience sharing, but they have also challenged different aspects of our practice. Faced with an increasingly complex world and changes that have affected the structure of demand, we must open to other ways of looking at the world and human interaction. We must deepen our understanding of these changes so that we can adjust our practice and our training when needed.

Yet, how do we take into consideration the effects of technological transformations, among them, the ways in which images are invading our minds and our world and the apparent cancellation of distance brought about by the immediacy of online communication? New cultural patterns favor speed and immediacy, affecting the way we deal with mental suffering. In an era that demands rapid changes, how can we successfully work with a mode of knowledge that deals with the non-chronological time of the unconscious so that we may continue to ponder, and work with, a different internal time? We need to develop our creativity to find our place in current reality, for the latter oscillates between the apparent certainties of modernity and the dizzying speed and unpredictability of postmodernity.

In this context, analytic training also becomes a focus of debate. Diverging opinions have existed for quite a while within the psychoanalytic field regarding what facilitates and fosters the evolution of our field and what impedes and halts it. Various authors have referred to the shortcomings of our training, emphasizing its rigidity. In 1982, Bob Wallerstein pointed out the threats posed by our unwholesome tendency to fall into an excessive conservatism that leads to ossification and a lack of receptivity to surrounding changes.

These changes force us to rethink our practice; we must take them into account in all their significance without renouncing our principles. Freud himself stated in "Lines of advance in psycho-analytic therapy", read in Budapest in 1918, that analysts

> have never prided ourselves on the completeness and finality of our knowledge and capacity. We are just as ready now as we were earlier to admit the imperfections of our understanding, to learn new things and to alter our methods in any way that can improve them. (Freud, 1919a, p. 157)

In other words, we must pay attention to emerging treatment and setting requirements so that we can respond to the challenges they pose.

Gradually, and often imperceptibly, analysts around the world have already modified their frame of reference and the analytic setting. Sharing ideas with colleagues worldwide will allow us to benefit from such modifications while maintaining the basic requirements that are essential for analysts to face the difficult task of helping patients relieve their mental pain. In addition, we cannot rethink our training model and practices without considering the socio-historical and cultural context in which each institution is immersed.

The consequences of these transformations for our training process

The training of new analysts and analytic continuing education constitute one of the most significant aspects of our discipline. For years we have been discussing psychoanalytic training and education in various meetings and conferences, which evinces our ongoing concern and our wish to improve them in view of current challenges. I believe that implementing changes to our educational system will contribute to transforming the future of psychoanalysis as a profession and as a science, enabling it to respond to the new obstacles it faces. The course psychoanalytic training will take is tied to our view of the ideal future psychoanalysts. These must be open-minded, flexible, and alert to the world outside the office and the institution in order to respond to new pathologies and new needs.

The shortening of distances and the new sense of immediacy created by technological transformations offer new possibilities for the training process—the ability to establish a frequent, albeit remote, contact. New teaching and treatment options urge us to develop novel conceptions of training that take these options into account so that we can use technology to improve and deepen knowledge production and transmission. For instance, we need to look further into practices such as condensed analysis and its specific features, which are the intensity of regression and resistance and the particular characteristics of the transference–countertransference dynamics. At the same time, the use of Skype raises its own questions: is the transference generated the same as the one that prevails in in-person analysis? What, if anything, remains concealed behind the image? Are we interpreting what we see and/or listen to as if analyst and patient were sharing the same space? Do we perceive any specific traits in a dialogue that seems to develop in an "in-between" space? (Sara Popovsky de Berenstein and Pablo Grinfeld (2009) have discussed their experience with analysis via Skype.)

In this context, several questions come to mind when pondering our training process: do we want to develop a capacity for theoretical thinking disconnected from clinical work? Do we believe our graduates should make psychoanalysis known to the community through their participation in it? Or, rather, should we integrate all these features? It is my contention that our graduates should be well situated in the real world, should possess a solid theoretical formation, should be able to think critically and creatively, and should be able to create, along with their patients, an analytic situation that will facilitate the unfolding of the analytic process. Yet, do these qualities suffice to make our graduates good teachers? Or good supervisors? These questions open up a necessary debate.

Another issue to be considered here is that psychoanalytic institutes worldwide are experiencing a significant drop in applications. According to Marcelo Viñar (2002), this crisis is the product of economic globalization and its effects on the choice of "long-term vocations". We know that the tendency among patients today is to opt for short psychotherapies with limited goals and quick results and for the use of psychotropic drugs rather than for treatments like psychoanalysis, which require a long-term commitment and whose results can take time to become evident.

Changing toward growth

Only an in-depth analysis of our history and of the reality in which we are training, growing, and doing will make it possible for us to implement the necessary changes that will preserve the basic psychoanalytic tenets while further developing psychoanalytic knowledge and training. Insisting on the need to maintain utter uniformity, be it in our theoretical teachings or in training in general, facilitates the emergence of closed groups rather than the development of scientific knowledge.

In his many works on analytic training and transmission, Otto Kernberg (1986, 1992, 1996, 2001) has underscored the need to make changes so that psychoanalysis can develop and grow. This author encourages institutions to embrace critical views of classic psychoanalytic texts, teach new and alternative ideas and methods, and foster interdisciplinary learning, among others. Along this line, I believe that, in order to develop the enabling environment essential for learning, we need democratic institutions that are open to dialogue within and without them, can interact with the healthcare and academic worlds on a regular basis, and are alert to what happens in the social context where they operate.

The future development of our field and its training process should lead to the transformation of analytic learning into a kind of external object that metabolizes what is experienced as "bad" and gives back to candidates new knowledge, new ideas, and new possibilities. Our training should tend less toward the establishment of a new and strong superego, and more to the creation of the conditions for candidates to feel free and to build a strong ego that can be both critical and plural. As early as 1948, Balint claimed that "what we consciously intend to achieve with our candidates, is that they should develop a strong critical ego, capable of bearing considerable strains, free from any unnecessary identification, and from any automatic transference or thinking patterns" (Balint, 1948, p. 166).

These goals are also appropriate for trained analysts, who should devote themselves to a continuing learning process as part of their professional identity. That is why it is vital to assess every so often whether our training institutes and societies actually "maintain and develop Freud's creation". How can we improve our training system? Should we not strive to understand why a discipline as creative as psychoanalysis promotes rigidity and stagnation?

To determine the course we should follow in renewing our training system, we should look into (a) the admission process; (b) the psychoanalytic institution, knowing that, due to its structure, it holds power over its members and ought to act as a container during the training process; (c) the training institute, which I think should shift from offering conventional courses to becoming a space where intrapsychic and interpersonal growth is fostered; (d) supervision, which should be the privileged site of analytic teaching and learning; (e) the candidates' personal analysis; (f) last but not least, the development of a continuing education program that combines studying, research, and the sharing of experiences and ideas. Here, I focus on the admission process, the institution and its Institute, supervision, and continuing education.

The admission process

Admission procedures are generally taken for granted in our field. While the training process has been amply discussed, admission procedures and criteria have not received enough attention. To be able to develop an analytic identity and ability, applicants must have the necessary emotional and intellectual capacity to face analytic work, and must be receptive toward the complexities of the psyche. We expect them to have a capacity for introspection and emotional maturity in their relationships. They have to be open to new ideas and to understanding and integrating outlooks that differ from their own.

Kohut (1968) already highlighted the significance of analysts' response and sensitivity to the other's emotions as well as their integrity, humaneness, creativity, and ego autonomy. To these qualities, we should add the ability to listen, empathy, and a desire to learn. Widlöcher (1976), in turn, underscores that analysts must build an interpersonal encounter that favors certain types of processes. I believe that interviews are the best predictors of the future performance of applicants. For this reason, it is essential that the two or three interviewers analyze and discuss their impressions. Careful discussions will prevent interviewers' projections from affecting their appraisal of the applicants.

Furthermore, admission to a psychoanalytic institute is the first link in the training chain, and requires that we consistently assess the admission committee's work. Deciding whether or not to admit an applicant is an arduous job. Committee members must carefully study each applicant's background. Moreover, they must have enough experience to define admission criteria that must evolve and change to adjust to a changing social environment. In her essay "Acerca de la admisión a la formación psicoanalítica en el contexto socio-económico y cultural actual" (On admission to psychoanalytic training in the current socioeconomic and cultural context), Berta Mantykow de Sola (2004) highlights that the admission process is the first nexus between the institution and its context. For this reason, our assessment of applicants also involves the institution, its philosophy, its prevailing theoretical frameworks, and its interaction with its environment. These factors will affect how applicants are evaluated.

Are we aware of the criteria we apply in deciding whether or not to admit new candidates? Are we taking into account applicants' prior training and experience? Should we not distinguish between those who have taken courses and seen patients from those who have not? Furthermore, we should review our requirements so that the curriculum may be adjusted according to new candidates' knowledge and experience. In this way, the training process could be more flexible and respond to individual needs. When the institution cannot adjust and, instead, constrains and sets boundaries, it is failing to convey to the candidates an indispensable aspect of psychoanalytic work. I am referring to the ability to take into account the uniqueness of each patient and to adjust to it.

Our institutions and institutes

I agree with Dr. Bolognini (2014) that our training rests actually on four pillars, and I made a similar claim in a discussion about the future of psychoanalysis (Zac de Filc, 1998). In his Presidential Address, "Towards a quadripartite model?", Bolognini states that a fourth element should be added that is

> essential to the future training of analysts: the acquisition of the ability to work together with colleagues and to become an integral part of scientific exchange activities and institutional life, as a permanent constitutive function of the psychoanalytic identity. (Bolognini, 2014)

The psychoanalytic institution is a necessary facet of the training process. Consequently, we need to become familiar with the different ways in which institutional dynamics can hamper this process. These include the distortion of power relations, where power in terms of potency to create and do becomes power as subjection, as well as the emergence of charismatic leaders who give rise to forms of idealization among candidates and members that affect their freedom to think and act. The way an institution incorporates candidates and makes them feel part of it will shape their sense of belonging, which can provide them with the stability and grounding necessary to think creatively and grow.

We should also keep in mind that institutions are embedded in a social, political, economic, and cultural milieu and traversed by transferences, idealizations, resistances, and countertransferences that account for the presence of the unconscious and its effects. Cross-transferences emerge with the supervisor, with the institution as a whole, with course instructors, and this process tends to be neglected. Sometimes, conflict develops among the different actors participating in candidates' training—unconscious competition that is counterproductive for the candidates. There have been cases of open confrontation between the training analyst and the supervisor because of differing theoretical perspectives.

Another issue we need to address is the rigidity of our training system. Such rigidity promotes an emotional environment that inhibits thought production and, at the same time, prevents us from discussing underlying causes and how to tackle them. Limited thought and debate and the lack of freedom to introduce necessary changes are two of the problems that plague our institutions today. They cause us to think the same issues over and over without daring to move forward. Our training system, and, hence, our institutions, tend to be dogmatic and rigid, thus contradicting the essence of psychoanalysis, which seeks truths that will enable us to go deeper into the human mind. We need to analyze the conditions that might modify candidates' subjection to an authoritarian, dogmatic treatment so as to create a training environment that will facilitate their ability to think critically, to offer containment, and to metabolize tensions. Instead of accepting thought patterns through automated transferences, candidates should be able to introject permissive figures with which to identify.

Examples of the negative atmosphere we create are the segregation of candidates—future colleagues—and our grouping in "castes" that determine the reproduction of negative attitudes toward other psychoanalytic or psychotherapy groups and societies. When we create a strong organizational system to set standards and monitor their observance, we do not realize that we are establishing a paternal authority that strongly pressures candidates and new members to identify with the "official" views. These unnecessary tensions, often based on a hierarchical system, give rise to the formation of new groups that develop their own ideals and control systems, which lead, in turn, to the narcissistic overestimation of small differences. Such an attitude conceals or minimizes the essential agreements that define psychoanalysis as a science, a therapeutic method, and a theory of the unconscious, and prevents us from understanding and confronting the problems engendered by our allegiances and loyalties.

Candidates' transformation into proselytizing followers of the ideas or theories of their analysts and supervisors is a clear illustration of the pressure to which they are exposed. (Bernardi (2003) points out that course bibliography in analytic training is geared toward strengthening the Institution's views rather than toward discussing the course content in a more general way.) In the same way, any questioning or criticism candidates might express places them in the uncomfortable position of the group's dissenter, a position not everybody is capable of enduring, thus leading them to engage in conformist behavior. Our respect of differences will not affect the quality of psychoanalytic training; conversely, it is the range of ideas and their debate that guarantees the production of solidly trained graduates.

Courses and supervisions are indispensable to analytic training, yet they should be reoriented to ensure that our candidates feel free to develop their own thoughts and ideas in a creative way. This involves a careful revision of our training system, our methodology, and, particularly, the nature of supervision. We have to make sure that we help our candidates develop the ability to reflect on their own time and place so that they learn to review and modify their way of thinking and working and to identify their resistance to change. Only if we are capable of doing so ourselves, and if we see change as a reorganizing rather than a disorganizing force, shall we be successful in our task as teachers.

A discrepancy often exists between what is explicitly stated and what is implicitly conceived of as the goals of training and the organizing structure of our psychoanalytic institutes. We say that we must act creatively, but what is creativity? In Spanish, to create means to make, to engender, to originate, to shape, to conceive. The Spanish philosopher Ferrater Mora states that

> when trying to understand the notion [of creativity] in its most radical sense, we must conclude that it does not refer simply to creating something, but also to creating the potential for the creative ability, and so on and so forth. (Ferrater Mora, 1994, pp. 716–717, translated for this edition)

It is precisely this potential for the emergence of a variety of possibilities that we must incorporate into our training and practice.

Perhaps we should agree on the need to leave aside sweeping utopias and hard morals that rest on authoritarian views. The very notion of being an analyst implies not to advocate authoritarian ethics, but to seek a healthy balance between a demanding superego and an utterly lax ego. We must search for new paths and fight against the lack of normative guidance that characterizes our times, for this lack leads to a loss of meaning.

Another aspect of the creative process is the possibility of dealing with the manifold psychoanalytic theories before us, not through disorder and chaos, but by conceptualizing and accepting their differences. In this way, our field will be perpetually open to a theoretical plurality while avoiding the trivialization of theory. Such an openness to new ideas raises the need to discuss critically instead of brandishing theories that act as emblems for identification. Access to a variety of perspectives enables us to reach individual interpretations, a process that is, in itself, rich and innovating.

Every training process entails constant learning, creativity, and discovery, and part of our task and our role as teachers and supervisors is to facilitate the emergence of these features. As Moustapha Safouan (1987) has stated, dogmatism leads to the emergence of an authoritarian institutional structure whose goal is often to protect ignorance. Only a flexible process that can simultaneously set limits and welcome creativity will bring about development and growth.

Supervision

The gradual prevalence of personal analysis as the key factor in the process of becoming a psychoanalyst—a very significant advance that warrants its worldwide persistence—has situated supervision in a sort of intermediate space between this analysis and the clinical and theoretical courses, and between psychoanalytic knowledge and its application in clinical practice. In recent years, however, a thorough rethinking of the supervision process has begun to take place: it is starting to be viewed as a complex precipitate of experiences that, like any practice linked to psychoanalysis, calls for the conjunction of theory, art, common sense, and a set of values.

I believe that because it brings together psychoanalytic theory, practice, and ethics, framed by the differing experiences of supervisor and supervisee, supervision constitutes the key site for the teaching and learning of psychoanalysis. There, we can witness candidates' application of what they have learned and true integration takes place through identification. Both candidate and supervisor, moreover, learn from this process.

The transmission of an ethics of psychoanalysis is, in my view, an essential aspect of analytic training. This ethics has three main components:

1. The search for truth, but the truth of the patient, not of the analyst.
2. The principle of abstinence, which does not mean emotional distance but, rather, refraining from becoming personally involved in the patient's life. It is worth recalling here Freud's words, quoted by Balint:

> We reject most emphatically the view that we should convert into our property the patient who puts himself into our hands in seek of help, that we should carve his destiny for him, force our own ideals upon him, and with the arrogance of a Creator form him in our own image and see that it was good. (Freud, 1918, p. 398)

3. Ensuring that our presence acts as a container for the patient.

Supervision is the locus for the convergence of two different teaching roles: the transmission of knowledge and experience, on the one hand, and the act of containment, on the other. Candidates need to develop particular ways of processing the anxiety produced by their experiencing supervision as a rite of passage in the arduous process of legitimizing their psychoanalytic identity. In conceiving of supervision as a space for teaching and learning, several questions emerge:

1. Is it closer to an analysis or to a clinical exercise?
2. Is it a specific transference–countertransference context?
3. Is it pertinent to bring to light emotional (transference) situations that we detect through supervision?
4. And if so, should we refer them explicitly to the candidate's personal analysis?

The philosophy of supervision as an educational process comprises the goals, frames of reference, techniques, and expectations of supervisors and institutions. Supervision weaves complex interrelations among all the actors that participate in candidates' training. First, supervisors, with their knowledge and experience; second, supervisees, affected by the persecutory anxieties that usually accompany the supervision process; third, the patient and the transferences emerging in the analyst/patient relationship; fourth, second or third supervisors; finally, the institution, which acts both as a containing framework and as a persecutory figure. We must understand the network of exchanges generated by these dyadic, triadic, and tetradic relationships if we want the supervisory process to become an enriching experience for all involved.

In every supervision process, we must construe, along with the candidates, the right framework for our shared task, a framework that includes a set of agreed-upon guidelines. Even though it is crucial to look at the unfolding of one particular case and at candidates' evolution throughout this process, I think that candidates should also be able to bring up doubts and difficulties posed by other cases. In this way, we will have a chance to assess their way of thinking and of handling difficulties and to identify the origin of such difficulties.

As the work of supervision unfolds, candidates will be increasingly able to integrate theory, perception, and intuition, and supervisors will devise the right ways to intervene and determine what they must discuss with their supervisees. Finally, candidates should succeed in identifying the focus of the treatment, the dynamic interplay of their transference with the patient's, and the changes that take place in the latter. Understanding these changes, in turn, should also lead to transformations in the analyst as well as in the supervisor.

Supervising entails an understanding of how we learn from clinical practice and the ability to do so, as well as the capacity to convey such knowledge to the candidate. It is in the supervision process that one's theoretical background, knowledge of the unconscious, and technical skills come together. Through their interaction with experienced analysts and their exposure to various theoretical approaches, candidates may integrate these approaches and introject the experience of analytic work.

Supervisors' role is to be guarantors of meaning and values, for professional authority in psychoanalysis derives, to a large extent, from the quality of training and the criteria we establish to assess professional competence. Supervisors are the ones who must evaluate the candidates' learning needs concerning both their theoretical knowledge and their clinical experience, so that they may fulfill the requirements to become analysts. While supervisors should understand candidates' views about the case and point out the theoretical assumptions underlying such views, they should also bring into play their own creative thinking. This contribution will enrich their shared work with the candidates, and, therefore, it will lead to the integration of the candidate into analytic work, thus creating a continuous upward spiral.

Another crucial aspect of supervision is the transmission of supervisors' experience; they have already gone through this process, and have had to visualize and understand the problems they have encountered throughout their ongoing learning and inquiry. The obstacles we face when we try to convey this experience often lead us to let our understanding of candidates' development be guided by our theoretical preconceptions. In this sense, we should apply to the work of supervision the same significance Bion (1970) attributes to clinical lived experience. Moreover, we must always keep in mind supervisors' and candidates' omnipotent fantasies and our tendency to focus on theoretical assumptions out of fear of the new and unknown that emerges in our joint work.

Given that supervision brings about anxiety, conflict, and personal questioning, it is advisable to have it coincide with candidates' personal analysis. Many believe that there is an inexorable "persecution" inherent in supervision, a persecution that characterizes any learning process and is, therefore, independent of the individuals involved and of the circumstances of each supervision process. That is why we must work through the structural and contextual aspects of supervision. In this interactive process, supervisor and supervisee build a relationship based on the former's experience and the latter's desire to learn that enables them to develop a shared approach to understanding the dynamics that unfold between candidates and their patients. Supervision work entails understanding not only patients and their reactions, but also candidates (as both analysts and students) and their feelings, which appear in the context of the supervisory relationship and of their participation in the analytic institution.

When we wonder about supervisors' role and influence, we must recall that, in almost all social relations, an individual or group may affect the behavior of other individuals or groups. According to Max Weber, we are both subjects of power and subjected to it (Bobbio et al., 2000), but in order to endure, command and obedience relations must be based on legitimacy. We designate as "authorities" those who hold legitimate power, and a legitimate power relationship facilitates the growth of those who participate in that relationship by applying agreed-upon rules and grounding authority on knowledge and experience.

The risk posed by power relations, however, is the emergence of a charismatic leader invested by the group whose power is deemed unlimited. Those subjected to it become passive and follow the commands or guidance of the subject in power without assessing its content. Supervisors run the risk of engaging in this form of power relation due to their role. By means of idealization and identification, authority as a source of knowledge and containment may be transformed into authority as imposition. Thus, a power relation emerges that might lead to the abuse of the transference and the primacy of supervisors' preconceptions. Candidates' otherness is, thus, cancelled and they are transformed into the same, and legitimate authority becomes authoritarianism.

In every clinical material we present, we show not only who the patient is, but also who we are as analysts—our frame of reference and theoretical background, what we consider to be good or bad analytic behavior, and so on. In the same way, supervisors should make themselves present in the supervising process, especially in what concerns interventions and interpretations. Each participant should offer his or her particular perspective in order to create an interactive process.

While I consider that supervision is the space for psychoanalytic learning *par excellence*, personal analysis plays a key role in this process. We do not teach psychoanalysis through personal analysis, but it is in that particular space where we live it; we try to analyze and retrace or deconstruct the multiple transferences we engage in and, thus, find new answers to our certainties. That is why we must keep in mind that supervision is not the space for the identification and interpretation of transferences. This should take place within each candidate's treatment, which should remain outside, and yet facilitate, the learning process.

Furthermore, we need to establish the goals we ought to achieve for both supervisor and supervisee in order to promote and strengthen candidates' analytic abilities, which include:

- the ability to wait;
- tact and conviction to traverse the patient's various resistance layers, without avoiding psychic pain, yet modulating it;
- the ability to be surprised without becoming undone, since surprise may generate uneasiness;
- the ability to process insidious counter-resistances that stem largely from the will to power and narcissism and that both candidate (in his or her personal analysis) and supervisor must examine;
- the ability to overcome dejection and, ultimately, their fantasies of terminating analytic work. Like any "negative" affect, dejection must be understood in relation to that particular moment in the analysis and to the analytic process as a whole;
- supervisors have to respect differing work styles. I am using the term style to refer to the combination of theoretical framework, analytic attitude, and manner and timing of interpretations that characterizes each analyst's work. A variety of styles could emerge and be integrated into the work of supervision as long as supervisors are able to promote and welcome change in its movement of transformation/creation.

We do not know how the supervising process affects the analytic process—whether we as supervisors are actually listening both to the candidate and to the candidate's patient, or whether we are projecting our own preconceptions on the case under supervision. This difficulty to assess the effect of supervision is due to the fact that each patient–analyst couple constitutes a unique dyadic (triadic, tetradic) relationship shaped by the sessions, the therapeutic situation, the supervisor–supervisee relationship, and the institution where candidates are training.

Is it possible to find indicators of a "good-enough supervisory technique"? Supervisors simultaneously practice the three impossible professions discussed by Freud; they analyze, educate, and govern (as agents of the analytic institute). What should we ask of them? To begin with, they must have undergone a "good enough" successful personal analysis and must possess knowledge, intuition, talent, empathy, and teaching skills. We should note, however, that for them to achieve the major goal of integrating theory and clinical practice, we must teach our supervisors how to teach.

We know that evaluation is indispensable, not just for the sake of institutional organization but also from the deeper perspective of the objectification of the supervisory task. Supervisors must be willing to talk to candidates about the latter's limitations. For this to happen, a suitable and pre-existing institutional support is needed that will protect both supervisor and supervisee. This support system requires that supervisors be open to reciprocal evaluations within the style and procedural methodology characteristic of each institution. We must be able to show what we do, which should coincide with what we preach, for the discrepancy between saying and doing is damaging both to the institution and to its members.

We should think of developing *ad hoc* advisory systems according to candidates' needs and demands. Institutions should establish competence criteria for the appointment of supervisors; nothing should automatically grant us that status. Moreover, it is my contention that personal analyst and supervisor are autonomous roles and should, therefore, remain separate, thus preventing the excessive concentration of power that occurs in analytic institutions. In Uruguay, the 1974 amendment of the bylaws gave rise to the creation of three groups with different roles, which are institute analysts (who conduct personal analysis with candidates), supervising analysts, and teaching analysts. (For a more detailed description of the amendment, see Bernardi (2010).)

Moreover, we should develop a training curriculum for supervisors and promote open collective supervisions that would also make it easier for candidates to choose their supervisors. In addition, the supervision of supervisors would serve to improve supervising practices and provide research material for further learning and would contribute to the necessary revalidation of the status of supervisor, avoiding its perpetuation.

Continuing education

We always talk about training new analysts, about the role of institutions, and even about the latter's interaction with the community and the academic world, but we forget that our analytic training does not end with graduation. We should discuss the need to instate a system of continuing education that will help us face the evolving requirements of clinical practice. I am referring to an ongoing training process that entails not only updating our knowledge, but also opening our minds to information and ways of knowledge production that are indispensable to understanding the complexity of our present-day world.

Such an endeavor implies both going deeper into the study of specific psychoanalytic theories and techniques, and looking into the world around us. In other words, we should resort to other disciplines to understand the socioeconomic and cultural context in which our institution and our practice are developing. In this way, our institutions will become living entities that grow and evolve with their members and their environment. To do so, we should encourage the creation and development of new research groups and programs.

Another problem that we have neglected is the role of elderly colleagues in psychoanalytic institutions. When they do not enjoy a high hierarchical status, they tend to be relegated. We should try to make the most of the knowledge and experience they have accumulated by resorting to them as consultants or advisors. I have referred to this problem elsewhere (Zac de Filc, 2012). Continuing education could become a space for knowledge sharing where we could make the most of the experience of elderly analysts, thus serving two purposes at once.

Final considerations

We might have reached the point where we need to rethink our work and determine to what extent we are dealing with new developments and realities that demand adjustments within our field. This does not mean renouncing our principles, but, rather, seeking new paths for growth and knowledge production that will serve to maintain these principles and, thus, facilitate the progress of psychoanalytic science and training.

Just as we need to develop a continuing education strategy, so do we need to internalize that, in order to survive, institutions must maintain an ongoing exchange with their environment. This means keeping abreast of advances in other sciences, but also of the vicissitudes of the socioeconomic and cultural context where they operate. Only by being open-minded and receptive to the outside *and* to the inside—by giving all our members and candidates a voice—shall our institutions continue to be living, dynamic entities.

References

Balint, M. (1948). On the psychoanalytic training system. *International Journal of Psychoanalysis, 29*: 163–173.

Bernardi, B. de León de (2010). La formación psicoanalítica en un contexto de pluralismo teórico y técnico. *Revista latinoamericana de psicoanálisis, 9*: 119–137.

Bernardi, R. (2003). What kind of evidence makes the analyst change his or her theoretical and technical ideas? In: M. Leuzinger-Bohleber, A. U. Dreher, & J. Canestri (Eds.), *Pluralism and Unity? Methods of Research in Psychoanalysis* (pp. 125–136). London: The International Psychoanalysis Library.

Bion, W. R. (1970). *Attention and Interpretation*. New York: Basic Books.

Bobbio, N., Matteucci, N., & Pasquino, G. (2000). *Diccionario de política*. México, DF: Siglo XXI editores.

Bolognini, S. (2014). Towards a quadripartite model? *IPA E-Newsletter*, May.

Ferrater Mora, J. (1994). *Diccionario de filosofía*. Barcelona: Editorial Ariel.

Freud, S. (1918). Turnings in the ways of psycho-analytic therapy. Paper presented to the International Psychoanalytical Conference, Budapest. Published in *Collected Papers, 2* (pp. 396–399), J. Riviere (Trans.). London: Hogarth, 1946.

Freud, S. (1919a). Lines of advance in psycho-analytic therapy. *S. E., 17*: 157–168. London: Hogarth.

Kernberg, O. (1986). Institutional problems of psychoanalytic education. *Journal of the American Psychoanalytic Association, 4*: 799–834.

Kernberg, O. (1992). Authoritarianism, culture, and personality in psychoanalytic education. *Journal of the International Association for the History of Psychoanalysis*, 341–354. Reprinted in: *Ideology, Conflict, and Leadership in Groups and Organizations* (pp. 230–237). New Haven, CT: Yale University Press, 1998.

Kernberg, O. (1996). Thirty ways to destroy the creativity of psychoanalytic candidates. *International Journal of Psychoanalysis, 77*: 1031–1040.

Kernberg, O. (2001). Some thoughts regarding innovations in psychoanalytic education. Presented to the International Psychoanalytical Association (IPA) Executive Council Meeting in Puerto Vallarta, Mexico, January 7.

Kohut, H. (1968). The evaluation of applicants for psychoanalytic training. *International Journal of Psychoanalysis, 49*: 548–554.

Mantykow de Sola, B. (2004). Acerca de la admisión a la formación psicoanalítica en el contexto socio-económico cultural actual. *Psicoanálisis, Revista de la Asociación Psicoanalítica de Buenos Aires, 27*: 763–774.

Popovsky de Bereinstein, S., & Grinfeld, P. (2009). Análisis telefónico, análisis por Skype. Presented to the 46th IPAC, Chicago, July.

Safouan, M. (1987). *La transferencia y el deseo del analista*, I. Agoff (Trans.). Buenos Aires: Paidós.

Viñar, M. (2002). Sobre admisión al Instituto. Presented to the XX FEPAL Training Analyst Pre-Congress, Guadalajara, México, September. Available at http://fepal.org/images/2004precongreso/sobre_admision_al_instituto.pdf. Accessed on 17 February 2015.

Wallerstein, R. (1982). Beyond lay analysis: pathways to a psychoanalytic career. *Journal of the American Psychoanalytic Association, 30*: 701–715.

Widlöcher, D. (1976). Psychanalyse aujourd'hui: un problème d'identité. In: E. D. Joseph & D. Widlöcher (Eds.), *L'identité du psychanalyste* (pp. 43–58). Paris: Presses Universitaires de France.

Zac de Filc, S. (1998). Psicoanálisis y futuro. Presented to the 21st FEPAL Conference, Cartagena de Indias, Colombia, August.

Zac de Filc, S. (2012). Envejecimiento del analista. Presented to the 29th FEPAL Conference, Sao Paulo, Brazil, October.

CHAPTER FOURTEEN

Theses on the heart of darkness

The unresolved Oedipus complex of psychoanalytic institution formation*

Peter Zagermann

> Since of the gathering bitter of years our people have drunken,
> Bitterness all the more dreadful because such fair hope had been blighted
>
> (Goethe, 1798, p. 478)

If this chapter is not a polemic one, it certainly has traits of it. It tries to depict a situation which, as I see it, is primarily responsible for the fact that psychoanalysis is so much under pressure on the plane of societal acceptance, and which urgently has to be altered if it wants to survive. This problematic is a consequence of fatal miscarriages of its construction as an organization. Against this backdrop, this chapter is the description of a catastrophe that could destroy one of the finest inventions of the human spirit.

The three columns of training, according to the worldwide prevalent Eitingon model, are the training analysis, the supervision, and the

*An abbreviated version of this paper was read at the 49th Congress of the International Psychoanalytical Association, Boston, 25 July 2015 and at the Congress of the German Psychoanalytical Association (DPV), Bad Homburg, 22 November 2014.

theoretical teachings. Within this model, the institutional sub-formation consisting of all training analysts, that is to say, the training committee, occupies the central role within the institution, as both training analysis and the supervision of the educational analyses—and, in some institutes or societies, also key theoretical seminars—are tied to the function of training analyst. The training committee is, therefore, the identity-giving moment of a psychoanalytic institute. The mode of coming into being of the personnel makeup of this committee is, in principle, the same worldwide: a cooption procedure within which the reshuffle is effected by nomination from within the training committee itself.

The mode, as such, is a discrete institutional background mechanism which, *de facto*, becomes hugely important as it determines not only the concrete makeup of the training committee itself, but also influences, in particular, the climate under which an institute lives and works. For the training committee trains future analysts, and its institutional character, as defined by the mode of its constitution, imprints on their analytical socialization.

In this chapter, I refer to the training committee, for short, when I mean the totality of the training analysts of an institute, although I am aware of the fact that, in many reformed institutes, officials of that institute who are not training analysts are members of the training committee for the duration of their tenure and by statute.

It is a fundamental sociological law of the psychoanalysis of organizations that the moment an examination or examination-like proof of qualification or other restriction is put up before access to a certain function within an institutional structure, this very function acquires hierarchical importance, even if, rationally, one would consider this unfounded. From a psychoanalytic perspective and diction, the moment of examination or restriction, respectively, in this structure introduces the theme of inclusion and exclusion, and, thus, together with hierarchization, the oedipal moment, in the sense of a transference automatism. This is as unavoidable as the Oedipus complex itself; it is the manifestation of the Oedipus complex in the institutional domain, for the oedipal complex is constituted by the moment of the exclusion from the primal scene. Each exclusion thus provokes, unconsciously and automatically, the oedipal phantasmatization, and this all the more so the more unjust and arbitrary this exclusion is experienced as, which—as the case may be—might reflect the actual truth.

Within the psychoanalytic institution formation which comprises the constitution of training committees in line with the Eitingon model, the importance of this hierarchization and its consequences is further emphasized by the fact that the function of training analyst is the only function after graduation and after acceptance into the society (in some psychoanalytic societies, this last step is tied to a special qualification), the access to which is barred by a distinct and separate examination. Through this oedipal transference automatism which exists because of the characteristic of examination, the psychoanalytic institutional structure acquires an inner dynamic aimed at the function of training analyst, and, because of the ubiquity of the oedipal theme, this dynamic also applies to all those colleagues who decide not to undergo the qualifying examination for the function as training analyst.

This argument is being countered by the statement that the climate of an institute is just as importantly determined by the self-esteem of those members who do not belong to the training committee. The train of thought that underlies this argument can be continued in the direction of fundamentally questioning the importance of the moment institutionally characterizing a training committee, which is its generativity—in the sense of the training of future analysts.

Generativity, however, cannot be considered outside of oedipality. As the oedipal transference to the training committee exists because of the examination that is placed before access is gained to the function of training analyst, and generativity, as discussed, cannot be seen outside of oedipality, the questioning of generativity within the framework of psychoanalytic institutes is directed against oedipality itself. One cannot dismiss oedipal transference at will. Within a decidedly oedipal institutional structure like that of a psychoanalytic institute, agenerativity, in the psychoanalytic view, which regards the Oedipus complex as the governing basic law for the functioning of the psyche, is not a possible value *per se*, but a symptom: it is one of the forms of narcissistic defense against being bound to the oedipal principle.

Apart from that, however, and with a view to the sociologic aspect of institution formation, it is totally impossible to accord an equal rank to agenerativity in comparison with generativity, for agenerativity, as a principle, would be a sociographic synonym for self-dissolution, meaning the dying of the institution. An institution, if it wants to survive, is dependent on generative reproduction, otherwise it will die out in consequence of a lack of members. In addition, generativity in a psychoanalytic institute is bound to the training committee: more specifically, to the training analysts. There is, therefore, in addition to the psychological reason for the heightened importance of the training committees (key words: examination/restriction placed before the function of training analyst and resulting oedipalization) also the sociological dimension, which lies in the importance, for the continued existence of the institution, of the generativity being tied to the training committee.

Furthermore, both moments—oedipalization and generativity—are, however, relating to each other in a way that they mutually potentiate each other: oedipalization gains its fullest possible force exactly because generativity is exercised by the training committee only; in turn, the moment of inclusion and exclusion—that is to say, oedipalization—brought about by the examination places the generativity that is bound to the training committee squarely into the oedipal context. Through this specific institutional construction, a fit of forces has come about which combines the two most energetically charged psychic themes in the sense of creating a reciprocal potentiation that is unsurpassable in its emotional power.

The combination of these factors is an absolute specific of psychoanalytic institutes. I would like to impart maximum importance to this line of thinking, for one would not find this anywhere else, that the generativity of an institution is tied to a certain sub-formation of this institution, exclusively, and that access to this formation in the form of an examination or other proof of qualification is so clearly oedipalized. Psychoanalysis has, in this way, installed a representation of the creative primal scene at the centre of its institutionalization. This means a representation of the Oedipus complex with all its destructive possibilities, drive-related wishes, and demands of abstinence which come with it. In the constitutional set-up of the training committees and in how they are related to, all complications that are linked to the Oedipus complex will come to bear.

Psychoanalysis, therefore, within the framework of human institution formation, represents and manifests the oedipal complex explicitly. If we consider it in a social and sociological frame of reference, psychoanalysis has a curative mandate here, too, in the sense of having to react to the complications of this situation according to its own principles, even if it has not recognized this mandate.

Generativity, for instance, actually also means sexuality. In the unconscious experience, the training committee represents the sexual instance in an institute, and this in exclusivity: sexual activity in the sense of generativity is exercised only by the members of the training committee. This is why all archaic mechanisms come into play here which are linked with sexuality: castration as an attempt to secure the sexual–procreative monopoly, and, equally, the huge difficulty of allowing each successive sexual generation to come into its own, let alone to withdraw from the training committee age-appropriately and to leave decisions to those who currently carry the generative responsibility, because this is being equated with the end of the sexually active phase. This being so, it is engrained in the dynamic of this institutional organization that psychoanalytic institutes have a tendency towards gerontocracy, as—on the unconscious plane—the sharing in the power of the training committees comes with the illusion of still belonging to the sexually active procreative generation, of still having the ability to live sexually. In addition to the internal complications this causes, it also leads to a distortion of the public image of psychoanalysis.

This sexual monopoly is also the cause of the high transference barrier which is linked with access to the training committee, an issue that is relevant for both sides: for the members of the training committee who want to secure their sexual monopoly position *vis-à-vis* the younger generation, and for the applicants, who find themselves confronted with the whole range of complications resulting from their claim to their own sexual–generative activity with respect to their oedipal parents. A vicious circle begins: once the oedipal transference has been established through hierarchization and the theme of inclusion and exclusion, this oedipal barrier, which has thus been established, has the tendency to be inflated from both sides in escalating excesses through the mutual transferences, continually fed by the sexual, generative prerogative of the training committee. What has come into existence here is the maximum stimulation of transference potentials that are at all conceivable in the area of institutional structures.

It has to be kept in mind that this organizational stimulation of oedipal transference potentials takes place within institutions the aim of which is to train young psychoanalysts who, for this reason, undergo their own personal training analyses. Psychoanalysis, as a science, is centered around the Oedipus complex, and the future psychoanalysts are both in an intense intellectual involvement with psychoanalytic theory—and this is to say, with the Oedipus complex—as they are, in their training analyses, confronted with their personal oedipal complications. This goes to show that in psychoanalytic institutes we find an exquisitely oedipal organizational structure within an intellectual and emotional climate entrenched with oedipality. In other words, fuel is added to the fire. Form and content go hand in hand. The oedipal properties of psychoanalytic institution formation meet with a mental setting that is expressly and specifically geared to just those properties and that, therefore, seizes them in lock and key fashion. This is the big difference from any other organization that would have the same institutional set-up. It is difficult to imagine a situation where oedipal transferences would and could be more enhanced than here.

Taking into account that oedipality is not only the most highly invested psychic content but is, in fact, the centerpiece, the bedrock of the structural organization of the psyche, this combination of maximum investment, unconscious meaning, and lock and key articulation between the institutional structure and the mental set-up of its members leads to a situation where psychoanalytic institutes function as a psychic trap that tends to imprison both training and non-training analyst faculty, non-faculty members, as well as candidates, for life. This is not what you would wish for in the sense of a healthy identification with an institution, instead being a malign situation that is draining away enormous amounts of life energy and is juxtaposed to the libertarian and self-determined spirit of psychoanalysis.

Depending on the degree of the neurotic deformation of the oedipal transferences on the part of all involved, this fundamentally opens up the total potential of the human propensity for conflict, including intrigue, that is linked with sexuality and oedipal inclusion and exclusion. It is no surprise, then, that, in our psychoanalytic institutes, we are frequently confronted with conflicts breaking out and, unfortunately, with an indisputable dimension of perfidy and vileness when these conflicts are in process or are being suppressed.

If the above thoughts on the high degree of oedipal structure of psychoanalytic training committees are correct, it comes as no surprise that they instantly became the target of the attack of oedipal transgression, and this attack is, in my opinion, the co-option mode of personnel replacement in the training committees. Within the procedure, which, in variants, is practiced throughout the IPA, proof of the clinical and theoretical qualification of the aspiring applicant—that is to say, the examination proper—is the precondition for entry. It then becomes the basis for the actual appointment—more exactly, nomination—through the current members of the pertinent local training committee, whereby the qualification itself gives no entitlement whatsoever. In other words, the nomination leading to appointment lies entirely with the autonomous exercise of power by the respective training committees.

In all traditionally organized psychoanalytic training institutes, training analysts are nominated in this manner by the local training committee, that is to say, they are co-opted. The nomination procedure in this context has—among other things depending on the size of the institute—various degrees of elaboration. However, upon taking a closer look, it is a co-option procedure in each and every case. This nomination must then be confirmed by the meeting of members and, in constituent organizations that have a federal structure, by the central national training committee and by the central executive board of the constituent organization.

In terms of the law governing associations, this is the appointment proper, the crucial step, however, is the nomination through the local training committee; meetings of members, central executive board, and central training committee do not, as a rule, and within the existing power structure, oppose the local training committee. In the case of the pure co-option mode, there is no provision for even the possibility of an application. If, in principle, the application procedure were to be accepted, no application for which prior internal approval had not been indicated would be presented anyway, so as to avoid public shaming. But even if there was the possibility to apply, the nomination is done exclusively through the autonomy of the training committee, which is not obliged to bind itself to formalized, reproducible criteria.[1]

If an application is filed without explicit consent, or even against the training committee's advice and under the condition of the co-option mode, this, more likely than not, would be equivalent to institutional suicide of the applicant. Following the organizational logic of the co-option mode, the training committee would deny such an application that challenges its monopoly, the applicant having no opportunity to appeal against the decision as there are no objective criteria on which to base such an appeal. What we are dealing with here is, thus, no real deviation from the co-option mode, and it is astonishing that considerate and serious colleagues mention the possibility of applying as convincing and compelling evidence for the reformability of the Eitingon model and, specifically, for the neutralization of the detrimental implications of the co-option mode. One cannot escape the conclusion that, here, powerful institutional defense mechanisms must be at work which produce a prohibition on thinking.

In any case, in dealing with the problematic of psychoanalytic training, I consider it necessary to accord special attention to the subject of institutional, large-group production of extraordinarily effective prohibitions on thinking. This cannot be understood in any other way, if a whole society of intellectually and scientifically highly trained, enlightened personalities subjects itself, for decades on end, to a system which has such obvious self-damaging and self-limiting implications. In my view, this is to do with the system's oedipal gratifications which are so strong once one has managed to push through to the—as Kernberg (2007, p. 186) names it—"power elite" of the training committee, at which point such achievement would equal a direct satisfaction of the oedipal phantasm. It is very difficult to question the system itself from this position of gratification, and a long period of development had to take place before things began to drift apart and further and further away from external reality (key words, the current danger of the social and scientific unimportance of psychoanalysis), so that the delusional character of this system could become evident.

The co-option mode of renewing the training committees is, therefore, as far as my analysis goes and which places the lack of mandatory and objectivising external criteria in the foreground, a more or less veiled endogamy, as it occurs without the option of an independently guaranteed application and without external control, from within the training committees themselves. This is what is referred to as co-option mode: the training committee appoints its new members at its own discretion. From the point of view of organizational psychoanalysis, this leads to a pathological concentration of power within the training committees which tends to paralyze the institutes, as well as to their tendency to narcissistically isolate and encapsulate themselves within themselves, for the training committee in this way not only has the generative and, thus, sexual prerogative, but, what is more, it has the privilege of autogenesis, hence it represents a completely closed-off, narcissistic universe. No wonder that membership in this institutional *perpetuum mobile* holds such a huge narcissistic seductive power. From the perspective of the psychoanalysis of organizations, and institutions, this is a fatal constellation, the worst that can be imagined.

Add the thought that this kind of internal problematic structure of psychoanalytic institutes does not remain internal, but transfers to the relationship with the outside world and the public perception and impact of psychoanalytic institutes. The training committee relates to the institute in the same way as the institute as a whole relates to its environment, for the relationship of the training committee with the institute is the only institutional object relationship within a psychoanalytic institute structured in line with the Eitingon model. This object relationship is picked up by the collective countertransference of the social field in which the institute operates. Society reacts to the object relations quality which emanates from psychoanalytic institutes and identifies them with it, just as the institute as a whole involuntarily and unavoidably is bound to identify itself with this inherent institutional object relationship which is its own, and relates to the outside world correspondingly. The accusation of being an arrogant, self-secluding power elite that we are notoriously confronted with is, thus, unfortunately, no unjust ascription, but the exact description of the flawed construction of our institutions' formation.

The problems with this endogamous autogenesis have been well noted by the authors who critically examined the subject. Kernberg, in this context, refers to a "self-proliferating", "self-selected", and "self-perpetuating power elite" (1986, p. 956, 2006, p. 1661, 2007, p 186) as do also Wallerstein (2007) and Auchincloss and Michels (2003). Kernberg, as well as the other authors, however, lists this characteristic descriptively in a series with all the other shortcomings of the training structure according to the Eitingon model, whereas I am going to show that this characteristic is the central problematic criterion from which all other problems derive.

A self-referential vicious circle results, which provides an underlying, factually existing reality for the neurotic phantasy which, in its turn, further potentiates the phantasm: the pathological, oedipal phantasmatization of the concentration of power and of the absolutist, narcissistic inclusion and exclusion is, thereby, institutionally confirmed as reality and retrospectively reinforced, that the training committee does indeed renew itself only from within itself—endogamously. The dangerousness of this solipsistic concentration of power lies in it being, on the one hand, something factual, and, on the other hand, and predominantly so, something phantasmatic, carried by unconscious oedipal transferences which are provoked by the pathological institutional structure. This is an incentive toward a delusional distortion of reality.[2]

One must not look at this, however, from the point of view only of the oedipal "children", that is to say, the "common" members of the institute and the candidates, who project to the training committee the theme of exclusion from the primal scene. A much more consequential aspect and more difficult to discern, because it is disguised by the claim of authority, is that the members of the training committee, based on that same oedipal theme, elevate the training committee to the rank of self-contained parental nobility, detached from the "children".

From the perspective of the psychoanalysis of organizations, the driving unconscious motive on the part of a training committee which functions according to the endogamous co-option mode is to be seen in the triumph of having reversed the oedipal situation: the fact of being excluded is turned into active exclusion, under the guise of the rationalization phantasma of keeping the teachings "pure". The unconscious phantasy behind this is, therefore, that of equation with the primal scene: the training committee takes the place of the procreative parental couple. This self-equation is psychically synonymous with incest. Incest—because of the exclusion of the third—is the psychic signature of infertility, and, thus, of agenerativity and anti-generativity.[3]

In consequence of this analysis, one might say that the classical structure of psychoanalytic institutes and their training virtually represent a seduction that invites oedipal transgression. It is not of decisive import in these considerations whether a concrete training committee succumbs to this structurally laid down aspect of seduction in a concretely abusive sense or whether it resists it. The problem lies buried in the institutional structure itself and is communicated unconsciously, or implicitly, even without any actually directed or enacted transgression. One must, in all consequence, hold to the insight of organizational psychoanalysis that the structure of an institution constellates and manifests its unconscious. The structure of an institution *is* its unconscious.

The co-option mode adds to the oedipal exclusion from the sexual function the moment of arbitrariness, and more specifically, of endogamous—and, thus, incestuous—selection. The background model of this form of procreation is the abuse, that is to say, submission to sexual coercion, exercised by the older generation: the training committee equates itself with the primal scene and, in exchange for granting inclusion in this oedipal circle, demands unconditional submission from those filling the vacancies.

This situation, once established, raises the very danger of adaptation opportunism which all authors who have engaged with the problematic nature of the Eitingon model note and lament, starting with Balint (1948) and Bernfeld (1962) to Auchincloss and Michels (2003), Wallerstein (2007), and Kernberg (2006, 2007, and *passim*). For one's only chance to be accepted as "peer" by the training committee and be nominated would then consist in some sort of subservient behaviour and mentality so that in one's head one already belongs, as it were, and the training committee, in the sense of an asexual procreation, can then easily confirm this belonging by an act of grace. It does not surprise that psychoanalysis, under these conditions of enforced adaptation, suffers from the ascription of ideology and indoctrination in its public perception.

The unconditionality of submission directly and unavoidably results from the arbitrariness of the nomination, independent of any possible good will. The process is so unavoidable as to be fateful. At the same time, this inclusion into the circle is, however, equivalent to incestuous transgression, as the training committee does, after all, represent the primal scene, and, therefore, it carries the price of oedipal guilt. The members of the training committee are, thus, linked to each other through an unconscious bond of guilt, which makes them, in this sense, members of a complot.

With this, a situation is constituted, unconsciously, where the training committee rejects those very oedipal rules of regulation of sexual activity for itself which would be its duty to represent in accordance with its function within the training. From the perspective of the psychoanalysis of institutions, this creates a situation that, in the sense of its organizational logic, can only be regarded as corrupt, carrying fateful traits of a group-dynamic enactment of the constellation that Rosenfeld (1971) described as the narcissistic pathological organization. This establishes, in principle, the readiness of a considerable measure of malignant reaction against anybody who disturbs this narcissistic satisfaction arrangement. This is an aspect that, quite understandably, in the social countertransference, deters the public.

As said, the abuse laid out in the co-option mode, the transgression of the incest taboo and the problematic of infertility it contains, are communicated as mere potentialities, independent of the question of their concrete actualization. In other words, because of the pathological mode of their own regeneration, the training committees that are operating under the co-option mode come into conflict with their institutional task, which is generativity. In my mind, this is one of the most important reasons for the negative external representation of institutionalized psychoanalysis, for this problematic field of meanings communicates itself to the outside world.

As long as institutionalized psychoanalysis does not solve this problem, it is subject to a blockade of its own making that restricts its institutional manoeuvering space and creative freedom, for what has constituted itself here, with reference to the training committees, is nothing else but what, under the perspective of the psychoanalysis of organizations, has to be defined as institutional pathology: the conscious task of the institution is, from several aspects (e.g., generativity and adherence to the oedipal laws), in contradiction and conflict with its organizationally implicit, and, to that extent, unconscious structural dynamics.[4]

At the level of consequences of the endogamous co-option mode, a further vicious circle establishes itself which caters to these problems: the more infertile and paralyzed a training committee and an institute *de facto* are, the more massively the narcissistic exclusion theme is set in motion in order to hush up creative poverty and replace it with narcissistic fiction. What happens then is a self-strangulation of our institutes, which blindly perish in haughty arrogance because, for reasons of defense, they are unable to link the lack of attractiveness for the outside world with their own endogamous exclusion pathology. If a malignant escalation results, this exclusion pathology, as we know from many institutes and cases, can go as far as enacting active abortion scenarios with reference to members who will not submit to the endogamous rules.

Apodictic statements of the kind that are to be heard within the framework of the usual procedure as matter-of-fact and unquestionable principle, that, even if qualification standards are met, there is no claim for an applicant to be appointed because the highest criterion for an appointment as training analyst is a personal fit with the local training committee, are, from the point of view of these considerations, a definite no go. They are the pseudo-rational reasoning for maintaining the endogamous nomination mode. It may be called unconscious cynicism, or sadism, when leading institutional representatives bring forth the argument, in defense of this principle and with the claim that this would obviate any further discussion, that only locally would there be the most knowledge available about an applicant for the function of training analyst as to his or her character and competence. This is a denial—bordering on open hypocrisy—of any knowledge about the fact that "locally" there can be considerable pathological group dynamics which might have the character of unconcealed power schemes, and that, in addition, nothing encourages such regressive group processes more than the dynamic of small, self-contained groups. What is more, in the case of psychoanalytic training committees, this existing dynamic of small groups is so maximally stimulated and expressly provoked by the factors described (i.e., narcissistic self-seclusion through the sexual and autogenetic privilege), in fact, as much as is at all possible within the framework of institution formation, that one is bound to assume irrational dynamics at work as the rule.

In the light of the fact that a member who has attained the formal qualification as training analyst has, as a rule, participated in the institute's life for many years and most of the time has also held functions within the institute, it must be regarded as a phantasm with symptom characteristics, to proceed as a rule from the assumption of the imminent danger that through this member the work of the training committee could be paralyzed, and to make this danger the fundamental reason for the endogamous mode of nomination. At the same time, this phantasm comes with a ban on thinking so that it does not occur to the majority of colleagues to seriously question it. In my opinion, this ban, or prohibition, on thinking is one of the clearest pieces of evidence for the pathological character of our institutional structure and the resulting highly active defense mechanisms.

Paradoxically, it has to do with this paranoid phantasm and the associated ban on thinking that, on the other hand, within a social milieu thus constituted, very serious pathologies might remain unrecognized for a long time, as if under a scotomization or a dissociative split, once the respective individuals have reached the status as members of the training analyst body. In his paper "The coming changes in psychoanalytic education" of 2006, Otto Kernberg, in this context, under the heading of "Paranoiagenic aspects of psychoanalytic education", wrote the following:

> As president of the IPA, I was also privy to individual concerns, complaints, and revelations of a broad variety of difficulties faced by members and candidates. What came as a shocking surprise was the discovery that seemingly isolated cases of mismanagement, mistreatment, unethical behavior, or gross unfairness as causes of individual and group complaints in various societies and institutes throughout the three regions proved to reflect more general, chronic ways of institutional malfunctioning that seemed detrimental to the tasks of psychoanalytic education, to the morale of the corresponding institution, and to the professional and scientific creativity of both faculty and candidates. Anne-Marie Sandler's (2004) dramatic, tactful and concerned analysis of a long-lasting tolerance within the British Psychoanalytic Society and Institute of a notorious case of corruption of psychoanalytic principles and ethics, unfortunately, is not about an isolated incident: I have been involved in similar situations in all three regions. While in all human institutions it is unavoidable, I believe, that such situations emerge, the question is, to what extent is a dysfunctional institutional structure contributing to trigger them and to prevent their correction. (Kernberg, 2006, p. 1653)

In my opinion, this "dysfunctional institutional structure" is to be found primarily in the structurally incestuous—endogamous—degeneration of our training committees which function in accordance with the co-option mode. Together with the lifelong appointment of training analysts and the federal autonomy of the institutes, a follow-on effect of the endogamous nomination practice is a kind of absolutist immunity that, of course, is exceedingly compatible with narcissistic personalities. This interconnection has been pointed out by Kernberg, starting with his first publication (1986) on this matter. Narcissistic personalities and endogamous training committee structure relate to one another in a correspondence relationship, linked by their joint motive of narcissistically motivated exclusion and inclusion. An institutional structure, especially within the framework of psychoanalysis, should work to counter its abuse by pathologically organized personalities instead of encouraging it.

The argument that harmony is important in the personnel makeup of the training committee is the gateway for an arbitrariness that is beyond regulation. Whoever yields to this argument basically makes the decision to choose open intrigue or unconsciously directed regressive group dynamics as the governing principle, even if this principle is not applied in all cases. Unholy alliances are part of the unavoidable weaknesses we encounter in human coexistence, and the members of the training committees are not exempt. What is not acceptable, however, is to officially invite such behaviour.

The necessary reform of the appointment procedure for training analysts, in a first step, can only consist of complete and instant cancellation of the local privilege of nomination and, thus, of the endogamous procedure as such. It must be demanded that colleagues who qualify for the function of training analyst are nominated based on this qualification, and that they must be deployable in each institute of a national association and that each institute must be able to integrate them. Anything else would be tantamount to admitting, *a priori*, that training committees chronically and fundamentally do not function, in Bion's words, in the mode of a work group, but in that of a primary assumption group.

In this context, a further aspect plays an important role. In most constituent organizations of the IPA the local institutes enjoy far-reaching autonomy. They are joined together under the federalist principle into the national organization. The, in principle, autonomous local institute is endowed by the national association to carry out the training in compliance with the rules and regulations of the IPA.

This local autonomy is the actual institutional background for the endogamous nomination mode of training analysts, and the question is whether recourse to the alleged necessity of fit of a new training analyst with the local training committee is mostly a, predominantly unconscious, rationalization in order to avoid the conflict about federal autonomy. This federal structure is principally not agreeing with the contractual responsibility to protect psychoanalysis and its principles that the respective constituent organizations have taken on towards the IPA and which is laid down in their statutes. For, in the case of conflict, the chair of the constituent organization has no easy and established opportunity to interfere with the federalist autonomy of the institutes, even if there are occurrences at a particular institute which are acute and which damage the public standing of psychoanalysis and threaten the psychological welfare of patients and candidates. The only means that are available to the central executive board in this case is the threat to withdraw the license to train, which, however, presupposes nothing short of a maximum escalation.[5]

Dependency from the object characterizes the psychic constitution of the human being. Conflict with this dependency leads to the oedipal structure and is, thus, the fire in which analysts are baptized. It would be the wrong step to want to avoid or soften this conflict. It must, however, be carried out on a fair basis. The danger is that psychoanalysis is being turned into a system of narcissistic exploitation of those dependency relationships on which the analytic training, and, thus, secondarily, the structure of the psychoanalytic institutes rests. This exploitation may take on varying degrees of concretism, up to the consummated analytical incest. The absolute concentration of power and the narcissistic self-seclusion under both the endogamous and federal constitution of the Eitingon model, which have no intrinsic possibility of being corrected, maximizes this danger to a degree that one cannot help but call plain seduction.

To sum up my argument: according to the logic of the pathological institutional structure of the endogamous, autogenetic training analyst system, a new member can be admitted into the circle of the training committee only if he or she has assimilated him- or herself to a degree that it must not be feared any more that he or she uncover the fiction of the superiority of the members of the training committee. This fiction cannot be questioned as there is no rule-giving regulatory body of power outside the training committees. In that, it bears a delusional character. This theme holds a demonic power, which, once erupted, can hardly be tamed, for, *nota bene*, this is the institutional fallout of the most elemental emotional relationships of the psyche.

Of course, I do not mean to say that each individual training analyst who has been appointed within such an institutional structure, would, of necessity, have concretely acted in this way. The same applies at the level of the institutes, which have taken up very diverse positions on the subject. But this is what the implicit pathological intelligence of this structure and group dynamics requires and wants, and there is surely no one whom the angel of temptation has passed by in this respect. This is about the confrontation with the oedipal illusion of power. Is this what we want to be associated with against the background of the ethos of psychoanalysis? Certainly not.

We are dealing here with the unresolved Oedipus complex of our institution. Psychoanalysis, furthermore, in its current institutional shape, represents and defines the unresolved Oedipus complex of human institution formation in general, in as far as it has at its center the theme of exclusion, or inclusion, respectively, in a sub-formation endowed with the sexual–generative monopoly and the privilege of autogenesis. The institutional overcoming and resolving of this conflict would release the creative potential of psychoanalysis on a large scale.

We are aware today in our clinical theory that the early good/bad split of object representations is overcome by the oedipal triangulation. In the same vein, we know that the incestuous attack on the oedipal triangle regressively reconstitutes this primary splitting anew. I have shown that the endogamous co-option mode, by its nature, is directed against the triangular aspect of oedipality and, thus, against the oedipal law and the oedipal order, and that it represents a realization of the incest phantasy. In the institutional framework, it is, thus, a psychotic defense in Bion's sense. This goes beyond the general observation that large groups, and organizations and institutions, tend to function according to the paranoid–schizoid mode. It is much more specific. I fear we have to envisage that from the point of view of the psychoanalysis of groups and organizations, we find ourselves in a structure with psychotic characteristics. One must realize that the psychotic moment in organizations does not reveal itself with the same clear symptoms as in the individual: organizations do not hallucinate, and they hear no voices. Definitely more questionable is the occurrence of delusions, and the function of reality testing, which can certainly go amiss in organizations. As said, the delusional oedipal bubble of the training committees has been drifting out of touch with reality, to the detriment of psychoanalysis as a whole.

The attack of an unconscious psychotic structure expresses itself in the individual as well as in organizations primarily in the attack on thinking and on the ability of symbol formation, and also in the formation of systems of dependency and subjugation that are, by their very nature, organized in a dual mode. It speaks via a pervasive destructiveness and hostility toward development, and it shows itself in the moment of a narcissistic self-segregation, as it is symptomatic of a structure that claims for itself the sexual–generative privilege and the privilege of autogenesis. We must ask how, in principle, analyses are to work within a structure based on submission, dependency, and absolutistic concentration of power, with training analysts who, willing or unwilling, are inherent parts of this system? The training of young psychoanalysts is the main goal of our institutes. What has come about here is a terrible double-bind situation by which the structure of our institutes goes against their purpose. We have to envisage that the endogamous mode of nomination has a large-scale negative effect on the standard of our science and that it installs a way of institutional functioning which is dually organized and creates a closed system which, in principle, excludes the position of the third, triangularity, based on the very properties of this organizational system. What has been set in motion here are desublimating dynamics.

We have, therefore, *horribile dictum*, installed the heart of darkness, the transgression of the incest taboo, in the midst of our institutes and have laid it down by our statutes. Must we not assume, based on the knowledge we have about the reliable precision of emotional transmission of unconscious group processes, that this internal problem communicates itself to the outside and has a far greater effect than we might think? And that it is directly related to our declining numbers of candidates because, one might suggest, infertility combined with moral corruption and suppression is just not particularly attractive?

If, in the psychoanalytic literature dealing with this subject, from Balint (1948) and Bernfeld (1962) to Kernberg (1986) and Auchincloss and Michels (2003), missing objective training and evaluation criteria, missing criteria for scientific truth, and a missing task-oriented work group attitude is deemed to be responsible for the regressive overvaluation of the training analyst function and its idealization, one must also add the *argumentum e contrario* that the institutional establishment of the Eitingon model retroactively prevents the formation of those same criteria and of an adequate and effective work attitude, exactly because the regressive idealization of the training analyst function inherent in the Eitingon model takes the place of reasonable factual and functional criteria. One cannot escape the conclusion that this institutional structure has an unconscious, that is, structurally implicit, interest to not define the criteria, both of its training and of its own scientific truth, for only in this way can the pressure to comply with idealization of the training analysts be maintained.

For this reason, the institutional structure of psychoanalysis according to the Eitingon model has an unconscious, that is, structurally inherent, interest to not define the criteria, for this is the only way to uphold the idealization of the training analysts. This implies an unconscious antirational and antiscientific tendency resulting from the structural characteristics of psychoanalytic institution formation.

Auchincloss and Michels (2003) put the interrelation between the personality cult of the Eitingon model and the tendency to make criteria superfluous this way:

> This condensation of all routes to power and prestige into a single 'monolithic career path' (Kernberg 2001b) cannot help but create the experience of an overwhelming gap in professional status between the training analyst faculty and non-training analyst faculty. . . . (In) our present system . . . our candidates are educated to believe that the training analyst is not only all powerful but all knowing. In a world where we have no agreed upon strategy for deciding who possesses knowledge, and where a single professional role is so venerated, ambitious students are socialized to imagine that they can close the gap between their relative ignorance and the omniscience of the training analyst not by enquiring into the nature of mental life, but by striving to become training analysts themselves. As scientific curiosity collapses into professional ambition, the 'authority' of the training analyst position is further exalted and the intellectual life of our field becomes impoverished. (Auchincloss & Michels, 2003, p. 396 fn)

Mystification of the training analyst function is factually and functionally unjustified, transforms the psychoanalytic institutes into a two-classes society, reduces the intellectual and scientific standard of our institutes, and binds incredibly large amounts of psychic energy in a completely useless manner. It is the symptom of unresolved training transferences, fatefully restricting and tying up the creative potential of psychoanalysis. What has become of Freud's "wild horde"?

In their 2003 paper, Auchincloss and Michels go on to describe the dangerous consequences of the Eitingon model that block scientific creativity:

> [In our profession] . . . control over educational structures is by far the dominant strategy for those seeking to establish some measure of influence. In contrast to other clinical or medical sub-specialties, most psychoanalytic treatment is decentralized and independent of hospitals or other organized structures for the delivery of care. . . . In contrast to the more traditional natural sciences, psychoanalysis does not, as yet, measure success in terms of research or even scholarly output. . . . while writing and publication are important sources of status, the lack of an agreed upon method for determining the validity of our theoretical propositions complicates the quest for recognition in the intellectual domain. . . . In any case, because of these special features of psychoanalytic clinical and intellectual life, control of the educational structures of local institutes and societies remains, for the majority of psychoanalysts, the most important measure of intellectual and/or professional success. (Auchincloss & Michels, p. 387 fn)

In conclusion, we should reform our statutes in the sense of putting a stop to the endogamous co-option mode. This is an instant measure we must take. The second step would be, unavoidably, to follow Kernberg's proposal (2006, 2013) and tie the functions of training analyst and of supervisor to a general certification which, ideally, should be acquired by all members of psychoanalytic societies within a time frame of three to five years post graduation. This would be a basic requirement for a reformed psychoanalytic training system.

Epilogue

There are also other models in the IPA, such as, for instance, that of the Association Psychanalytique de France, an institution recognized by the IPA in 1964, whose members are, or have been, well-known analysts such as Anzieu, Laplanche, Pontalis, and Widlöcher, and in which, as Michel Gribinski (1997) described, centralized control over the didactic curriculum is suspended, and the training analyses take place as personal psychoanalyses before the beginning of the training, with an analyst whom the prospective candidate freely chooses. In the application, the aspiring applicant has to make the case that a genuine psychoanalytic process had come about in his or her analysis. When this is positively decided, this analysis is then recognized as a training analysis and the candidate is admitted for training. Gribinski has underlined this as the central aspect of the French model by the fact that he titled his presentation "In favour of personal analysis". The position and function of training analyst is, thus, relinquished in this model. It is replaced by supervision as the only means of quality control.

The motive of this institutional change is described by Gribinski as follows:

> Mistrust of power . . . explains the specificity of our training methods: we were for quite some time the only Psychoanalytical Society of the IPA to have ended training analysis, judging that the institute should not interfere in the candidate's personal analysis. And we are still the only society to have done away with the category of training analysts, and to allow admission of candidates in analysis with an analyst who is, for example, a member of another society . . . and who may indeed be a candidate; sometimes we consider an application coming, as our reports amusingly put it, from an "unknown couch". This does not mean that we ignore the candidate's analysis. *ON THE CONTRARY, THIS MEANS THAT WE REFER ONLY TO WHAT THE CANDIDATE CAN (OR CANNOT) SAY ABOUT IT*, or only to what he is aware of. . . . It is an *ANALYTICAL CONSIDERATION OF HIS PERSONAL ANALYSIS* which is thus sought. (Gribinski, 1997, p. 2, original capitals and italics)

Gribinski ends his description of the "French model", which is used also by Francophone institutes in Belgium, Switzerland, and Canada, with the statement: "The question for analytical training could be: *HOW TO HAND DOWN WHAT WE CANNOT PRETEND TO POSSESS*" (Gribinski, 1997, p. 11, original capitals and italics). One can look upon this, by all means, as a very thought-worthy, very psychoanalytical maxim, the observing of which, as an inner attitude of abstinence from the seductive qualities that lie in the exercise of power, would correct the "excessive authoritarianism" (Kernberg, 2001a, p. 198). It must, however, be critically noted—as Kernberg (2000) and Auchincloss and Michels (2003) have done before—that in this case the supervision analysts move up to the very position of power occupied by the training analysts in the Eitingon model. But at least there is not the specific regressive and transferential problem of an analysis of the candidate that runs parallel to training. Yet, the problem cannot be solved merely by abolishing the training analyst function, even though the French model provides a series of safety measures against the power of supervision analysts growing excessive. Decentralization of the didactic aspect of the training and the dissolution of the training analyst function, in any case, emphatically attempt to counter "excessive authoritarianism".

In this model, there is, therefore, no formation of a training committee in the sense of the Eitingon model. Also, as the "training analysis" (which here does not have this didactic aspect any more) takes place as a personal analysis basically before the training starts, there is also no transference of the regressive dynamics of training analyses on to the structure of the institute, as is otherwise the case. But this model also has obvious practical disadvantages, in as much as the beginning of clinical training and, with it, the emotional resonance of the candidates from the contact with patients is not accompanied by their own simultaneous analysis. This also contributes to the specific overvaluation of supervision in the French model and to the difficulty of keeping supervisions free from a therapeutically oriented field of interaction with the candidate and its respective transference dynamic, once the candidates, in their first analyses, are being confronted with the onslaught of transferences and the accompanying regressive potential.

The second alternative to the Eitingon model within the IPA's confines is the institutional concept developed by the Uruguayan Psychoanalytic Association from 1974 onwards, as Bernardi (2008) describes:

> The reform of 1974 sought to suppress the concentration of power in the training analysts; the "training analyst" category disappeared, and was substituted by "member of a group with training functions". Three groups were created: the Institute analysts, the supervisors and the professors. These designations were not granted for life; they had to be renewed periodically. An analyst could belong to all three groups, or only one of them, and had to go through clearly stipulated procedures in order to be accepted. . . . An analyst interested in acting as an Institute analyst, professor or supervisor, must present a personal application to the corresponding group, be interviewed by an ad hoc committee that evaluates her/his interests and qualifications, based on which the group decides if the analyst is to be accepted. . . . For example, to join the Institute supervisors' group, the presentation of clinical material is required; in the case of the professors' group, prior teaching assistance is necessary along with the presentation of a

> proposal for a seminar. This type of procedure prioritizes objective criteria. ... The group coordinators form part of the Education Committee that governs the Institute, which is also comprised of representatives of candidates and graduates. ...
>
> Power is located in group procedures. ... The general opinion is that the result is better than it would be with other possible alternatives. The worst excesses are avoided because the functioning of the groups is always ruled by explicit and transparent procedures and because all members participate, avoiding the excessive concentration of personal power. The entry of candidates is decided by a specific committee, the Institute's Admissions Committee, in which the candidate's analyst does not participate. An analysis of at least three times a week is accepted, both for candidates and for supervised analyses, while revision of the frequency of the sessions is advised, according to the patient's characteristics. (Bernardi, 2008, p. 236)

For the train of thought developed in this paper, I consider it especially important to point out that both alternative models—the French and the Uruguayan one—arose explicitly as a reaction to the problem of power concentration in the Eitingon model. Therefore, they relate to it in negation, reflecting its problems, whereby the French model does away with the training analyst function totally, while the Uruguayan concept attempts a kind of democratic basis alternative. With regard to the model of the Uruguayan association, a closer analysis reveals that the difference from the classical Eitingon concept lies in the fact that, for one, the nominations are fixed term. Second, according equal rights in the institute's leadership between coordinators of the working groups, graduated members, and candidates surely contributes to counteract the concentration of power within the ranks of the training analysts. Also, the Uruguayan model offers the possibility of disconnecting various functions which, in the classical Eitingon model, "self-evidently" are tied to the appointment as training analyst: the right to supervise, and the right to teach, that is to say, the right to lead theoretical seminars. In my view, the central phrase in Bernardi's description is, however, the following: "The worst excesses are avoided because ... all members participate, avoiding the excessive concentration of personal power" (Bernardi, 2008).

Kernberg's (2006, 2013) demand that, in principle, all graduates of an institute, thus, summarily, all members of a constituent organization, acquire a certification and, thus, qualification to conduct training analyses without any further additional nomination within three to five years after graduation—as Kernberg suggests—and that in principle the individual functions are to be kept separate, actually makes a connection between the essential characteristics of the French model, on the one hand, with its emphasis on a strictly personal, uninterfered analysis, and the Uruguayan model, on the other. Such a range of access, as wide as possible, to the functions of training analyst as well as supervisor would also have the advantage of not needing to introduce further safety measures against uncontrolled power concentration, as, for instance, a fixed-term nomination for training analysts or an institutional separation of the function of training analyst and supervisor. Each certified member would be a training analyst and supervisor in so far as fulfillment of that function was demanded of him or her at a specific moment in time.

Notes

1. With regard to criteria, it is especially problematic that, in many societies, one of the central conditions for nomination is the requirement that aspirants declare they have carried out several parallel high-frequency analyses in the years preceding their nomination. Such declaration is not verifiable due to the privacy and protection accorded to patient data. Not only is this a corrupting influence which invites one to misrepresent the facts, but it must also be pointed out that, from a normative and legally regulatory perspective, one cannot choose as a decisive criterion for nomination a self-declaration which cannot be verified; this is especially true if this criterion—rightly so—is the shibboleth of classical psychoanalysis.
2. It could be described as one of the general tasks of a psychoanalytic training to offer to the candidate a situation which stimulates transference and which is as intense as possible, creating evidence about the existence of the unconscious—and specific unconscious content, especially of the Oedipus complex—while referring to the immediate emotional experience of the candidate. This can be assumed to be an important aspect of the original, most likely unconscious, motive for the specific Eitingonian construction of psychoanalytic training institutes, with their invention of a training committee where the sexual and procreative function is exclusively located, in so far as nothing else corresponds so exactly to the oedipal phantasmatization on the

institutional plane. In order to fulfill this task, it should be ensured, though, that the oedipal constellation of the training committees does not turn into a one-sided manifestation of the castrating, excluding aspects of the Oedipus complex, as this prevents the sublimative impulse inherent in a healthy oedipal situation. This, however, with unconscious precision, is the very effect that we see taking place through the traditional constitution of the training committees according to the co-option mode.

3. Perhaps psychoanalytic societies have such difficulties providing an institutional answer to real sexual boundary transgressions within the framework of training—that is, real incidents of analytic incest—because the factual sexual enactment corresponds so strongly to the unconscious background characteristics of the institution.
4. From these considerations it also follows why the co-option mode proves especially deleterious in the case of psychoanalytic institutes. For it can rightly be pointed out that this mode is equally widespread in other areas of the social arena—from scientific institutions to art academies—and has, in fact, been copied from there. In psychoanalysis, however, this mode, with its unconscious implications, directly contradicts the central themes and tenets of psychoanalytic science and psychoanalytic training, so much so that it was able to become the mode of self-blockade of this science and of the training leading to it. In addition, in pointing out the ubiquity of this proliferation mode of social institutions, it is not said that this mode does not have negative consequences elsewhere, too, along the lines of the corrupting effects on psychoanalytic institution formation. Not for nothing do universities traditionally have the principle to rule out in-house appointments, and not for nothing is this principle being traditionally evaded with great ingenuity.
5. Here, the passing of the "Ethical Principles" of the IPA in 1999 resulted in a largely unrecognized and unacknowledged institutional problem, which is due to the collision of the institutes' federal autonomy with the regulations in paragraph 2,A,1 of the "Principles":

> *General Obligation to Maintain Ethical Standards.* Each IPA Constituent Organisation shall take reasonable measures to ensure that every psychoanalyst, and each training facility and other activity operated by or for the Constituent Organisation, maintains high ethical and professional standards, which are consistent with the IPA's Principles and with applicable laws and customs.

The federal principle which has applied so far is in open contrast with the "obligation to maintain ethical standards" as it hinders the constituent organizations to take the "appropriate measures" addressed in the ethics guidelines of the IPA.

That is to say that the suspension of the endogamous mode of nomination cannot be enforced in the existing constitution against the opposition of the institutes that consider themselves autonomous. In other words, in the same breath in which we talk about ending the endogamous nomination procedure, we are also, for necessary reasons inherent in the rules governing psychoanalytic associations and which primarily have nothing to do with the practice of nomination but pertain to the obligation to protect psychoanalysis and its principles, talking about the end of the federalistic principle of organization within the framework of the IPA.

References

Auchincloss, E. L., & Michels, R. (2003). A reassessment of psychoanalytic education: controversies and changes. *International Journal of Psychoanalysis, 84*: 387–403.

Balint, M. (1948). On the psychoanalytic training system. *International Journal of Psychoanalysis, 29*: 163–173.

Bernardi, R. (2008). Letter from Uruguay. *International Journal of Psychoanalysis, 89*(2): 233–240.

Bernfeld, S. (1962). On psychoanalytic training. *Psychoanalytic Quarterly, 31*: 453–482.

Goethe, J. W. (1798). Hermann und Dorothea. In: *Goethes Werke* (Hamburger Ausgabe). Hamburg: Christian Wegner. Translated and published by Harvard Classics.

Gribinski, M. (1997). In favour of personal analysis. Training at l'Association Psychanalytique de France. *Bulletin of the European Psychoanalytic Federation, 48*: 102–107.

Kernberg, O. F. (1986). Institutional problems of psychoanalytic education. *Journal of the American Psychoanalytic Association, 34*: 799–834.

Kernberg, O. F. (2000). A concerned critique of psychoanalytic education. *International Journal of Psychoanalysis, 81*: 97–120.

Kernberg, O. F. (2001a). Presidential Address: given at the 42nd International Psychoanalytic Congress, Nice France. *International Journal of Psychoanalysis, 83*: 197–203.

Kernberg, O. F. (2001b). Some thoughts regarding innovations in psychoanalytic education. *International Psychoanalytical Association Newsletter, 10*: 6–9.

Kernberg, O. F. (2006). The coming changes in psychoanalytic education: Part 1. *International Journal of Psychoanalysis, 87*: 1649–1673.

Kernberg, O. F. (2007). The coming changes in psychoanalytic education: Part 2. *International Journal of Psychoanalysis, 88*: 183–202.

Kernberg, O. F. (2013). The twilight of the training analysis system. Plenary address at the annual conference of the American Psychoanalytic Association. *Psychoanalytic Review*, April 2014.

Rosenfeld, H. (1971). A clinical approach to the psycho-analytical theory of the life and death instincts: an investigation of the aggressive aspects of narcissism. *International Journal of Psychoanalysis, 52*: 169–178.

Sandler, A.-M. (2004). Institutional responses to boundary violations: the case of Masud Khan. *International Journal of Psychoanalysis, 85*: 27–42.

Wallerstein, R. S. (2007). The optimal structure for psychoanalytic education today: a feasible proposal? *Journal of the American Psychoanalytic Association, 55*: 953–984.

INDEX